Advances in
Neuromuscular Disorders

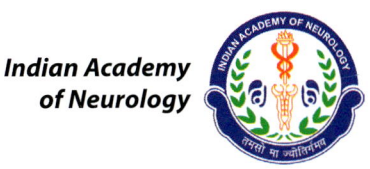

Indian Academy of Neurology

Advances in Neuromuscular Disorders

Editor-in-Chief
Debashish Chowdhury
DTCD MD(Medicine) DM(Neurology) FIAN FRCP(Edinburgh)
Commonwealth Fellow in Stroke Medicine(Edinburgh)
Director–Professor and Head
Department of Neurology
GB Pant Institute of Postgraduate Medical Education and Research
New Delhi, India

Editors

Atchayaram Nalini DM PhD
Professor
Neuromuscular Specialist
Department of Neurology
National Institute of Mental Health and Neurosciences (NIMHANS)
Bengaluru, Karnataka, India

Vishnu VY MD DM
Additional Professor
Department of Neurology
All India Institute of Medical Sciences (AIIMS)
New Delhi, India

Foreword
Satish Khadilkar

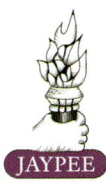

JAYPEE BROTHERS MEDICAL PUBLISHERS
The Health Sciences Publisher
New Delhi | London

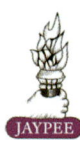 **Jaypee Brothers Medical Publishers (P) Ltd**

Headquarters
EMCA House
23/23-B, Ansari Road, Daryaganj
New Delhi 110 002, India
Landline: +91-11-23272143, +91-11-23272703
+91-11-23282021, +91-11-23245672
E-mail: jaypee@jaypeebrothers.com

EU GPSR Authorised Representative
Logos Europe, 9 rue Nicolas Poussin
17000, La Rochelle, France
Phone: +33 (0) 6 67 93 73 78
E-mail: Contact@logoseurope.eu

Corporate Office
Jaypee Brothers Medical Publishers (P) Ltd.
4838/24, Ansari Road, Daryaganj
New Delhi 110 002, India
Phone: +91-11-43574357
Fax: +91-11-43574314
E-mail: jaypee@jaypeebrothers.com

Overseas Office
JP Medical Ltd.
83, Victoria Street, London
SW1H 0HW (UK)
Phone: +44-20 3170 8910
Fax: +44(0)20 3008 6180
E-mail: info@jpmedpub.com

Website: www.jaypeebrothers.com
Website: www.jaypeedigital.com

© 2025, Jaypee Brothers Medical Publishers

The views and opinions expressed in this book are solely those of the original contributor(s)/author(s) and do not necessarily represent those of editor(s) or publisher of the book.

All rights reserved. No part of this publication may be reproduced, stored or transmitted in any form or by any means, electronic, mechanical, photocopying, recording or otherwise, without the prior permission in writing of the publishers.

All brand names and product names used in this book are trade names, service marks, trademarks or registered trademarks of their respective owners. The publisher is not associated with any product or vendor mentioned in this book.

Medical knowledge and practice change constantly. This book is designed to provide accurate, authoritative information about the subject matter in question. However, readers are advised to check the most current information available on procedures included and check information from the manufacturer of each product to be administered, to verify the recommended dose, formula, method and duration of administration, adverse effects and contraindications. It is the responsibility of the practitioner to take all appropriate safety precautions. Neither the publisher nor the author(s)/editor(s) assume any liability for any injury and/or damage to persons or property arising from or related to use of material in this book.

This book is sold on the understanding that the publisher is not engaged in providing professional medical services. If such advice or services are required, the services of a competent medical professional should be sought.

Every effort has been made where necessary to contact holders of copyright to obtain permission to reproduce copyright material. If any have been inadvertently overlooked, the publisher will be pleased to make the necessary arrangements at the first opportunity.

Inquiries for bulk sales may be solicited at: jaypee@jaypeebrothers.com

IAN Advances in Neuromuscular Disorders / Debashish Chowdhury, Atchayaram Nalini, Vishnu VY

First Edition: 2025
ISBN: 978-93-6616-198-3
Printed in India at Purewall Ventures Pvt Ltd

Indian Academy of Neurology

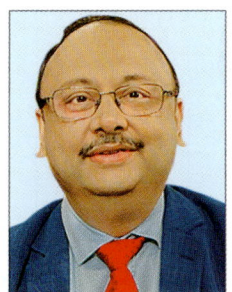

PRESIDENT
Debashish Chowdhury
New Delhi, India

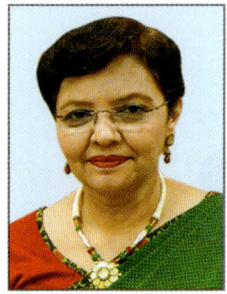

PRESIDENT-ELECT
Sangeeta Ravat
Mumbai, Maharashtra, India

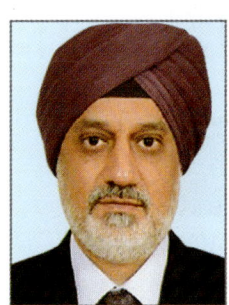

IMMEDIATE PAST PRESIDENT
Gagandeep Singh
Ludhiana, Punjab, India

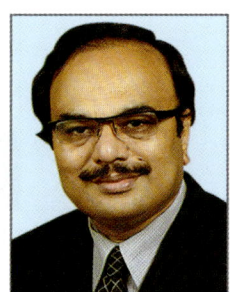

PAST PRESIDENT
Nirmal Surya
Mumbai, Maharashtra, India

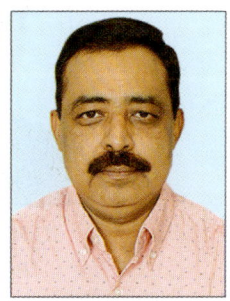

TREASURER
Achal Srivastava
New Delhi, India

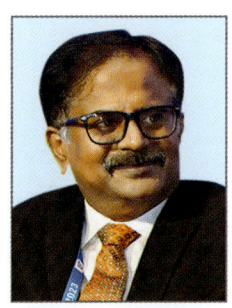

SECRETARY
U Meenakshisundaram
Chennai, Tamil Nadu, India

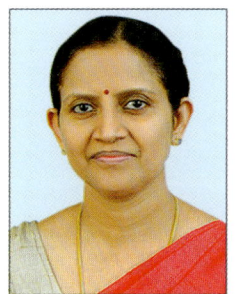

EDITOR, ANNALS OF IAN
PN Sylaja
Thiruvananthapuram, Kerala, India

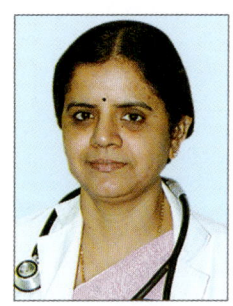

CME CONVENER
Sita Jayalakshmi
Hyderabad, Telangana, India

Executive Members

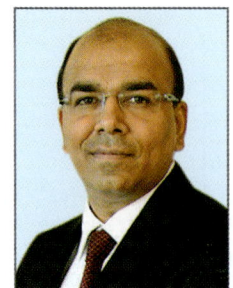

Arvind Sharma
Ahmedabad, Gujarat, India

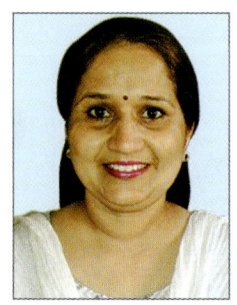

Bhawna Sharma
Jaipur, Rajasthan, India

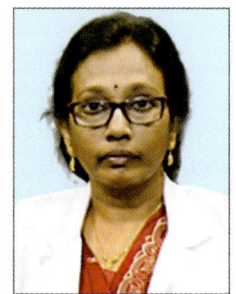

Atchayaram Nalini
Bengaluru, Karnataka, India

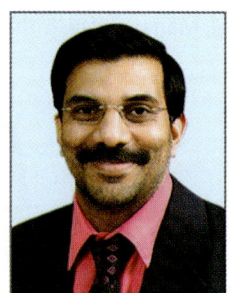

JOINT TREASURER
Pradeep VG
Kozhikode, Kerala, India

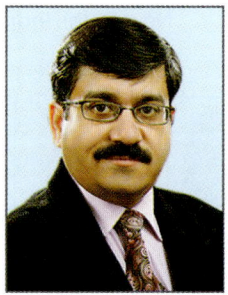

JOINT SECRETARY
Sumit Singh
Gurugram, Haryana, India

Contributors

Abhijeet K Kohat MD(General Medicine) DM(Neurology)
Associate Professor
Department of Neurology
DKS Post Graduate Institute and Research Center
Raipur, Chhattisgarh, India

Aditya Nair MD(General Medicine) DM(Neurology)
Associate Professor
Department of Neurological Sciences
Christian Medical College
Vellore, Tamil Nadu, India

Ajith Sivadasan MD(General Medicine) DNB(General Medicine) DM(Neurology) DNB(Neurology)
Postdoctoral Fellowship in Neuromuscular Disorders (University of Toronto)
Professor
Department of Neurological Sciences
Christian Medical College
Vellore, Tamil Nadu, India

Alisha Reyaz MSc(Medical Biochemistry)
PhD Scholar
Department of Neurology
All India Institute of Medical Sciences (AIIMS)
New Delhi, India

Ann Agnes Mathew MRCPCH FRCPCH Fellow Pediatric Neurology(GOSH, London) Fellow Pediatric Epilepsy(London) Fellow Pediatric Neuromuscular Disorders(GOSH, London) Fellow Paediatric Neurovascular Disorders(GOSH, London)
Consultant Pediatric Neurologist and Neuromuscular Specialist
Head, Synapse Neuro and Child Development Centre
Head, Neuromuscular Services
Bangalore Baptist Hospital
Bengaluru, Karnataka, India

Anuradha Mahto MD
Senior Resident
Department of Neurology
Government Grant Medical College, Sir JJ Hospital
Mumbai, Maharashtra, India

Atchayaram Nalini DM PhD
Professor
Neuromuscular Specialist
Department of Neurology
National Institute of Mental Health and Neurosciences (NIMHANS)
Bengaluru, Karnataka, India

Deepak Menon MD DM(Neurology)
Associate Professor and Neuromuscular Specialist
National Institute of Mental Health and Neurosciences (NIMHANS)
Bengaluru, Karnataka, India

Deepti Narasimhaiah MD PhD
Addtional Professor
Department of Pathology
Sree Chitra Tirunal Institute for Medical Sciences and Technology
Thiruvananthapuram, Kerala, India

Dhananjay Bhat MS MCh(Neurosurgery)
Former Professor
Department of Neurology
National Institute of Mental Health and Neurosciences (NIMHANS)
Bengaluru, Karnataka, India

Dipti Baskar MD DM(Neurology)
PDF in Neuromuscular Disorders
Research Associate
Neuromuscular Specialist
National Institute of Mental Health and Neurosciences (NIMHANS)
Bengaluru, Karnataka, India

Jharna Mahajan MD
Chief Resident
Department of Neurology
Bombay Hospital Institute of
Medical Sciences
Mumbai, Maharashtra, India

Karthik Muthusamy
MD(Pediatrics) DM(Neurology)
DNB(Neurology) Fellow of American
College of Medical Genetics(FACMG)
Senior Associate Consultant
Department of Clinical
Genomics, Mayo Clinic
Jacksonville, Florida, USA

Lokesh Bathala DM(Neurology)
RPNI(ASN)
Senior Consultant
Aster CMI Prime Hospital
Bengaluru, Karnataka, India

Madhu Nagappa MD DM
Additional Professor
Department of Neurology
National Institute of Mental
Health and
Neurosciences (NIMHANS)
Bengaluru, Karnataka, India

Manoj Kumar Goyal MD DM
Additional Professor
Department of Neurology
Postgraduate Institute of
Medical Education and Research
Chandigarh, India

Nupur Pruthi MS
MCh(Neurosurgery)
Professor of Neurosurgery
National Institute of Mental
Health and Neurosciences
(NIMHANS)
Bengaluru, Karnataka, India

Ragavendar Bhuvaneswaran
MD(General Medicine)
Senior Resident (DM)
Department of Neurology
Jawaharlal Institute of
Postgraduate Medical Education
and Research (JIPMER)
Puducherry, India

Rakesh K Singh MD
DM(Neurology) DNB
Honorary Assistant Professor
Department of Neurology
Government Grant Medical
College
Sir JJ Hospital
Consultant Neurologist
Jupiter Hospital
Mumbai, Maharashtra, India

Ritu Shree MD DM
Assistant Professor
Department of Neurology
Postgraduate Institute of
Medical Education and Research
Chandigarh, India

Samim MM DM
Senior Resident
Department of Neurology
National Institute of Mental
Health and Neurosciences
(NIMHANS)
Bengaluru, Karnataka, India

Saranya B Gomathy MD DM
DrNB(Neurology)
Assistant Professor
Department of Neurology
Jawaharlal Institute of
Postgraduate Medical
Education and Research
(JIPMER)
Puducherry, India

Saraswati Nashi DM
Postdoctoral Fellowship
Neuromuscular Disorders
Associate Professor
Department of Neurology
National Institute of Mental
Health and Neurosciences
(NIMHANS)
Bengaluru, Karnataka, India

Satish Khadilkar MD DM DNBE
FIAN FICP FAMS FRCP
Dean and Professor and Head
Department of Neurology
Bombay Hospital Institute of
Medical Sciences
Mumbai, Maharashtra, India

Seena Vengalil MD DM
Postdoctoral Fellowship
Neuromuscular Disorders
Associate Professor
Department of Neurology
National Institute of Mental
Health and Neurosciences
(NIMHANS)
Bengaluru, Karnataka, India

Sruthi S Nair MD DM
Additional Professor
Department of Neurology
Sree Chitra Tirunal Institute
for Medical Sciences and
Technology
Thiruvananthapuram, Kerala,
India

Vaibhav Wadwekar
MD(General Medicine)
DM(Neurology)
PDF(Neuromuscular Disorders)
Professor
Department of Neurology
Jawaharlal Institute of
Postgraduate Medical
Education and Research
(JIPMER)
Puducherry, India

Varsha Patil MD DM
Consultant Neurologist
Department of Neurology
Bombay Hospital Institute of
Medical Sciences
Mumbai, Maharashtra, India

Vishnu VY MD DM
Additional Professor
Department of Neurology
All India Institute of Medical
Sciences (AIIMS)
New Delhi, India

Y Muralidhar Reddy
DM(Neurology) Associate FAMS
Lead Consultant
Renova Institute of
Neurological Sciences (RINS)
Renova Century Hospital
Hyderabad, Telangana, India

Foreword

The knowledge explosion in the fields of neurology and neuromuscular medicine continues. A huge body of evidence has been accumulating with respect to the understanding of the disease processes, and newer therapy paradigms are evolving. The fields of genetics and immunology have been the torchbearers and every few days, new pieces of information get added in these areas. With the new knowledge, new vistas open for therapeutic interventions. Neurologists in India cater to a very large population, are largely involved with service neurology and to be effective, information of the ongoing therapeutic advances becomes very important.

This book, entitled *IAN Advances in Neuromuscular Disorders*, is a very welcome effort to update the neurologists of the current therapeutic developments. The editors Dr Atchayaram Nalini and Dr Vishnu VY have designed the table of contents very carefully and you will see that it covers the contemporary issues in neuromuscular disorders exhaustively. The book contains 15 chapters which cover a wide range of neuromuscular topics beginning with myopathies and going up to the anterior horn cell diseases. Immunological diseases take the major share, understandably so, but the editors have taken care to include the genetic and developmental diseases which are becoming amenable to interventions. The thrust of discussion is on therapeutics and has been discussed in detail in all the chapters; particularly the newer concepts have been well explained. Keeping to the theme of the book, pathophysiology and other aspects of the diseases find limited space.

This volume is a very welcome addition to the libraries and individual academic collections. I congratulate the Indian Academy of Neurology for conceptualizing this series, the editors Dr Nalini and Dr Vishnu for bringing together a comprehensive volume, and all the authors for their exhaustive and authoritative deliberations.

Satish Khadilkar
MD DM DNBE FIAN FICP FAMS FRCP
Dean and Professor and Head
Department of Neurology
Bombay Hospital Institute of Medical Sciences
Mumbai, Maharashtra, India

Message from Editor-in-Chief

Dear Readers,

The Indian Academy of Neurology (IAN) has been at the forefront of neurology education and has a rich history of publications which rank high in terms of academic and scientific content. As President, it has been my pleasure to team up with my Executive Committee members, who are experts in various neurological subspecialties and high-quality and prolific authors with an impressive track record of publications, as editors and bring out a series of books which continue to hold high the tradition of IAN in terms of high-impact scientific content.

As Chief Editor of IAN *"Advances in Neuromuscular Disorders"*, it is my pleasure to bring to you a book which sets the bar high for content—accurate, updated, and relevant—and at the same time presents it in a reader-friendly manner, which makes the book an ideal companion for everyone interested in the subject. I thank my colleagues and editors of this book, *Dr Atchayaram Nalini and Dr Vishnu VY*, for the shared vision of high-quality, focused content as well as excellent support rendered during the making of this book.

This has been our collective effort, and we sincerely hope that each of you will like reading this book as much as we loved bringing this out.

Debashish Chowdhury

Preface

We, the contributors to this book, warmly welcome you to this Indian Academy of Neurology textbook entitled *"Advances in Neuromuscular Disorders"*, prepared with great diligence as a comprehensive resource and designed to illuminate the recent advances in diagnosis and management of neuromuscular disorders encountered frequently. The complexities and nuances of neuromuscular conditions are documented elegantly. This book is intended for medical professionals, researchers, students, and anyone with a keen interest in the field of neurology and neuromuscular disorders.

Neuromuscular disorders encompass a diverse array of inherited and acquired diseases and have profound effects on an individual's mobility, quality of life, and overall health. From the well-known conditions like Duchenne muscular dystrophy to complex neuromuscular disorders, the spectrum of disorders is vast and complex and intricate.

This textbook is structured to provide a thorough understanding of the diagnostic and management strategies in neuromuscular disorders and some basic clinical knowledge of the disorders covered.

Each chapter is meticulously crafted to offer both foundational knowledge and cutting-edge advancements in the field. Our aim is to bridge the gap between clinical diagnosis and gain a comprehensive grasp of both advanced diagnosis and practical management aspects.

In preparing this textbook, we have drawn upon the expertise of a diverse group of specialists from India. Their contributions ensure that this book reflects the latest research, clinical guidelines, and evolving treatment strategies. We have also included case studies and clinical scenarios to help contextualize the material and facilitate practical learning.

We hope that this book serves as a valuable tool in your professional journey, enhancing your understanding and ability to manage the complexities of neuromuscular disorders. As our knowledge and technologies continue to evolve, it is our hope that this text will contribute to the ongoing dialogue and advancements in the field, ultimately improving patient outcomes and fostering a deeper appreciation of the intricacies of neuromuscular health.

Thank you for choosing this book as your guide through the fascinating and challenging world of neuromuscular disorders. We are excited to embark on this journey with you and look forward to the advancements and discoveries that behold each one of us.

Atchayaram Nalini
Vishnu VY

Acknowledgments

I, Dr Atchayaram Nalini, would like to dedicate this book on neuromuscular disorders to the founding members who strived to establish this domain of neurology into an important specialty. I am indebted to Professor M Gourie-Devi, my teacher and mentor who introduced and encouraged me to continue with her legacy of working on monomelic amyotrophy/Hirayama disease and primary muscle diseases. I am obligated to remember Late Dr Anisya Vasanth Taly for her teaching on muscle diseases which made them appealing to me. I am thankful to all my current and former team members (Dr Seena Vengalil, Dr Saraswati Nashi, Dr Kiran Polavarapu, Dr Veeramani Preethish-Kumar, Dr Priya Treesa Thomas, and Dr Keertipriya) and students who have been the pillars of support for me to pursue this specialty to great heights, thus matching international standards in India. I deeply appreciate my neurosurgical colleagues, Dr Nupur Prusty and Dr Dhananjay Bhat, who made it possible to find great success in the surgical intervention of Hirayama disease.

I, Dr Vishnu VY, dedicate this book to my wife, Dr Aishwarya Krishnamurthy, and my two sons, Nandan Vishnu and Agastya Vishnu, who have been my greatest strength and motivation. I would also like to thank Professor Padma Srivastava, who motivated me to take up the neuromuscular field along with stroke as a research field. Finally, I would like to thank my teachers at PGI Chandigarh, especially Professor Sudesh Prabhakar and Professor Vivek Lal, and at JIPMER Puducherry, Professor TK Dutta and Professor T Kadhiravan, for instilling the clinical skills in neurology and medicine.

We would like to deeply thank all the authors who responded with great enthusiasm and kept up with the deadlines. We are also thankful to the publisher, M/s Jaypee Brothers Medical Publishers (P) Ltd, New Delhi, India, and the team for continued and persistent support and co-operation. Lastly, we would like to profusely thank the enthusiastic and highly motivated IAN President, Dr Debashish Chowdhury, and all IAN team members for giving us this opportunity to contribute on this important subspecialty book.

Atchayaram Nalini
Vishnu VY

Contents

CHAPTER 1: **Disease-modifying Therapies in Spinal Muscular Atrophy and Duchenne Muscular Dystrophy: A Rapidly Changing Scenario**   1
Ann Agnes Mathew

CHAPTER 2: **Refractory Myasthenia: Management Strategies**   10
Deepak Menon, Seena Vengalil, Saraswati Nashi, Atchayaram Nalini

CHAPTER 3: **Congenital Myasthenic Syndromes: Genetic Spectrum and Management**   20
Seena Vengalil, Samim MM, Saraswati Nashi, Deepak Menon, Atchayaram Nalini

CHAPTER 4: **Idiopathic Inflammatory Myopathies and Current Immunology**   33
Sruthi S Nair, Deepti Narasimhaiah

CHAPTER 5: **Updates on Limb–girdle Dystrophies and Gene Therapies**   52
Vaibhav Wadwekar, Abhijeet K Kohat, Ragavendar Bhuvaneswaran

CHAPTER 6: **Clinical Utility and Interpretation of Genetic Testing in Neuromuscular Disorders**   64
Ajith Sivadasan, Karthik Muthusamy, Aditya Nair

CHAPTER 7: **Facioscapulohumeral Dystrophy: Update on Treatment**   80
Alisha Reyaz, Vishnu VY

CHAPTER 8: **Riboflavinopathies: Potentially Treatable Disorders**   93
Saraswati Nashi, Seena Vengalil, Dipti Baskar, Deepak Menon, Atchayaram Nalini

CHAPTER 9: **Mitochondrial Disorders: A Neuromuscular Perspective**   103
Madhu Nagappa

CHAPTER 10:	**Therapeutic Advances in Nodoparanodopathies**	113
	Satish Khadilkar, Varsha Patil, Jharna Mahajan	
CHAPTER 11:	**Chronic Inflammatory Demyelinating Polyradiculoneuropathy and its "Variants": Current Treatment Recommendations**	124
	Rakesh K Singh, Anuradha Mahto	
CHAPTER 12:	**Neuromuscular Imaging: MRI and Ultrasound**	136
	Lokesh Bathala, Y Muralidhar Reddy	
CHAPTER 13:	**Hirayama Disease/Monomelic Amyotrophy: Recent Advances and Surgical Management**	152
	Atchayaram Nalini, Dipti Baskar, Nupur Pruthi, Dhananjay Bhat, Seena Vengalil	
CHAPTER 14:	**Recent Classification and Emerging Therapies in Charcot–Marie–Tooth Disease**	167
	Ritu Shree, Manoj Kumar Goyal	
CHAPTER 15:	**Genetics of Amyotrophic Lateral Sclerosis and Implications for Therapy**	178
	Saranya B Gomathy, Seena Vengalil, Atchayaram Nalini	

Index   191

Disease-modifying Therapies in Spinal Muscular Atrophy and Duchenne Muscular Dystrophy: A Rapidly Changing Scenario

Ann Agnes Mathew

ABSTRACT

The neuromuscular world has seen an explosion of newer treatments that have changed the way we look at these groups of diseases that were previously considered untreatable. Duchenne muscular dystrophy (DMD) and spinal muscular atrophy (SMA) are protypes for many of these diseases. The advent of newer therapies, be it protein level correction for SMA and DMD or even DNA level correction with gene therapy, has reawakened interest in the management of these conditions. But standards of cares (SOCs), established by the entire neuromuscular fraternity remain the backbone for the management of individuals affected by these conditions and become even more important today as the paradigm of their prognostication and management seems to be shifting very rapidly and they ultimately help us as clinicians deliver better care, quality of life, and outcomes to affected families.

Keywords: Duchenne muscular dystrophy, Spinal muscular atrophy, Disease-modifying therapies, Standards of care, Newer treatments.

■ INTRODUCTION

Spinal muscular atrophy (SMA) and Duchenne muscular dystrophy (DMD) are classical prototypes of inherited neuromuscular disorders (NMDs), a diverse group of monogenic disorders that cause progressive weakness, leading to increasing difficulty in ambulation, breathing, and swallowing. Disease severity and progression is determined by the deleterious effect of the affected protein on the function of the motor unit. This in turn is linked to the gene defect responsible and its repercussion on protein production and function. Mostly these conditions leave the central nervous system unaffected and consequently cognition is often intact. Although increasingly, it is recognized that dystrophin protein (Dp) has a major isoform expressed in the brain which is the basis for the 19 country European union and Japanese[1] collaboration called the BIND (Brain Involvement in Dystrophinopathy) project that is working toward ameliorating this. Advances in our understanding of these conditions have vastly changed survival and their natural history. Where previously they were considered untreatable, they have now become an exciting field in medicine, thanks to the explosion of available potential therapies, many of which work on more than one pathway.

To understand these advances, it is important to look at the basic underlying disease process, especially at the molecular level. While a one-step cure for these disorders is unlikely, available disease modifying therapies (DMTs) have revolutionized their care.

Advances in protein expression that translated to therapeutics may be divided into two categories:

1. Technology that ensures some production of functional, albeit truncated protein. This could further be classified as:
    i. At the protein level—at the mRNA level, e.g., nusinersen
    ii. Those at the DNA level—onasemnogene abeparvovec-xioi
2. Technology targeting downstream effects occurring due to the absence of the said relevant protein. These include newer steroids such as deflazacort or steroid analogs such as vamorolone and givinostat—a histone deacetylase (HDAC) pan inhibitor inhibitor.[2]

■ SPINAL MUSCULAR ATROPHY

Classical SMA is caused by homozygous functional loss of the survival motor neuron 1 *(SMN1)* gene located on the chromosome 5q13 locus. The *SMN1* gene is known to be critical for the survival of motor neurone[3] and is a widely expressed housekeeping protein in the cell. SMA is the leading cause of inherited death in infancy and is the second most common autosomal recessively inherited disease. It is characterized by progressive loss of lower motor nerve (anterior horn cells) in the spinal cord. It has an estimated prevalence of anywhere between 1 in 6,000 and 1 in 10,000[4] with concerns of a higher prevalence in regions with raised consanguinity given its autosomal recessive nature.

5qSMA, the most common SMA accounts for 95% of all SMA with a wide plethora of ever-increasing causes of non-5q types of SMA with many varied causative genes such as *TFG, HEXB, GLE1, EXOSC3, VRK1, ASAH1, SLC52A3, SLC52A2, VAPB, SETX, TRPV4, DYNC1H1, LMNA, AR, BICD2,* and *UBA1* to name a few. Many of these have other phenotypes such as that seen in the riboflavin transporter deficiency neuronopathy caused by mutations in the solute carrier gene *SLC52A2* that is amenable to treatment with riboflavin and may also have concomitant sensorineural deafness.

Types of Spinal Muscular Atrophy

Based on the age of onset as well as clinical severity, affected individuals were historically classified into SMA1, SMA2, SMA3, and SMA 4. There is a smaller subgroup of SMA 0 patients who have antenatal onset of disease, evidenced by contractures at birth resulting from fetal akinesia. Despite all the current advances, this subgroup is still very challenging to treat. SMA1, 2, and 3 may also be broadly classified into nonsitters, sitters who do not walk, and walkers. This pragmatic classification becomes handier particularly as DMTs have changed their natural history **(Table 1)**.

Current Classification[5]

- Non-sitters
- Sitters
- Walkers

Disease-modifying Therapeutics in Spinal Muscular Atrophy

These are classified into two categories:
1. *SMN2* dependent
2. *SMN2* independent
   SMN independent agents which are still in the research phase.

Nusinersen

Nusinersen an *SMN2* targeted antisense oligonucleotide (ASO) approved in both

TABLE 1: Previous clinical classification of spinal muscular atrophy (SMA).[3]

SMA type	Age of onset	Mobility	Life expectancy
0	Prenatal	Fetal hypokinesia	<2 months
1a	<2 weeks	No head control	<2 years
1b	<3 months	Never rolled or sat unsupported	<2 years
1c	3–6 months	Never sat unsupported	<2 years
2	7–18 months	Sat, but never stood unsupported	Variable
3a	18 months–3 years	Walked but later loss of ambulation	Normal
3b	>3 years	Walk but later could lose ambulation	Normal
4	Onset after 10 years age	Stand and walk during adulthood	Normal

children and adults works at the mRNA level. This intrathecally administered ASO, was the first effective and pioneering therapy for SMA. We know that SMN protein is crucial for the functioning of anterior horn cells. It is encoded by the *SMN1* gene, but a paralog gene *SMN2* also produces SMN protein inefficiently with only about 10% functional protein production. This is due to a naturally occurring skipping of exon 7 of the *SMN2* gene, resulting in a nonfunctional protein. Nusinersen helps include exon 7 at the mRNA level with this ASO technology, consequently resulting in more stable protein, thus utilizing naturally occurring *SMN2* gene to its best potential.

Nusinersen exploits the differences between *SMN1* and *SMN2* genes. The homologue *SMN2* differs from *SMN1* in that there is a C to T exchange in exon 7 of the *SMN2* gene leading to altered splicing at exon 7 of the *SMN2* gene. This leads to transcription of an mRNA where exon 7 is missing, resulting in an unstable and nonfunctional protein. This naturally occurring exon skipping noted at the turn of the century, geared research toward undoing this, thus reducing *SMN2* exon skipping and consequently increasing SMN protein expression. This trendsetting drug gained Food and Drug Administration (FDA) approval in December 2016, and patients in India gained access by late 2019.

Mechanism of Action of Spinraza

Antisense oligonucleotides target the intronic splicing silencer N1 (ISSN1) and increase inclusion of exon 7 in *SMN2* mature mRNA transcripts followingly—nusinersen uses a synthetic strand of nucleic acids linked together with a 2'-O-methoxyethyl backbone. This then functions by recognizing and binding to RNA in the cells, thus correcting the gene splicing. So it uses the nucleotide base pairing (adenine-thymine and guanine-cytosine) as in the Watson and Crick model to bind specifically to the ISSN1. Consequently, there is an increase exon 7 inclusion in *SMN2* leading to more mature mRNA transcripts. ISSN1 is a major inhibitory element regulating exon 7 splicing. These ASOs enter the cell through endocytosis after being intrathecally injected. Once inside the nucleus, they bind to *SMN2* pre-mRNA transcripts correcting exon 7 splicing **(Flowchart 1)**.

There is a lot of on-going work being done to increase and improve ASO penetration, duration of action, efficacy, safety, and side effect profile. We are beginning to understand that when dealing with neurodegenerative diseases such as SMA, the timing of intervention matters a lot as this determines how much functionality is maintained. Neuronal loss is irreversible after a certain point, hence earlier interventions have better outcomes.

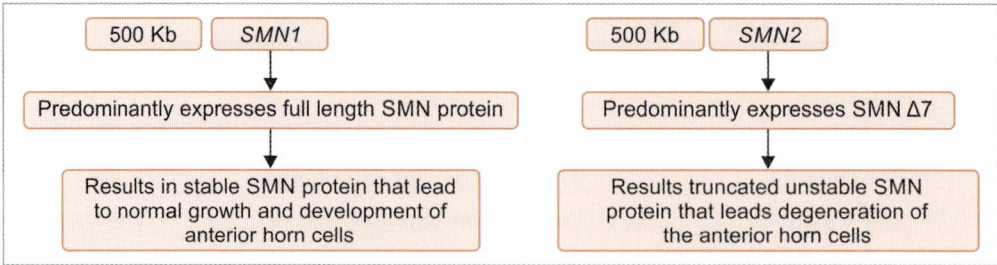

FLOWCHART 1: Some differences between survival motor neuron 1 (*SMN1*) and *SMN2* genes and their transcripts.[6]

Enhanced Understanding of SMN Genetics

The statement that increased *SMN2* gene equals less severe SMA would be mostly true, although it is an oversimplification. For example, an individual with four copies of *SMN2* gene and no copies of the *SMN1* gene having less severe disease is usually the norm but there are exceptions to this, including in siblings within the same family, with the same copy numbers, but with varying disease severity. This begs the question as to whether there are other disease modifiers that need consideration.

Some known modifiers of the *SMN* gene are *PLS3* encoding plastin 3,[7] and *NCALD2* (neurocalcin delta 2).[8] The c.859G>C variant within the *SMN2* gene is a protective positive disease modifier that reduces its severity resulting in a milder *SMN2* allele with reduced severity of SMA. Presence of some negative modifiers means that we sometimes see SMA1 patients, albeit rarely with 4 *SMN2* copy numbers. This leads us to the point that the classification of SMA types cannot be made genetically and remains a clinical one. Studying 303 sibships from the Cure SMA database is a point in case for this phenotypic divergence in 15.2% patients.[7]

Administration of Nusinersen

It has a loading phase followed by a maintenance one. The loading phase has intrathecal injections administered on day 0, 14, 28, and 63 and is maintained at 4 monthly intervals thereafter. A fixed dose of 12 mg in 5 mL is administered to individuals of all weights and ages. Maintenance interval was calculated based on the duration fully functioning SMN protein started waning in the CSF. A well-tolerated drug, its usual side effects are those of lumbar puncture with some systemic ones such as thrombocytopenia and elevated transaminases along with rare proteinuria, a class side effect of most ASOs.

Risdiplam/Evrysdi in Spinal Muscular Atrophy

Risdiplam (Evrysdi), a small molecule pre-mRNA splice site modifier of the *SMN2* gene, is orally administered and systemically distributed. Both nusinersen and risdiplam have different targets, though they both increase the amount of functional SMN protein.

Mechanism of Action

Risdiplam like nusinersen includes exon 7 in the *SMN2* gene mature mRNA transcript, by enhancing U1-pre-mRNA.

Administration of Risdiplam

It is administered once daily orally, and the dose is calculated as 0.2 mg/kg body weight for infants under 2 years of age and 0.25 mg/kg daily dosing for infants over 2 years of age. The ceiling maximum daily dose is 5 mg for anyone over 20 kg. It is generally well tolerated with occasional adverse effects such as thrombocytopenia along with some proteinuria and elevated transaminases.

Onasemnogene Xioi (Zolgensma)

This revolutionary purported one-off medication and "cure" came on the field of SMA, as the most expensive medication known until recently, when gene therapy for DMD overtook it in terms of cost.

It uses recombinant adeno-associated virus (AAV) vectors to target the absence of the *SMN1* gene. Onasemnogene abeparvovec-xioi is licensed in the USA for infants younger than 2 years with biallelic mutations of *SMN1* and in the European Union for those with biallelic *SMN1* deletion but with up to three copies of *SMN2* with the weight cut off not being specified. There have been recent studies that have shown the usefulness of this DMT even in older children up to 13.5 kg.[9] It is a self-complimentary AAV vector with serotype 9 (scAAV-9) that carries a cDNA of a full-length *SMN1* under the control of hybrid enhancer/chicken β-actin promoter.[7] This is a nonreplicating virus and so on intravenous administration, the viral vector/capsid (scAAV9) crosses the blood brain barrier, entering the CNS and the motor neuron by endocytosis finally moving into the nucleus. Once the scAAV9 is inside the nucleus, the capsid is lost and the single stranded cDNA of the *SMN1* uses the machinery of the nucleus to make itself a double-stranded DNA copy of itself.

Administration of Onasemnogene

This is administered at a dose of 1.1×10^{10} viral vector genomes (vg) per kg of body weight intravenously over 60 minutes as a single injection after being immune primed with corticosteroids 24 hours previously. Steroids are continued thereafter to help mitigate the immune-mediated adverse events, primarily the hepatic ones. The other key adverse effects of administering onasemnogene are thrombocytopenia, elevated troponin I (although its significance is still not well known) and rarely thrombotic thrombocytopenic purpura. By far the most common adverse effects are increased transaminases and some flu-like illness.

The major drawback of onasemnogene is that transduction efficiency is age dependent, reflecting on importance of reaching the irreversible pool of motor neurons that cannot be gained back once lost if not delivered in a timely fashion. This strongly highlights the need for early intervention to maximize clinical benefit. So intuitively early recognition and treatment would have maximum benefits as seen in the best cohort so far, those of presymptomatic patients with three copies of SMN2 who have achieved age appropriate milestones.[11]

■ DUCHENNE MUSCULAR DYSTROPHY

Duchenne muscular dystrophy, the most common muscular dystrophy, affects approximately 1 in 3,500 newborn boys. With progressive weakness, it has calf muscle hypertrophy as its hallmark. Children with the disease, tend to walk on their toes and often present with frequent falls.

The DMD is caused by a loss of function mutation (frame shift mutation) in the *DMD/dystrophin* gene that codes for the Dp, a cytoskeletal protein. *DMD* gene is located on the X chromosome. Dp is key for the functioning of skeletal and cardiac muscles and is expressed in the brain as well. It acts as a shock absorber in the skeletal muscle forming a link between the contractile apparatus of the cell with the muscle plasma membrane, as a key part of the dystrophin-associated protein complex (DAPC). DAPC dysfunction results in mechanical damage to skeletal muscle fibers. Hence absence of Dp results in abnormal forces of transmission during muscle contraction resulting in skeletal muscle damage. This leads to muscle weakness and wasting as well as exhaustion of the skeletal muscle's ability to regenerate. Chronic inflammation follows, resulting in the fibrofatty replacement seen externally as calf hypertrophy.

Standards of Care and Advances in Cardiac Care

Cardiac involvement is ubiquitous in DMD. This was previously thought to occur in the second decade. But we are increasingly detecting them early through advanced cardiac imaging techniques such as cardiac magnetic resonance imaging (CMRI). A dedicated functional echocardiogram is as often as good as CMRI in picking up early involvement of the heart. This is helpful in resource limited settings and helps alter the course of the disease. The idea being that, by the time abnormal results are captured on routine 2D ECHO, cardiac involvement has already advanced. Functional studies clue us in on what is happening within the cardiac muscle, allowing us to intervene before they get translated to diastolic dysfunction, thus delaying disease progression. This is also why despite weak evidence most centers have adopted the current standards of care (SOC) of starting angiotensin-converting enzyme inhibitors (ACEI) usually perindopril into their guidelines for all boys regardless of their cardiac imaging status by the age of 10 years.[12]

Antisense Oligonucleotides in Duchenne Muscular Dystrophy

Antisense oligonucleotides have long played a big role in the DMD therapy armamentarium. It is believed that nearly 80% of all DMD mutations are skippable. The first approved product targeted skipping of exon 51 of the dystrophin gene, which was extrapolated to benefit at least 14% of all boys affected with DMD. The situation currently is that there we have four licensed products that skip exons 51, two for 53 and 45, that can help manage 30% of boys affected by DMD by restoring the translational reading frame of DMD through specific exon skipping. Personalized medicine such as this depends on individual patient mutations. There are many more such DMT under development in the pipeline such as those for 52 and 44 skipping.

Eteplirsen (Exondys)

The *DMD* gene the longest human gene spans 2.4 Mb is in the Xp21 region, has 79 exons and produces a 14 kb transcript. Due to its sheer length, it is susceptible to mutations. But certain mutational hotspots, account for nearly 60% of all mutations. Majority of mutations are deletions with some duplications and a smaller percentage of point mutations. In most cases, these mutations disrupt the *DMD* reading frame, resulting in absent dystrophin production.

Exon skipping aims to fix this using nucleic acid-based drugs. Eteplirsen was the first such therapy which gained FDA approval in September 2016.

The inspiration for exon skipping comes from nature through observing the milder dystrophinopathy Becker muscular dystrophy (BMD), in which the dystrophin reading frame is not disrupted. Understanding and replicating these naturally occurring variants with shortened albeit functional Dp then became the goal for a cure. So, researchers began working on making the *DMD* mutation less deleterious by changing it from an out of frame to an in-frame mutation, thus mitigating the severity. The translational reading frame is thus restored using synthetic nucleic acid analogs. These ASOs then interfere with mRNA splicing. An exon is targeted and through tweaking of the splicing machinery, the ASO ensures that the targeted exon is excluded from the final transcript.

Mechanism of Action

Eteplirsen is a 30-nucleotide long phosphorodiamidate morpholino oligomer (PMO) category of ASO. Unlike regular RNA or DNA,

PMOs are attached to a morpholino moiety. Their subunits are connected via phosphorodiamidate linkages. Eteplirsen hybridizes to exon 51 of DMD causing exon 51 to be skipped during splicing, thus restoring the reading frame. Another molecule drisapersen was also studied for exon 51 skipping but failed to gain FDA approval over safety concerns and lack of efficacy giving us an example of a lot of such investigational molecules that have fallen by the wayside.

The safety and tolerability of PMOs are based on their being neutral and of not having a negative charge that could potentially invite nuclease-mediated degradation.

Exon 53 Skipping

Two molecules have been currently approved. *Golodirsen* which was FDA approved in December 2019 and *viltolarsen* which gained FDA approval in August 2020. Both these target exon 53 skipping and can treat the subset of patients with mutations that are amenable to this skipping.

Exon 45 Skipping: Casimersen

Yet another ASO molecule developed, which targets exon 45 of the *DMD* gene for skipping and was approved in February 2021. This is a PMO type of ASO.

Ataluren: Stop Codon Read Through

This is a molecule used to treat DMD with nonsense mutation because of a premature stop codon. Currently, it has approval in the European Union for ambulant boys above 5 years of age. Ataluren makes ribosomes less sensitive to premature stop codons by an effect called as "read through".

Gene Therapy in Duchenne Muscular Dystrophy

Conventional gene therapy aiming to deliver functional copies of the *DMD* gene is problematic in DMD due to the large size of the *DMD* gene resulting in poor delivery and owing to the immune response against the vector. Despite many hurdles, there has always excitement about gene therapy in DMD. The first significant obstacle was the sheer size of the dystrophin gene with its 79 exons and the difficulty in finding a vector that could carry it. Recently, the first microdystrophin expressing gene therapy, delandistrogene moxeparvovec was approved for use in boys with DMD aged 4–5 years of age conditionally by the FDA and has been priced at 3.2 million USD. There have been safety concerns due to some mortality involved with subjects in the trial, particularly the older subjects. The current understanding is that older subjects have difficulty in weathering the immune storm and their impaired cardiac reserves often get in the way of their withstanding it.

■ ADVANCES IN STANDARDS OF CARE AND ETHICAL CONCERNS

Until recently and for most of the children in our country by and large, since these expensive therapeutic options are not easily available the management of SMA and DMD involved managing its complications, that is managing complications arising from weakness, such as breathing difficulty, swallowing, and feeding issues as well as the cardiac involvement in DMD.

The advent of newer therapies has caused a huge paradigm shift in the way we look at and treat these conditions. But we need to bear in mind that we have not cured, but just altered the natural history of these conditions. Hence even treated SMA children, would, depending on how old they were before we intervened with a DMT, still have lost anterior cells that could never be regained and hence need significant on-going care to manage these effects and their implications. So we once again come back to SOC. The first classic document that was drawn up by an international group of SMA experts was the 2007 Consensus guidelines for SMA,[13] which is still an elegant document on which the newer documents were later built upon.

Currently, the two-part consensus guidelines from 2018 are what are still in use.[12,13] These address various aspects such as diagnosis and genetics, physical therapy and rehabilitation, orthopedic care, bone health, nutrition, pulmonary care, acute care in hospital settings, other organ system involvement, and finally touch upon ethics and palliative care.[10,14]

These ethical issues loom large for all of us in the field as patients are increasingly become aware that there are available medications, which are inaccessible to them due to their exorbitant pricing. Previously before the advent of the newer therapies, decisions to palliate an affected infant was taken in conjunction with the family and though difficult, was still straight forward due to limited options. Hence invasive measures such as a tracheostomy where thought to be putting length of life above quality of life and were mostly unheard off. We are faced with an ever-evolving dilemma of providing care options in a balanced and fair way, all the while making families aware that the option for care or palliative care need not be an either-or option and could at various points include both being interlinked.[10] This was why even the SMA working group could not achieve any consensus on standards of palliative care and could only acknowledge the massive numbers of ethical dilemmas this changing landscape of SMA treatment called for.

These entire bundles of dilemmas are slowly getting transposed to DMD care as well and it should encourage all of us in the field to keep abreast of the newer developments and have healthy consensus in our own settings.

■ CONCLUSION

We live in exciting times where we can offer increasingly better outcomes due to newer DMTs.[15] But this comes with its own challenges, making selecting the right patient for the right therapy and delivering it at the right time crucial. Current DMTs work on various pathways and hence personalized medicine along with combinatory therapies will most likely be the norm. As evidenced by *DMD* gene therapy, where steroids for treated patients have not been stopped. And we now have agents such as givinostat being added to this mix. All these innovation demands that treating physicians keep abreast of all the issues involved to wield them in the best possible manner.

REFERENCES

1. Wijekoon N, Gonawala L, Ratnayake P, Amaratunga D, Hathout Y, Mohan C, et al. Duchenne muscular dystrophy from brain to muscle: The role of brain dystrophin isoforms in motor function. J Clin Med. 2023;12(17):5637.
2. Comi GP, Niks EH, Vandenborne K, Cinnante CM, Kan HE, Willcocks RJ, et al. Givinostat for Becker muscular dystrophy: A randomised placebo-controlled, double blind study. Front Neuro. 2023;14:1095121.
3. D'Amico A, Mercuri E, Tiziano FD, Bertini E. Spinal muscular atrophy. Orphanet J Rare Dis. 2011;6:71.
4. Nishio H, Niba ETE, Saito T, Okamoto K, Takeshima Y, Awano H. Spinal Muscular atrophy: The past present and future of diagnosis and treatment. Int J Mol Sci. 2023;24:11939.
5. Dubowitz. Spinal Muscular Atrophy revisited. Neuromusc Dis. 2019;29:413-4.
6. Cherry JJ, Androphy EJ. Therapeutic strategies for the treatment of spinal muscular atrophy. Future Med Chem. 2012;4(13);1733-50.
7. Abiusi E, Costa-Roger M, Bertini ES, Tiziano FD, Tizzano EF, Baranello G, et al; SMN2 Study group. 207th ENMC International Workshop: Consensus

for SMN2 genetic analysis in SMA patients 10-12 March, 2023, Hoofddorp, The Netherlands. Neuromusc Dis. 2024;34:114-22.
8. Gowda V, Atherton M, Murugan A, Servais L, Sheehan J, Standing E, et al. Efficacy and safety of onasemnogene abeparvovec in children with spinal muscular atrophy type 1: Real world experience from 6 infusion centre in the United Kingdom. Lancet. 2024;37:100817.
9. Bernal S, Also-Rallo E, Martínez-Hernández R, Alías L, Rodríguez-Alvarez FJ, Millán JM, et al. Plastin 3 expression in expression in discordant spinal muscular atrophy (SMA) siblings. Neuro Musc Dis. 2011;21(6):413-9.
10. Finkel RS, Mercuri E, Meyer OH, Simonds AK, Schroth MK, Graham RJ, et al. Diagnosis and management of spinal muscular atrophy: Part 2. Neuromusc Dis. 2018;28:197-207.
11. Ojala KS, Reedich EJ, DiDonato CJ, Meriney SD. In search of a cure: The development of therapeutics to alter the progression of spinal muscular atrophy. Brain Sci. 2021;11(2):194.
12. Birnkrant DJ, Bushby K, Bann CM, Alman BA, Apkon SD, Blackwell A, et al. Diagnosis and management of Duchenne muscular dystrophy, Part 2: respiratory, cardiac, bone health and orthopaedic management: DMD care considerations working group. Lancet Neurol. 2018;17:347–61.
13. Wang CH, Finkel RS, Bertini ES, Schroth M, Simonds A, Wong B, et al. Consensus statement for standard of care in spinal muscular atrophy. J Child Neurol. 2007;22(8);1027-49.
14. Mercuri E, Finkel RS, Muntoni F, Wirth B, Montes J, Main M, et al. Diagnosis and management of Spinal Muscular atrophy: Part 1:Update from the SMA care group. Neuromusc Dis. 2018;28:103-15.
15. Schorling DC, Pechmann A, Kirschner J. Advances in treatment of spinal muscular atrophy—new phenotypes, new challenges, new implications for care. J Neuromusc Dis. 2020;7(1):1-3.

CHAPTER 2

Refractory Myasthenia: Management Strategies

Deepak Menon, Seena Vengalil, Saraswati Nashi, Atchayaram Nalini

ABSTRACT

Refractory myasthenia gravis (MG) is a significantly disabling condition affecting 10–20% of patients with MG (pwMG) and presents numerous management challenges. Advancements in our understanding of MG immunopathology have identified several potential therapeutic epitopes that, if targeted, can reduce disease severity. While conventional agents such as cyclophosphamide (Cyc) and methotrexate (Mtx) remain integral to treatment, there is a growing shift toward newer targeted biological agents, which have demonstrated better efficacy and safety profiles, particularly in refractory MG. The current chapters explore these various aspects of refractory MG, including novel therapeutic agents and the current limitations within the Indian context.

Keywords: Myasthenia gravis, Refractory, Complement inhibitors, FCRN blockers, Rituximab.

■ INTRODUCTION

The development of immunosuppressive agents and advancements in therapeutics have heralded a significant transformation in the natural history of myasthenia gravis (MG). Mortality rates in patients with MG (pwMG), which once stood as high as 50–80% at the turn of the century, have now decreased to levels nearly comparable to the normal population in many regions worldwide.[1,2] Although the vast majority of pwMG respond to conventional immunomodulatory treatment, a moderate minority of patients experience inadequate response. This can be in the form of symptom persistence, worsening or frequent myasthenic crises despite adequate treatment, and the inability to taper immunosuppressive agents, especially steroid or in the form of intolerable treatment side effects.[3] The International Consensus Guidance for Management of MG defines MG as refractory when the postintervention status remains unchanged or worsens after corticosteroids and at least two other immunosuppressive agents, despite adequate dose and duration, with persistent symptoms or side effects that limit functioning as defined by patient and physician.[4] Data from across the world shows that approximately 10–20% of pwMG experience refractory MG. These patients in general tend to have more severe disease, bulbar symptoms, potentially life-threatening exacerbations, and poses serious management challenges.[5,6]

IMMUNOPATHOLOGY BEHIND REFRACTORY MYASTHENIA GRAVIS

Treatment strategies for MG are primarily derived from the understanding of the immunopathology that drives the disorder. The autoantibodies responsible for the failure of postsynaptic neuromuscular junction transmission belong to different immunoglobulin G (IgG) subclasses depending on the specific type of MG. In acetylcholine receptor (AChR) antibody-positive MG, the autoantibodies are mainly IgG1 and IgG3 subclass, while in lipoprotein receptor-related 4 (LrP4)-positive MG, they are IgG1 and IgG2, and in muscle-specific kinase (MuSK)-positive MG, they are IgG4. It is important to note that while IgG1 and IgG3 subclass antibodies bring about postsynaptic dysfunction through complement-mediated processes; this is not the case with IgG4 subclass antibodies.[7] These antibodies are secreted by plasma cells which in turn are derived from activated B cells and along with plasmablasts and memory B cells, sustain the MG immunopathogenesis. The upstream CD4+ T and B cell activations and interactions that lead to the generation of these antibodies are more complex and research have identified several immune targets that hold promise in treatment of MG, many of which are already available in the market.[8]

The immunopathological basis for why a minority of pwMG remain refractory to treatment is not fully understood. One of the drawbacks of conventional immunosuppressive agents is their broad and nontargeted action. Memory B cells and long-lived plasma cells can survive in bone marrow niches, out of reach of conventional immunomodulators.[9] These long-lived plasma cells may take up a pivotal role in pathogenesis, a role that is suboptimally targeted by conventional agents and can lead to relapse of MG or treatment resistance.[10] Additionally, patient-to-patient differences in genetically-mediated pharmacokinetics and pharmacodynamics can contribute to variations in drug tolerability and adverse effects. These differences may also limit the ability to titrate treatment to an optimal drug dosage.

"PSEUDO" REFRACTORINESS

Before a patient is deemed "refractory" the physician must suspect several alternative scenarios. First and foremost, would be a reconsideration of diagnosis, keeping in mind that several other neurological and non-neurological conditions can mimic the symptoms of MG.[11] The list is long and would include mitochondrial disorders, myopathies, polyradiculopathies, brainstem syndromes as well as medical conditions including endocrine or metabolic disorders, depression, toxins, and levator palpebrae dehiscence. Importantly, it must be borne in mind that congenital myasthenic syndromes can manifest even in third or fourth decade and can mimic an autoimmune myasthenia. Other causes for an apparent treatment responsiveness can be drug noncompliance, default or intolerance, intake of alternative medications liable to worsen MG, and undercurrent infections or medical conditions such as hyperthyroidism. Additionally, unrealistic expectations, insufficient knowledge about the disease, and biases from patients and their families can come across as treatment unresponsiveness. Using objective measures such as the quantitative MG (QMG) score, MG activities of daily living (MG-ADL), MG quality of life (MG-QOL), and MG impairment index (MGII) serially during clinic visits provide informative and well-documented assessments. However, the caveat is that these measures can be time-consuming and that most are not validated in Indian languages.

GENERAL TRENDS IN MYASTHENIA GRAVIS TREATMENT IN THE INDIAN CONTEXT

Although practices vary, the conventional strategy of MG treatment consists of first-line initiation of steroids alongside symptomatic treatment with pyridostigmine. In the setting of severe symptoms or impending crisis, intravenous immunoglobulin (IVIg) or plasma exchange (PLEX) is warranted. Additionally, a steroid-sparing agent is often introduced concurrently or when a patient is noted to be steroid-dependent.[4,12] Azathioprine (AZA) and mycophenolate mofetil (MMF) are the two most popular steroid sparing agents in use, especially in India. While relatively inexpensive, these two agents take a minimum of 4–6 months for their actions, during which steroids at least in low dose would have to be maintained.[12] If the patient remains treatment refractory to the earlier mentioned paradigm, there are alternate broad-spectrum immunosuppressants and novel biologicals that have showed promise in the treatment.

ALTERNATE CONVENTIONAL AGENTS AS TREATMENT OPTIONS IN REFRACTORY MYASTHENIA GRAVIS

Cyclophosphamide

Despite the emergence of several newer agents, cyclophosphamide (Cyc) remains one of the go-to second-line agents of immunosuppression in severe autoimmune disorders, especially in low- and middle-income countries (LMIC). There is sufficient evidence from prospective and retrospective studies to support use of Cyc in refractory MG with benefits in terms of improvement in MG as well as steroid tapering.[12] Monthly pulse of low-dose Cyc has shown to induce a response as early as 1 month but fails to maintain a long-term remission with patients often relapsing within a year.[13,14] While recommended in refractory MG, the potential side effects, especially in young people with higher cumulative doses, makes Cyc most suited for inducing remission in severe MG rather than as a long-term maintenance treatment.[4]

Methotrexate

The evidence favoring use of methotrexate (Mtx) in MG is less robust. A recent systematic review of two trials and one observational study noted mixed results but overall the efficacy of Mtx seems comparable to AZA as a long-term steroid-sparing agent.[15] Despite this, the International Consensus Guidance does recommend Mtx as a treatment option when alternate first-line agents are not tolerated or efficacious.[16]

Cyclosporine and Tacrolimus

The effectiveness of cyclosporine (Cys) in the treatment of MG is well established. In fact, one of the earliest drug trials in MG have been with Cys, where a rapid and significant improvement in immunosuppression naïve patients noted as early as 2 weeks into treatment.[17] More specifically, Cys resulted in significant improvement when used in patients refractory to high-dose steroids, AZA, IVIg, or PLEX with improvement as early as 3 weeks with maximum benefit by 6 months.[18] However, the unfavorable toxicity profile and the need for frequent monitoring of drug levels may make Cys less attractive in the Indian context. Nevertheless, Cys remains a viable option in refractory MG particularly due to its rapid onset of action.

Tacrolimus (FK506) has a mechanism of action that is nearly identical to Cys. A systematic review of prospective clinical trials from 1947 to 2014 revealed its benefits in refractory MG.[19] However, two recent randomized controlled trials (RCTs) failed to show a significant benefit in MG unresponsive to steroids.[12]

Immunoglobulins and Plasma Exchange

Chronic IVIg and therapeutic PLEX as monthly pulses have been well-recognized as beneficial in refractory MG and is recommended.[4] While effective, there are several drawbacks for their use in the Indian context. Beyond the obvious financial burden and resource limitations, the logistics involved in 3–4 weekly hospital visits and need for repeated venous access puts this beyond acceptability for most patients.

A compelling alternative to patients reliant on maintenance treatment with IVIg is transitioning to subcutaneous immunoglobulin (SCIG) and has gained much traction in developed countries.[20] Several studies have showed a sustained benefit in pwMG when transitioned to SCIG.[12] SCIG comes in 20% and 16.5% formulations distinct from intravenous formulations, and offers several pharmacokinetic and practical advantages in ease of administration. For one, it offers the choice of self-administration of medication in the comforts of home, 2- or 3-day a week, either by themselves or a family member. As the absorption is from the subcutaneous compartment, it offers a sustained, stable, and higher trough levels in the serum and has better tolerance compared with IVIg.[21] Other than affordability, setting up the infusion device does have a learning curve and may be difficult for patients experiencing upper limb weakness.

BIOLOGICAL AGENTS IN THE TREATMENT OF REFRACTORY MYASTHENIA GRAVIS

Rituximab

Rituximab (Rtx) is a chimeric monoclonal antibody that selectively depletes CD20+ B cells and thus bring about a favorable shift in MG immunology and has been accepted as a first-line agent in MuSK MG. However, Rtx currently occupies an enigmatic position concerning its use in AChR-positive generalized MG. This ambiguity arises from the discrepancies between some of the RCT data and international recommendations on one side, and the more recent real-world data on the other. Except for the first phase II BEAT-MG trial which showed lack of response, systematic reviews, meta-analyses, and subsequent case series have largely demonstrated an unequivocal beneficial effect in MG both in reducing the disease severity and in steroid sparing.[12,22] The more recent RINOMAX trial in 2022 showed that even low-dose Rtx (single 500 mg dose) had a significant benefit in MG advocating an early initiation of Rtx.[23] To make matters more obscure, the latest systematic review and meta-analysis in 2023 found that while anticomplement and Fc receptor (FcRn) inhibitors are effective, Rtx failed to prove beneficial in MG.[24] And finally, a systematic review and meta-analysis that specifically looked at Rtx in refractory MG concluded that Rtx reduced the MG severity, allowed steroid tapering and had minimal adverse effects and the benefit seemed to be independent of the dose of Rtx.[25] But the review did not incorporate any clinical trial as none was available in this context. Despite some ambivalence, overall, Rtx can be recommended as a definite treatment option for refractory MG, especially in India due to its ease of availability, accumulated experience, and the largely favorable side effect profile. Decade-long experiences with use of Rtx in other autoimmune disorders gives reassurance that threat of conditions such as progressive multifocal leukoencephalopathy (PML) or malignancy appears nominal.[26]

Complement Inhibitors

Complement inhibitors act by binding with variable affinities to C5 complement and preventing the downstream formation of membrane attack complexes which are one of the final effector pathways of MG immunopathogenesis. Eculizumab was the initial molecule in this category which was approved by the Food and Drug Administration (FDA) in 2017 for AChR positive generalized MG. REGAIN trial and its open label extension phase showed a rapid and sustained benefit in patients with AChR positive generalized refractory MG when treated with eculizumab.[27] In general, the onset of action is seen around 12 weeks of treatment. The adverse events are mostly minor and include headache, diarrhea, and respiratory tract infection but the principal safety concern is life-threatening infection with encapsulated organisms such as *Neisseria meningitidis* which is the class side effect and vaccination prior to initiation of treatment is mandatory.

The two other agents in this category that have been approved for AChR-positive generalized MG and are options in refractory cases are ravulizumab (approved 2022) and zilucoplan (approved 2023). Both agents have been shown to have a rapid and sustained benefit and offers advantages in dosing regime and mode of administrations. Ravulizumab has a dosing interval of 8 weeks compared to the 2 weekly dosing of eculizumab while zilucoplan has a daily dosing but can be self-administered subcutaneously. The side effects are minor and similar to that of eculizumab.

Fc Receptor Blockers

The long half-life that IgG enjoys in comparison to other proteins in the serum is to a great extend due to the FcRn which are beta-2 macroglobulin-associated proteins that bind to them and protecting IgG from lysosomal degradation.[28] FcRn inhibitors act by blocking these receptors which in turn leads to enhanced IgG breakdown and limits the IgG recycling. A dramatic drop in IgG levels thus ensues and hence treatment with this class of molecules has been referred to as "medical PLEX".

Two agents in this group, efgartigimod (approved 2021) and rozanolixizumab (approved 2023) has received approval for treatment in AChR or MuSK-positive generalized MG. A rapid fall in IgG levels has been noticed as early as 1 week with clinical improvement in 2 weeks and although the levels may reach baseline in 8 weeks, the clinical benefit usually lasts longer. The side effects are mild and include headache, nasopharyngitis, diarrhea, and asymptomatic fall in monocyte counts. Two other agents in this category, nipocalimab and batoclimab could soon receive approval.

Hematopoietic Stem Cell Transplantation

As mentioned earlier, the role of memory B cells and long-lived plasma cells in perpetuating the immunological milieu in MG has been recognized. As they lack CD20 expression and remain confined within the bone marrow compartment, they remain untargeted by conventional agents. Hematopoietic stem cell transplantation (HSCT) eradicates all autoreactive pathological T and B cells thus resetting the immunological memory and has remained an attractive concept for treatment of chronic refractory autoimmune disorders.[29] The initial conditioning regimen of cytotoxic therapy or irradiation for immunoablation is followed by infusion of previously harvested autologous stem cells. In a short case series of seven patients with refractory life-threatening MG, HSCT showed a tremendous response with all patients going into sustained stable remission and with successful tapering of immunosuppressive therapies.[30] Although a definite option in pwMG in whom all options have been exhausted, there are short- and long-term safety concerns which cannot be ignored.[31] These are largely dependent on the conditioning regimen and include risk of infection and gastrointestinal toxicity with long-term risks of infertility and secondary neoplasms.

Chimeric Antigen Receptor T Cell and Chimeric Autoantibody Receptor T Cell Therapies

Although not yet available for the clinical treatment of MG, chimeric antigen receptor T (CAR T) cell therapy warrants special mention. It has the potential to revolutionize the management of autoimmune disorders, much like it has completely transformed the field of hemato-oncology. Autologous T cells are harvested and genetically modified to express receptors that recognize tumor cell target antigens. These cells undergo ex vivo expansion and are infused back to the patient which would then bring about targeted destruction of malignant cells. As the CAR T cell remains and multiplies within the circulation they are also called "living drugs".[32] The T cells can also be engineered against autoreactive B cells [chimeric autoantibody receptor T (CAAR T) cells] which can specifically target the autoreactive B cells implicated in the immunopathogenesis.[33] The adverse effects include cytokine release which at times can become severe enough to cause cytokine storm syndrome. Currently phase I and II trials are underway exploring CAR T cell therapy in AChR MG.[20]

■ OTHER AGENTS WITH ANECDOTAL EVIDENCE

Benefits have been reported with tocilizumab, an interleukin-6 blocker, in two pwMG with high titers of AChR antibodies, refractory even after Rtx.[34] Similarly subcutaneous bortezomib, a proteasome inhibitor primarily used in myeloma, was found to induce rapid response in a patient with MuSK MG who remained symptomatic despite steroids, PLEX, IVIg, and Rtx. However, it may not be an ideal option for of long-term maintenance due to the limiting side effect of peripheral neuropathy.[33] Anecdotal case report of a patient with MuSK MG who had suboptimal response to Rtx having prolonged and sustained response to ocrelizumab highlights the role for alternate anti-CD20 agents in refractory MG.[35]

■ THYMECTOMY

Following the 2016 landmark RCT, thymectomy is advised in patients with AChR-positive generalized MG between 18 and 50 years of age, especially when there is inadequate response to immunotherapies, even in the absence of a thymic lesion.[16] Thymectomy is advised early in the course of the illness but should be performed electively only when the patient is stable, as attempting thymectomy during worsening or impending crisis poses significant risks of further deterioration and prolonged ventilation. The benefits of thymectomy are not immediate; it often takes months to over a year for patients to start experiencing the benefit. For patients who remain refractory or experience relapse after an adequate period post-thymectomy, the possibility of residual or ectopic thymic tissue should be considered, even if not identified radiologically. Studies that examined an extended repeat thymectomy in refractory MG have reported clinically significant improvement but less frequent chances of complete remission.[36,37]

■ PRACTICAL ASPECTS AND CLINICAL CONUNDRUMS

The treatment of patients with refractory MG is highly individualized and a uniformly applicable treatment escalation protocol cannot be recommended. It is essential to educate the patient about their disease, treatment options, potential adverse events and need for monitoring, financial burden, and the implications on the reproductive health. A treatment trial of sufficient duration must be tried before deeming ineffective unless the patient has intolerable side effects.

Globally the treatment trends in autoimmune disorders, including MG, are moving toward targeted biological agents that offer improved efficacy and safety. The systematic review and meta-analysis of innovative therapies in MG showed a unequivocally significant improvement with complement inhibitors and FcRn inhibitor class of agents.[24] However cost-benefit analyses and the long-term safety impact on pwMG are currently unclear. Moreover, the financial implications mean that these agents would currently remain out of reach for most patients in India. In addition, several questions remain with regards to interclass and intraclass switching and when to initiate early as soon as patient fails first-line agents or after exhausting other options.[20] Nevertheless, with recent advances, pwMG and their physicians have more safe and effective options and hopefully a parallel drop in percentage of refractory MG may be expected in the coming decades (**Fig. 1** and **Table 1**).

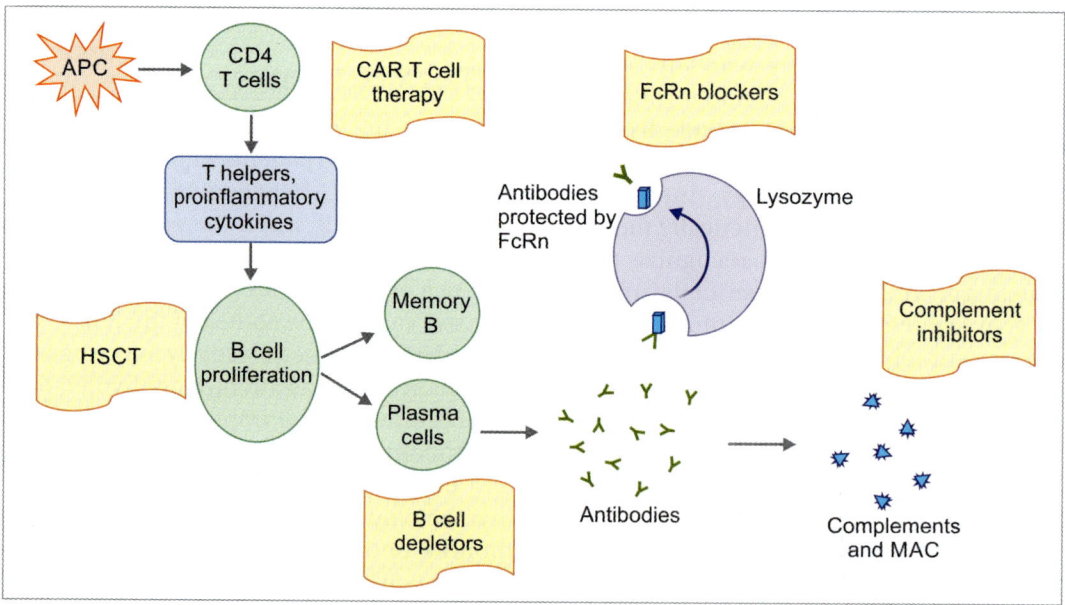

FIG. 1: Summary of the novel biological agents that and their targets in the MG immunopathology.
(APC: antigen presenting cell; CAR T: chimeric antigen receptor T; FcRn: Fc receptor; HSCT: hematopoietic stem cell transplantation; MAC: membrane attack complex; MG: myasthenia gravis)

TABLE 1: Summary of dose and most relevant adverse effects.

Agent	Dose	Adverse effects
Cyclophosphamide	IV, 1–1.5 mg/m^2 over 5 days, monthly pulse	Need for premedications, risk of infections, and bladder hemorrhage. Cumulative risk of gonadal toxicity and malignancies
Methotrexate	Oral, 10 mg weekly single dose, increased to 20–25 mg/week	Pancytopenia and elevated liver enzymes
Cyclosporine	Oral, starting at 3 mg/kg/day and increased to 6 mg/kg/day titration based on clinical efficacy and TDM	Nephrotoxicity, hypertension, paresthesia, gum sensitivity, altered taste, and hirsutism. TDM target 400–600 ng/mL
Tacrolimus	Oral, 3 mg/kg/day titration based on clinical efficacy and TDM	Similar to Cyc but less sever. TDM target 7–8 ng/mL
Rituximab	IV, 1,000 mg 2 weeks apart. Alternate 375 mg/m^2 weekly for 4 weeks	Infusion-related reactions, leukopenia, and infections
Eculizumab	IV, 900 mg weekly for 4 weeks followed by 1,200 mg every 2 weeks	Concern of *Neisseria meningitidis*, prevaccination, headache, and nasopharyngitis
Ravulizumab	IV, weight based 2,400–3,000 mg initial 2 weeks apart, subsequent once every 8 weeks	Concern of *Neisseria meningitidis* and prevaccination
Zilucoplan	SC, 0.3 mg/kg/day	Local injection site reactions and headache
Efgartigimod	IV, 10 mg/kg weekly	Headache, leukopenia, and nasopharyngitis
Rozanolixizumab	IV, weight based 420–840 mg weekly once	Headache

(Cyc: cyclophosphamide; IV: intravenous; SC: subcutaneous; TDM: therapeutic drug monitoring)

■ CONCLUSION

The treatment options for patients with refractory MG are rapidly expanded with the emergence of several novel biological agents in the recent years. While the future is optimistic, the treatment landscape continue to evolve demanding further studies to determine their positions in the real-world setting especially in low and middle income countries.

REFERENCES

1. Keesey JC. A history of treatments for myasthenia gravis. Semin Neurol. 2004;24(1):5-16.
2. Zhang C, Wang F, Long Z, Yang J, Ren Y, Ma Q, et al. Mortality of myasthenia gravis: a national population-based study in China. Ann Clin Transl Neurol. 2023;10(7):1095-105.
3. Schneider-Gold C, Hagenacker T, Melzer N, Ruck T. Understanding the burden of refractory myasthenia gravis. Ther Adv Neurol Disord. 2019;12:1756286419832242.
4. Sanders DB, Wolfe GI, Benatar M, Evoli A, Gilhus NE, Illa I, et al. International consensus guidance for management of myasthenia gravis. Neurology. 2016;87(4):419-25.
5. Mantegazza R, Antozzi C. When myasthenia gravis is deemed refractory: clinical signposts and treatment strategies. Ther Adv Neurol Disord. 2018;11:1756285617749134.
6. Cortés-Vicente E, Álvarez-Velasco R, Pla-Junca F, Rojas-Garcia R, Paradas C, Sevilla T, et al.

Drug-refractory myasthenia gravis: Clinical characteristics, treatments, and outcome. Ann Clin Transl Neurol. 2022;9(2):122-31.
7. Phillips WD, Vincent A. Pathogenesis of myasthenia gravis: update on disease types, models, and mechanisms. F1000Res. 2016;5:F1000 Faculty Rev-1513.
8. Menon D, Barnett C, Bril V. Novel Treatments in Myasthenia Gravis. Front Neurol. 2020;11:538.
9. Yi JS, Guptill JT, Stathopoulos P, Nowak RJ, O'Connor KC. B cells in the pathophysiology of myasthenia gravis. Muscle Nerve. 2018;57(2):172-84.
10. Kaminski HJ, Denk J. Corticosteroid Treatment-Resistance in Myasthenia Gravis. Front Neurol. 2022;13:886625.
11. Engstrom JW. Myasthenia gravis: diagnostic mimics. Semin Neurol. 2004;24(2):141-7.
12. Menon D, Bril V. Pharmacotherapy of Generalized Myasthenia Gravis with Special Emphasis on Newer Biologicals. Drugs. 2022;82(8):865-87.
13. Gomez-Figueroa E, Garcia-Trejo S, Bazan-Rodriguez L, Cervantes-Uribe R, Chac-Lezama G, López-Hernández JC, et al. Intravenous cyclophosphamide monthly pulses in refractory myasthenia gravis. J Neurol. 2020;267(3):674-8.
14. Nagappa M, Netravathi M, Taly AB, Sinha S, Bindu PS, Mahadevan A. Long-term efficacy and limitations of cyclophosphamide in myasthenia gravis. J Clin Neurosci. 2014;21(11):1909-14.
15. Prado MB, Adiao KJB. Methotrexate in generalized myasthenia gravis: a systematic review. Acta Neurol Belg. 2023;123(5):1679-91.
16. Narayanaswami P, Sanders DB, Wolfe G, Benatar M, Cea G, Evoli A, et al. International Consensus Guidance for Management of Myasthenia Gravis. Neurology. 2021;96(3):114-22.
17. Matsuda S, Koyasu S. Mechanisms of action of cyclosporine. Immunopharmacology. 2000;47(2–3):119-25.
18. Lavrnic D, Vujic A, Rakocevic-Stojanovic V, Stevic Z, Basta I, Pavlovic S, et al. Cyclosporine in the treatment of myasthenia gravis. Acta Neurologica Scandinavica. 2005;111(4):247-52.
19. Cruz JL, Wolff ML, Vanderman AJ, Brown JN. The emerging role of tacrolimus in myasthenia gravis. Ther Adv Neurol Disord. 2015;8(2):92-103.
20. Menon D, Urra Pincheira A, Bril V. Emerging drugs for the treatment of myasthenia gravis. Expert Opin Emerg Drugs. 2021;26(3):259-70.
21. Menon D, Sarpong E, Bril V. Practical Aspects of Transitioning from Intravenous to Subcutaneous Immunoglobulin Therapy in Neuromuscular Disorders. Can J Neurol Sci. 2022;49(2):161-7.
22. Vesperinas-Castro A, Cortés-Vicente E. Rituximab treatment in myasthenia gravis. Front Neurol. 2023;14:1275533.
23. Piehl F, Eriksson-Dufva A, Budzianowska A, Feresiadou A, Hansson W, Hietala MA, et al. Efficacy and Safety of Rituximab for New-Onset Generalized Myasthenia Gravis: The RINOMAX Randomized Clinical Trial. JAMA Neurol. 2022;79(11):1105-12.
24. Saccà F, Pane C, Espinosa PE, Sormani MP, Signori A. Efficacy of innovative therapies in myasthenia gravis: A systematic review, meta-analysis and network meta-analysis. Eur J Neurol. 2023;30(12):3854-67.
25. Zhao C, Pu M, Chen D, Shi J, Li Z, Guo J, et al. Effectiveness and Safety of Rituximab for Refractory Myasthenia Gravis: A Systematic Review and Single-Arm Meta-Analysis. Front Neurol. 2021;12:736190.
26. van Vollenhoven RF, Emery P, Bingham CO, Keystone EC, Fleischmann RM, Furst DE, et al. Long-term safety of rituximab in rheumatoid arthritis: 9.5-year follow-up of the global clinical trial programme with a focus on adverse events of interest in RA patients. Ann Rheum Dis. 2013;72(9):1496-502.
27. Mantegazza R, Wolfe GI, Muppidi S, Wiendl H, Fujita KP, O'Brien FL, et al. Post-intervention Status in Patients With Refractory Myasthenia Gravis Treated With Eculizumab During REGAIN and Its Open-Label Extension. Neurology. 2021;96(4):e610-8.
28. Bhandari V, Bril V. FcRN receptor antagonists in the management of myasthenia gravis. Front Neurol. 2023;14:1229112.
29. Alexander T, Bondanza A, Muraro PA, Greco R, Saccardi R, Daikeler T, et al. SCT for severe autoimmune diseases: consensus guidelines of the European Society for Blood and Marrow Transplantation for immune monitoring and biobanking. Bone Marrow Transplant. 2015;50(2):173-80.
30. Bryant A, Atkins H, Pringle CE, Allan D, Anstee G, Bence-Bruckler I, et al. Myasthenia Gravis Treated With Autologous Hematopoietic Stem Cell Transplantation. JAMA Neurol. 2016;73(6):652-8.
31. Mariottini A, Bulgarini G, Cornacchini S, Damato V, Saccardi R, Massacesi L. Hematopoietic Stem Cell Transplantation for the Treatment of Autoimmune Neurological Diseases: An Update. Bioengineering (Basel). 2023;10(2):176.
32. Aghajanian H, Rurik JG, Epstein JA. CAR-based therapies: opportunities for immuno-medicine beyond cancer. Nat Metab. 2022;4(2):163-9.

33. Nair SS, Jacob S. Novel Immunotherapies for Myasthenia Gravis. Immunotargets Ther. 2023;12: 25-45.
34. Jonsson DI, Pirskanen R, Piehl F. Beneficial effect of tocilizumab in myasthenia gravis refractory to rituximab. Neuromuscul Disord. 2017;27(6): 565-8.
35. Aljaberi KM, Mandalawi AN, Chirakkara SKP, Shatila AO. A Case of Myasthenia Gravis Treated with Ocrelizumab. Mult Scler Relat Dis. 2023;80: 105324.
36. Ng JKY, Ng CSH, Underwood MJ, Lau KKW. Does repeat thymectomy improve symptoms in patients with refractory myasthenia gravis? Interact Cardiovasc Thorac Surg. 2014;18(3):376-80.
37. Zieliński M, Kuźdżał J, Staniec B, Harazda M, Nabiałek T, Pankowski J, et al. Extended rethymectomy in the treatment of refractory myasthenia gravis: original video-assisted technique of resternotomy and results of the treatment in 21 patients. Interact Cardiovasc Thorac Surg. 2004;3(2):376-80.

CHAPTER 3

Congenital Myasthenic Syndromes: Genetic Spectrum and Management

Seena Vengalil, Samim MM, Saraswati Nashi, Deepak Menon, Atchayaram Nalini

ABSTRACT

The congenital myasthenic syndromes (CMSs) are a heterogeneous group of inherited disorders of neuromuscular transmission characterized by fatigable, fluctuating weakness of ocular, bulbar, or limb muscles. Nearly 35 genes have been identified as causative of CMS in the last couple of decades, though the most common have been postsynaptic defects involving the acetylcholine receptor (AChR). Impaired neuromuscular transmission is only one of the myriad manifestations of this disease, central nervous system, and other organs may be involved in many of the subtypes. Though phenotypic clues and electrophysiological tests may give hint to a subtype, genetic testing is the gold standard of diagnosis. CMS is treatable; however, identification of the gene defect is essential as the drugs benefitting one type may aggravate the symptoms in others.

Keywords: Congenital myasthenic syndromes, Neuromuscular junction, Acetylcholine receptor, Next-generation sequencing, Choline esterase inhibitors.

■ INTRODUCTION

Congenital myasthenic syndrome (CMS) constitutes a heterogeneous group of inherited disorders of neuromuscular transmission characterized by fatigable, fluctuating weakness of ocular, bulbar, or limb muscles. Mutations in the genes encoding for AChR are the most common form of CMS and were the earliest to be described in literature. The list has been ever expanding and variants in 35 genes have been identified as causative of CMS, as of January 2023.[1] CMSs are rare disorders with a prevalence of around 9.2 per million in children <18 years of age.[2] Diagnosis is difficult due to the rarity, lack of awareness, and wide spectrum of age of onset, severity, and clinical manifestations.

In this chapter, we focus on the recent genetic advances and management of CMS.

■ CLASSIFICATION

Congenital myasthenic syndromes are classified into presynaptic, synaptic, and postsynaptic depending on the location of the mutated protein. More than 50% of the CMS are due to mutations in the postsynaptic region[3] while the presynaptic and synaptic defects constitute around 6 and 13% of the cases, respectively. **Figure 1** demonstrates the genetic defects causing CMS. All CMS cases show autosomal recessive (AR) inheritance except slow channel CMS (SCCMS), PURA-CMS, SNAP25-CMS, and few cases of synaptotagmin-2 (SYT2-CMS).

CHAPTER 3: Congenital Myasthenic Syndromes: Genetic Spectrum and Management

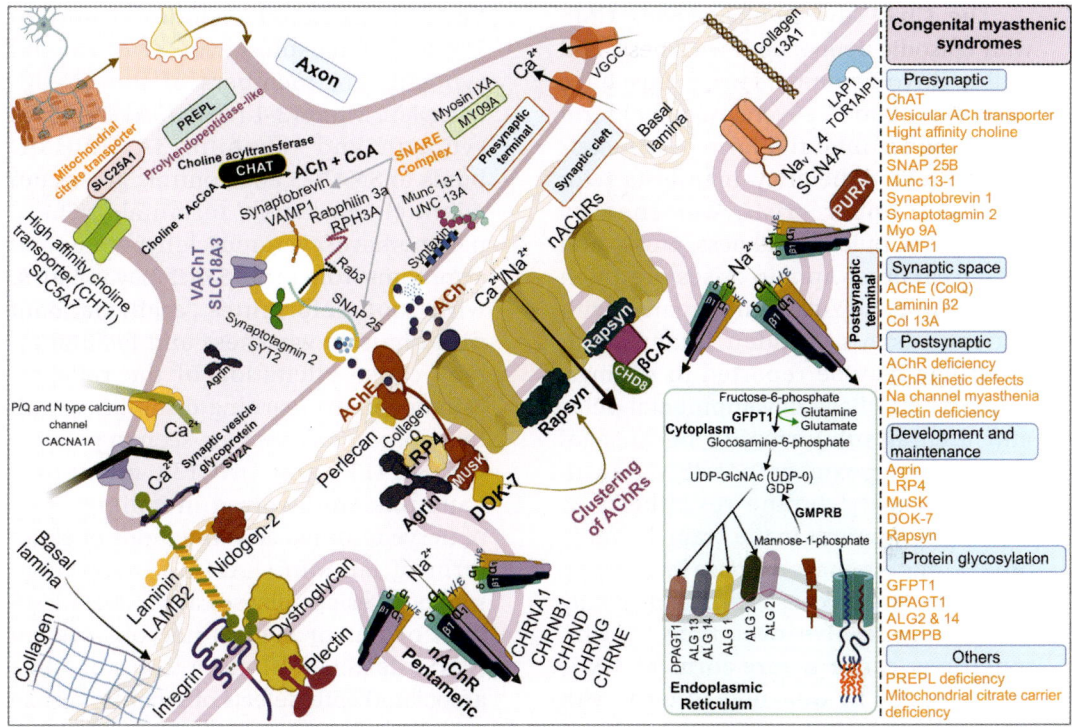

FIG. 1: The genetic defects causing congenital myasthenic syndrome (CMS).

Most of the patients preset with symptoms in infancy and early childhood but sometimes the symptoms may be delayed till adolescence or adulthood. CMS patients have fatigable weakness of ocular, limb, bulbar, or respiratory muscles. Diurnal fluctuation of muscle weakness may not be observed in CMS, unlike in myasthenia gravis and these patients may have seasonal variations or fluctuations over days. Diplopia is not reported usually as the external ophthalmoplegia is present since infancy and compensatory mechanisms occur. Patients who do not have ocular involvement are called limb-girdle CMS (LG-CMS). ChAT-CMS, SCN4A-CMS, and COLQ-CMS may have episodic apnea and history of sibling deaths. Developmental delay may be seen especially in presynaptic CMS. Based on pathophysiological mechanisms, CMS is divided into different groups. The clinical features of various CMS are described as follows:

- *Presynaptic CMS due to defective recycling of ACh*: This group includes mutations of choline acetyltransferase (ChAT), vesicular acetylcholine transporter (VAChT), SLC18A3, SLC5A7, and PREPL. ChAT is required for the synthesis of acetyl choline from choline and acetyl coenzyme A (CoA).[4] Synthesized ACh is transported to synaptic vesicle by VAChT. The first intron of ChAT encodes SLC18A3. SLC5A7, a choline transporter, is required for the uptake of choline at the nerve terminal. Prolyl-endopeptidase like (PREPL) is a serine peptidase required for refilling of ACh in the synaptic vesicle. Deficiency of PREPL causes reduced quanta of ACh release.

The ChAT deficiency causes CMS with episodic apnea, limb weakness, and bulbar involvement. Two forms have been described: A severe, neonatal form and a milder infantile form.[5] Neonatal-onset ChAT deficiency manifests with recurrent apneic crisis, worsened by fever/stress, bulbar weakness, ptosis, and limb weakness. Apneic crises are often mistaken as seizures and treated with anticonvulsants. Sudden infant death syndrome may be reported in siblings. Children may have developmental delay and mental subnormality because of recurrent hypoxia or possibly due to defective acetylcholine resynthesis in cholinergic neurons in the brain. Infantile onset forms may have exercise intolerance and muscle weakness, symptoms may completely resolve over time. VAChT mutations cause a rare form of CMS, characterized by weakness at birth with arthrogryposis and respiratory failure.[6] Cerebral atrophy and microcephaly may be seen.[7] SLC18A3 and SLC5A7 patients have a similar phenotype and may have arthrogryposis and congenital malformations. *PREPL* gene mutations have a milder phenotype with bulbar symptoms, fatigable limb weakness, and sometimes require ventilatory support. *PREPL-CMS* gene overlaps with *SLC3A1* gene, encoding hypotonia-cystinuria syndrome and patients may have combined features of both.[7] Endocrine abnormalities such as hypogonadotropic hypogonadism, growth hormone deficiency, and short stature have been reported.[8]

- *Presynaptic CMS causing Lambert–Eaton like myasthenic syndrome (LEMS) (SYT2, SNAP25, VAMP1, RPH3A, UNC13A, and LAMA5)*: Synaptotagmin (SYT2), a calcium ion sensor, sets off the formation of SNARE complex needed for the release of ACh into the synaptic space. Vesicle-associated membrane protein 1(VAMP1)/synaptobrevin, SNAP25, and syntaxin are members of the SNARE complex. Munc13-1 (UNC13A) stabilizes syntaxin and rabphilin 3A (RPH3A) binds to SNAP25 and controls potassium channels in nerve terminals. These patients have severe muscle hypotonia and symptoms from birth. SYT2 may manifest with foot deformities, areflexia, and distal muscle weakness and facilitation may cause elicitation of the reflexes. Microcephaly, learning disabilities, and thin corpus callosum are seen in patients with RPH3A and UNC13A mutations. Laminins are involved in maintenance of nerve terminal and mutations of alpha form of laminin (LAMA5) involved in synaptic vesicle release cause CMS-LEMS with ocular or central nervous system (CNS) defects.[9] All these forms of CMS, associated with defects of synaptic vesicle release, show decrement on low frequency repetitive nerve stimulation (RNS) but increment occurs on high frequency RNS or after maximal voluntary contraction, resembling LEMS.
- *Presynaptic CMS associated with deficiencies in nerve terminal formation (MYO9A and SLC25A1)*: Myosin 9A (MYO9A) and SLC25A1, a succinate transporter, are involved in the formation of nerve terminal and NMJ. They cause a presynaptic defect with phenotype like the other forms with ptosis, ophthalmoparesis, hypotonia, bulbar involvement, and sometimes respiratory insufficiency. Intellectual disability is reported with SLC25A1.[10]
- *Synaptic CMS (COLQ, COL13A1, and LAMB2)*: Collagen Q binds to acetylcholinesterase (AChE) in the synaptic space and anchors it to synaptic basal lamina, COLQ loss of function variants thus result in AChE deficiency. COLQ patients may present with poor cry and weakness at

birth. This form of CMS presents mainly with limb-girdle myasthenia (LGM), though half the patients may have ptosis or ophthalmoparesis. Delayed pupillary response, a characteristic of COLQ mutations, is seen in only 25% of the patients.[11] Beta-2 laminin (LAMB2) is present not only in the neuromuscular junction but also in the kidneys and eyes. LAMB2 mutations cause Pierson syndrome, characterized by nephrotic syndrome and eye abnormalities (changes in lens, retina, and cornea). COL13A1 has symptoms from birth and affects ocular, bulbar, and trunk muscles with relative sparing of limb muscles.

The following are the types of postsynaptic CMS:

- *AChR deficiency (CHRNA, CHRNB, CHRND, CHRNE, and rapsyn)*: Acetylcholine receptor is a pentameric unit comprised of 2α1, 1β1, 1δ, and 1γ subunit in embryo. In adults, the γ subunit is replaced by ε subunit. Biallelic variants causing CHRNE may be compensated to some extent by replacement with embryonic γ subunit. Lack of other subunits cannot be compensated and may be fatal. Missense variants affecting any of these subunits may cause AChR deficiency or kinetic changes. CHRNE variants are the most common reported, probably due to the compensatory mechanisms.[12] These patients present commonly in infancy or childhood with ptosis, ophthalmoparesis, bulbar, and limb weakness. They may have a fluctuating course and may have scapular winging or scoliosis.[13] They show a favorable response to acetylcholinesterase inhibitors (AChEIs).

  Rapsyn is needed for the clustering of AChR at the crests of junctional folds. Rapsyn mutations cause AChR deficiency. The most common variant reported is p.N88K. Patients have ocular, bulbar, or limb fatigue exacerbated by infections.[14]

- CHRNG mutations and Escobar syndrome: CHRNG mutations involving the γ subunit of AChR cause a syndrome of arthrogryposis multiplex congenita (AMC) and multiple pterygia due to decreased fetal mobility in utero. As the γ subunit is replaced by the adult ε subunit after 33 weeks of gestation, there are no significant myasthenic symptoms at birth.[15] Lethal forms of fetal akinesia deformation sequence (FADS) due to mutations in CHRNA, CHRND, MuSK, RAPSN, and DOK7 are known. They may have clubfoot, genital abnormalities, cardiac defects, kyphoscoliosis, and short stature.[16]

- *Kinetic defects of AChR causing SCCMS or fast-channel CMS (FCCMS)*: Mutations of any of the subunits may cause kinetic defects. SCCMS occurs due to prolonged opening of AChR due to mutations affecting the dissociation of ACh from AChR. Prolonged channel opening leads to desensitization of AChR or endplate myopathy due to excessive calcium influx. SCCMS follows autosomal dominant (AD) inheritance. FCCMS occurs due to missense variants causing narrow channel opening, destabilization of channel opening state, or affects ACh binding or ion channel gating. Weakness of wrist and finger extensors along with those of cervical and scapular muscles is a key feature of SCCMS.[17] Repetitive compound muscle action potentials (CMAPs) are seen due to prolonged open channel duration. FCCMS manifests at birth or infancy and is marked by severe respiratory crisis along with ocular, bulbar, or limb-girdle involvement.[18]

- Defects in clustering of AChR (agrin, LRP4, MuSK, and DOK7): Downstream-of-kinase (DOK7) activates MuSK along with agrin and LRP4, this complex being required for AChR clustering. DOK-7 CMS patients have onset in early childhood with limb girdle weakness, with sparing of extraocular muscles. Stridor and wasting of tongue muscles may be seen.[19] Worsening may occur with AChEI. Agrin and LRP4 CMS patients have LGM and tongue atrophy is a characteristic feature of MuSK.[20]

- *Sodium channel (SCN4A) CMS*: SCN4A loss of function variants cause accelerated hyperpolarization and reduced excitability of sodium channel to repetitive stimulus. The spectrum of clinical features ranges from severe symptoms at birth to mild weakness resembling a congenital myopathy with gradual improvement over time.[21] Episodic apnea and sudden infant deaths have been reported.

- *Plectin (PLEC1) CMS*: Plectin is an intermediate filament required for maintenance of structural integrity of muscle and neuromuscular junction. Plectin deficiency causes myasthenic syndrome with myopathy and epidermolysis bullosa.[22]

- *CMS due to glycosylation defects (GFPT1, DPAGT1, GMPPB, ALG2, and ALG14)*: Glycosylation of proteins is needed for protein folding and stability. Mutation of proteins associated with glycosylation such as glutamine-fructose-6-phosphate transaminase 1 (GFPT1), dolichyl-phosphate N-acetylglucosamine phosphotransferase 1 (DPAGT1), asparagine-linked glycosylation 14 homolog (ALG14), asparagine-linked glycosylation 2 homolog (ALG2), and GDP-mannose pyrophosphorylase B (GMPPB) are associated with LG-CMS. Ptosis and external ophthalmoplegia are rare. Tubular aggregates on muscle biopsy are seen with variants of GFPT1, DPAGT1, ALG2, and ALG14, but not in GMPPB. Creatine kinase (CK) is elevated around 3-fold in GFPT1 and about 2- to 20-fold above normal in GMBBP variant patients. GMPPB mutations can result in muscular dystrophy phenotype with replacement of muscles by fatty tissue in proximal limb muscles and axial muscles.[23] Intellectual disability and epilepsy are reported with DPAGT1 and ALG14 variants.

- *Other genes causing CMS (TOR1AIP1, CHD8, and PURA)*: Mutations of TOR1AIP1, a nuclear membrane protein, cause a milder form of LG-CMS.[24] CHD8, chromatin remodeling protein defect, may have neonatal onset with ocular and limb involvement. Patients may also have autism and intellectual disability.[25] PURA, purine-rich element-binding protein A, is present in many tissues and is required for DNA replication. Patients may have multisystem involvement with gastrointestinal symptoms, excessive somnolence, startle response, and endocrine abnormalities.[26]

■ NIMHANS COHORT OF CONGENITAL MYASTHENIC SYNDROME PATIENTS

About 156 patients from 141 families were confirmed to have CMS by whole exome sequencing.[27] Male:female ratio is 87:69. Mean age of onset was 6.6 ± 9.8 years (neonatal onset to fourth decade) with a diagnostic delay of 12.5 ± 9.9 years. 17 CMS genes were identified. 62.4% were postsynaptic, glycosylation defects (21.3%), basal lamina defects (4.3%), and presynaptic (2.8%) were the others. Most common variants were CHRNE (39.4%), DOK7 (14.4%), DPAGT1 (9.8%), GFPT1 (7.6%), MuSK (6.1%), GMPPB (5.3%), and COLQ (4.5%). **Figures 2A to J** shows clinical features of patients evaluated at the National Institute of Mental Health and Neurosciences (NIMHANS).

CHAPTER 3: Congenital Myasthenic Syndromes: Genetic Spectrum and Management

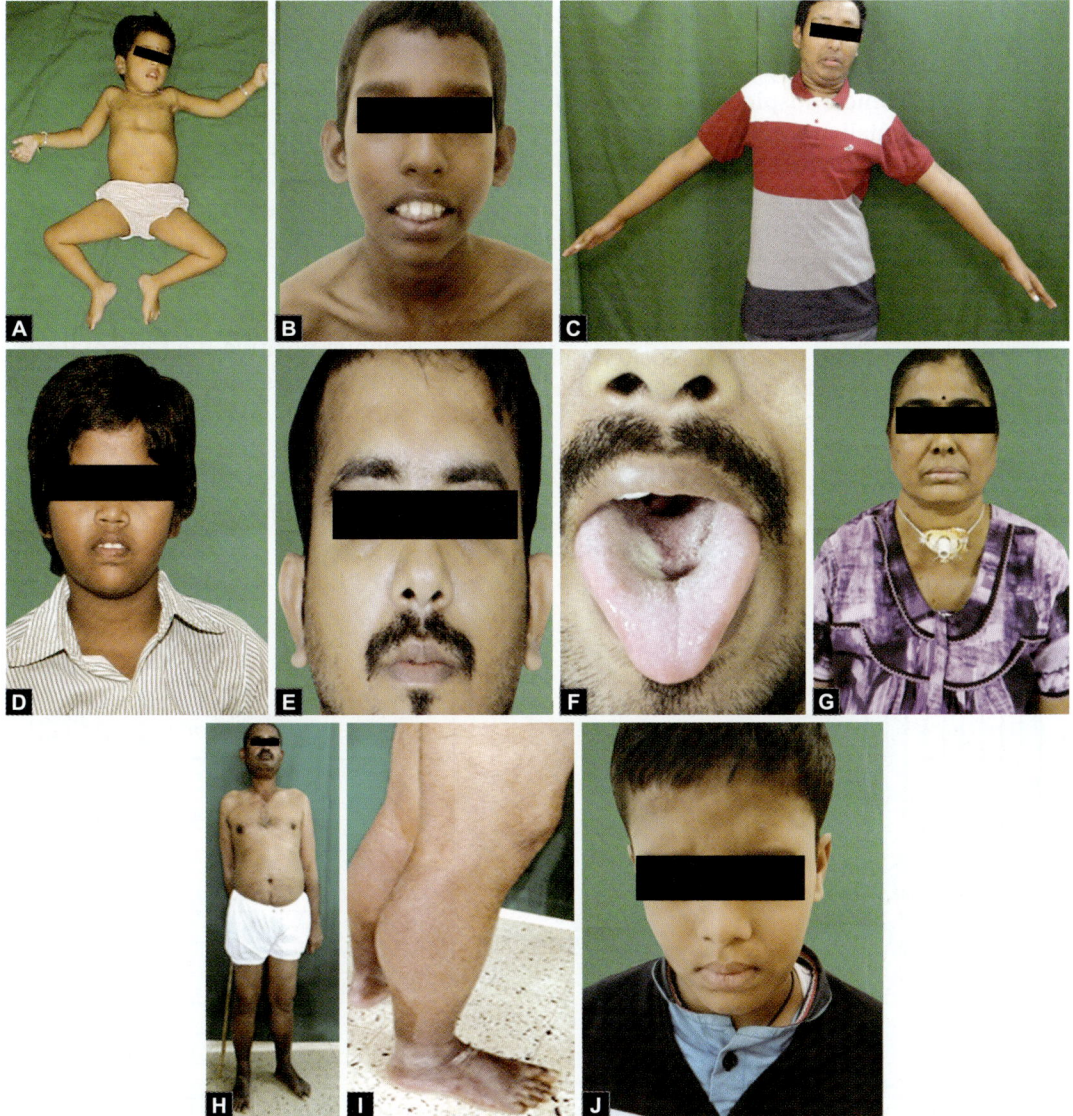

FIGS. 2A TO J: Clinical features of different types of congenital myasthenic syndrome (CMS). (A) VAMP1 [c.97C>T (p.Arg33Ter), homozygous]—a 2-year-old floppy child with bulbar symptoms and respiratory distress; (B) CHRNE—a 9-year-old child with ptosis, ophthalmoparesis, elongated facies, and low set ears; (C) Agrin—a 14-year-old boy with ptosis and limb fatigue; (D) DPAGT1—a 12-year-old child with mental subnormality, seizures, ptosis, and limb fatigue; (E and F) MuSK—a 24-year-old with mild ptosis, limb fatigue, tongue atrophy, and grooving; (G) COLQ—a 54-year-old lady fatigue from young age, respiratory distress in 50s, on bilevel positive airway pressure (BiPAP), improved well on salbutamol; (H and I) GMPPB—a 52-year-old man with limb fatigue and weakness, calf hypertrophy present; and (J) DOK7—11-year-old boy with bifacial weakness, ptosis and limb fatigue.

DIAGNOSIS OF CONGENITAL MYASTHENIC SYNDROME

High index of clinical suspicion is the key to diagnosis, especially in adults who present with limb-girdle symptoms. History of developmental delay or fatigue from early childhood may be elicited. Worsening of fatigue during fever, stress, menstrual cycles, and pregnancy may be present with seasonal fluctuations. Family history may be positive. Decremental response of >10% is elicited on low frequency 3 Hz RNS in most of the cases and single-fiber electromyography (SFEMG) may demonstrate increased jitter or blocking. Yield of 3 Hz RNS may be low, especially in CHAT, showing decremental response only in about 10% of the cases. Prolonged subtetanic stimulation at 10 Hz for 5 minutes increases the positive rate to 90%.[28] Repetitive CMAPs are elicited with single stimulation in AChE deficiency, SCCMS, and PURA-CMS.[29] Cholinergic hyperactivity and prolonged endplate potential causes re-excitation and repetitive CMAPs. In LEMS like presynaptic CMS, low-frequency RNS elicits decremental response while on high-frequency RNS, incremental response is noted. It is important to fix the recording electrodes properly to avoid erroneous positive decremental responses. **Figure 3** shows decremental response of 39% on stimulation of trapezius in a patient with CMS. CK levels show mild elevation of two- to three-fold in GFPT1, DOK7, and SCCMS and nearly 20-folds in GMPPB CMS. Tubular aggregates are seen on muscle biopsy in GFPT1, ALG2, and DPAGT1. Testing

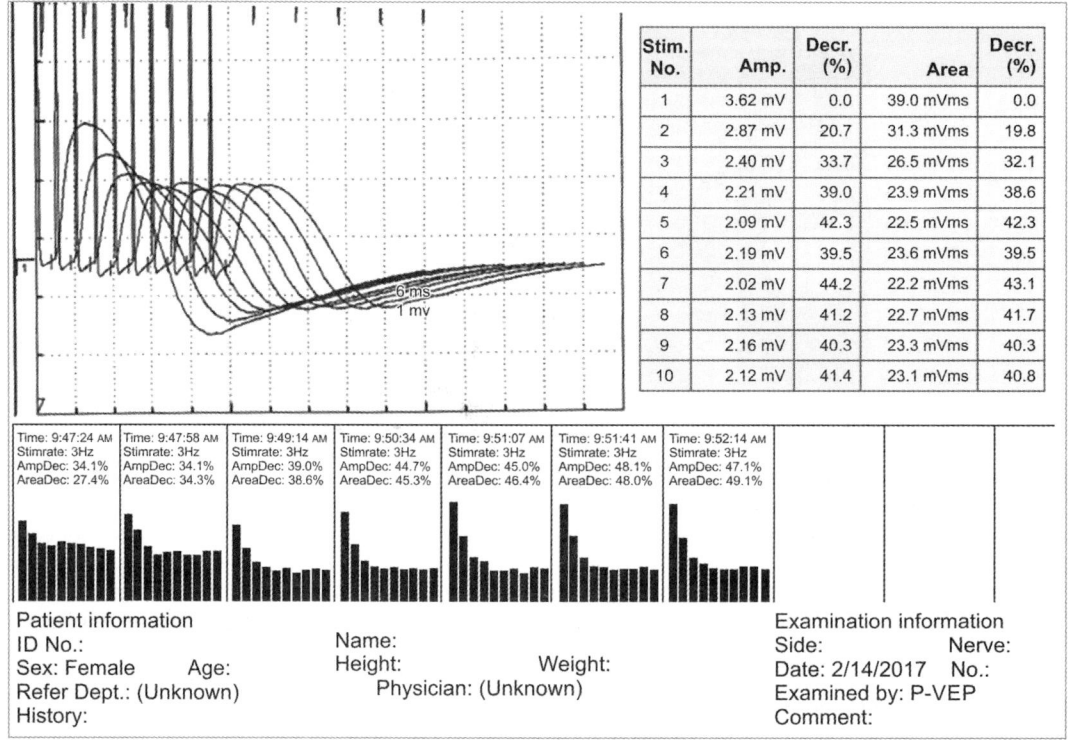

FIG. 3: Repetitive nerve stimulation (RNS) at 3 Hz on trapezius shows decremental response of 39%.

for antibodies against AChR and MuSK may be needed in sporadic cases.

An accurate molecular diagnosis is essential for confirming diagnosis and for optimal medical management. With genetic testing becoming widely available at a cheaper rate, next-generation sequencing (NGS) has become the cornerstone for diagnosis. Microarray-based comparative genomic hybridization helps in detecting large deletions or duplications which may be missed on exome sequencing.[30] 20–40% do not get genetic confirmation despite comprehensive genetic testing.[31] Functional studies of the mutated protein are required for confirming diagnosis in novel genetic defects.

■ TREATMENT

Congenital myasthenic syndrome is a treatable genetic disorder. There are many drugs available, and the treatment choice depends on the subtype, as drugs beneficial for one type may worsen another type of CMS. Mechanism of action includes increasing available ACh at the synaptic cleft (AChEI which prevent ACh breakdown and 3,4-diaminopyridine, a potassium channel blocker, which increases ACh release) or decrease the prolonged channel opening time in SCCMS (open channel blockers such as quinidine and fluoxetine).[32] β2 agonists such as salbutamol and ephedrine are useful in CMS, though their exact mechanism of action is unknown. They stabilize endplate structures and compensate for defective signaling in agrin-LRP4-MuSK pathway by second messenger pathway, preventing excessive cholinergic effects.[33] They are also beneficial in other forms such as AChR deficiency, probably by preventing the disruption of neuromuscular junction structures, which happens with long-term AChEI therapy. Unlike effects of other drugs, onset of action of β2 agonists is slow and may be discernible over weeks or months. **Table 1** shows the list of drugs used in CMS with their dosage, mechanism of action, subtypes in which they are used, and side effects.

■ DEVELOPING A TREATABOLOME

Congenital myasthenic syndrome is a classic example demonstrating requirement of specific treatment based on genotype. Developing a database called treatabolome, which will contain the variants and genes described, with their specific treatment.[32] The treatment recommendations may vary over time, with gain of additional experience and new gene discoveries. Diagnostic delay in these disorders, especially those with apneic spells can be detrimental. This treatabolome should be readily accessible to all users including nonexperts, with facility to flag the genes and variants, with relevant treatments and existing evidences.

■ SUMMARY OF CLINICAL, ELECTROPHYSIOLOGICAL FEATURES, AND TREATMENT RESPONSE IN CONGENITAL MYASTHENIC SYNDROME

Table 2 gives a summary of important features of CMS.

■ CONCLUSION

Congenital myasthenic syndromes are rare, inherited disorders of impaired neuromuscular transmission with varying manifestations. It is important to consider CMS as a differential diagnosis of inherited limb girdle syndromes as this disorder is potentially treatable. Look for phenotypic and electrophysiological clues and accurate phenotyping is needed prior to genetic testing.

TABLE 1: Drugs used in CMS.

Name of drug	Mechanism of action	Dosage	CMS subtypes in which they are useful	Side effects
Acetylcholinesterase inhibitors (pyridostigmine)	Inhibits hydrolysis of ACh	• *Pediatric:* 4–6 mg/kg/day (can go up to 7–9 mg/kg/day) in four to six divided doses • *Adults:* 60 mg 4–6 times/day (up to 500 mg/day)[34]	AChR deficiency, CHAT, fast channel syndrome, ALG2, ALG14, glycosylation defects, MYO9A, PLEC1, PREPL, Rapsyn, SCN4A, SLC18A3, SLC25A1, SLC5A7, and VAMP1	• Gastrointestinal—diarrhea, abdominal cramps, nausea. Cholinergic symptoms, increased bronchial secretions • Worsening of myasthenia in MuSK, SCCMS, DOK7, LRP4, and COLQ
Salbutamol (albuterol)	Activates cAMP protein kinase A,[35] compensates for reduced MuSK signaling in defects of DOK7, LRP4, agrin, MuSK complex, and stabilizes endplate structure	4 mg 2–3 times/day in adults, 0.05–0.2 mg/kg/day, start with 2 mg and increase to full dose slowly over 6 months[36]	COLQ, DOK7, COL13A1, LAMB2, LRP4, and MuSK	Palpitations, tremor, headache, restlessness, insomnia, hypertension, and hypokalemia
Ephedrine	β2 agonist, increases quantal release of ACh	25–50 mg 2–3 times/day and 1–3 mg/kg/day in three divided doses in children, starting with 1 mg/kg/day with gradual escalation[37,38] (limited availability in many countries)	COLQ, DOK7, COL13A1, LAMB2, LRP4, and MuSK	Like salbutamol
Fluoxetine	Open channel blocker of AChR	80–100 mg/day in adults	Slow channel CMS	Nausea, insomnia, nervousness, sexual dysfunction, hyponatremia, and increased suicidal tendency in children with depression

Continued

Continued

Name of drug	Mechanism of action	Dosage	CMS subtypes in which they are useful	Side effects
Quinidine	Reduces open channel state of AChR	15–60 mg/kg/day in children, 200 mg three times a day for a week in adults and then adjust the dosage to maintain serum level of 1–2.4 µg/mL or 3–7.5 µmol/mL	Slow channel CMS	Cardiac conduction abnormalities, gastrointestinal disturbances, hypersensitivity, drug interactions due to inhibition of cytochrome P450
3,4-diaminopyridine	Increases quantal release of ACh, blocks potassium current, and causes more calcium entry in presynaptic nerve terminal	1 mg/kg in four divided doses (5–20 mg 4 times per day in	AChR deficiency, fast channel syndrome, GFPT1, MUNC13-1, SNAP25, Rapsyn, SYT2, and variable effect on MuSK	Cholinergic side effects, precipitates seizure, and hence contraindicated in patients with history of seizure
Acetazolamide	Carbonic anhydrase inhibitor, prevents reabsorption of sodium	250 mg three to four times a day along with AChEI	SCN4A	Gastrointestinal symptoms, paresthesia, renal stones, bitter taste, hypokalemia, and hyponatremia

(AChEI: acetylcholinesterase inhibitor; CMS: congenital myasthenic syndrome)

TABLE 2: Summary of clinical features of congenital myasthenic syndrome (CMS).

Episodic apnea	CHAT, MuSK, SLC5A7, SLC25A1, RAPSN, and COLQ
Mental subnormality	VAChT, SLC25A7, DPAGT1, SNAP25, COL13A1, and MYO9A
Endocrine abnormalities	PREPL
LEMS like	SYT2, SNAP25, VAMP1, RPH3A, UNC13A, and LAMA5
Distal weakness and areflexia	SYT2
Delayed pupillary response	COLQ
Pierson syndrome	LAMB2
Escobar syndrome	CHRNG
Fetal akinesia deformation sequence	CHRNA, CHRND, MuSK, RAPSN, and DOK7
Weakness of cervical muscles, wrist, and finger extensors	Slow channel syndrome
Tongue atrophy	MuSK
Limb–girdle syndrome	COLQ, DOK7, MuSK, GFPT1, ALG2, ALG14, DPAGT1, and GMPPB
Vocal cord paralysis	COLQ and DOK7
Epilepsy	DPAGT1 and ALG14
Epidermolysis bullosa	Plectin
Cerebellar ataxia	SNAP25
Repetitive CMAPs	COLQ and slow channel syndrome
Worsening with pyridostigmine	MuSK, SCCMS, DOK7, LRP4, and COLQ

More than 35 genes have been listed as causative so far. The list has been expanding and whole exome sequencing may identify many more novel genes. Functional studies and knowledge of the pathogenic mechanisms are essential for newer drug discoveries and appropriate management of the cases. Individualized treatment approach is required depending on the genetic defect identified.

REFERENCES

1. Ohno K, Ohkawara B, Shen XM, Selcen D, Engel AG. Clinical and Pathologic Features of Congenital Myasthenic Syndromes Caused by 35 Genes—A Comprehensive Review. Int J Mol Sci. 2023;24:3730.
2. Parr JR, Andrew MJ, Finnis M, Beeson D, Vincent A, Jayawant S. How common is childhood myasthenia? The UK incidence and prevalence of autoimmune and congenital myasthenia. Arch Dis Child. 2014;99(6):539-42.
3. Engel AG. Congenital Myasthenic Syndromes in 2018. Curr Neurol Neurosci Rep. 2018;18:46.
4. Zhang Y, Cheng X, Luo C, Lei M, Mao F, Shi Z, et al. Congenital Myasthenic Syndrome Caused by a Novel Hemizygous CHAT Mutation. Front Pediatr. 2020;8:185.
5. Schara U, Christen HJ, Durmus H, Hietala M, Krabetz K, Rodolico C, et al. Long-term follow-up in patients with congenital myasthenic syndrome due to CHAT mutations. Eur J Paediatr Neurol. 2010;14(4):326-33.
6. Aran A, Segel R, Kaneshige K, Gulsuner S, Renbaum P, Oliphant S, et al. Vesicular acetylcholine transporter defect underlies devastating congenital

myasthenia syndrome. Neurology. 2017;88(11): 1021-28.
7. Régal L, Shen XM, Selcen D, Verhille C, Meulemans S, Creemers JW, et al. PREPL deficiency with or without cystinuria causes a novel myasthenic syndrome. Neurology. 2014;82(14):1254-60.
8. Yang Q, Hua R, Qian J, Yi S, Shen F, Zhang Q, et al. PREPL Deficiency: A Homozygous Splice Site PREPL Mutation in a Patient With Congenital Myasthenic Syndrome and Absence of Ovaries and Hypoplasia of Uterus. Front Genet. 2020;11:198.
9. Lorenzoni PJ, Scola RH, Kay CSK, Werneck LC, Horvath R, Lochmüller H. How to Spot Congenital Myasthenic Syndromes Resembling the Lambert-Eaton Myasthenic Syndrome? A Brief Review of Clinical, Electrophysiological, and Genetics Features. Neuromolecular Med. 2018;20(2):205-14.
10. Balaraju S, Töpf A, McMacken G, Kumar VP, Pechmann A, Roper H, et al. Congenital myasthenic syndrome with mild intellectual disability caused by a recurrent SLC25A1 variant. Eur J Hum Genet. 2020;28(3):373-77.
11. Mihaylova V, Müller JS, Vilchez JJ, Salih MA, Kabiraj MM, D'Amico A, et al. Clinical and molecular genetic findings in COLQ-mutant congenital myasthenic syndromes. Brain. 2008;131(Pt 3):747-59.
12. Ramdas S, Beeson D. Congenital myasthenic syndromes: where do we go from here? Neuromuscul Disord. 2021;31(10):943-54.
13. Finsterer J. Congenital myasthenic syndromes. Orphanet J Rare Dis. 2019;14(1):57.
14. Natera-de Benito D, Bestué M, Vilchez JJ, Evangelista T, Töpf A, García-RibesA, et al. Long-term follow-up in patients with congenital myasthenic syndrome due to RAPSN mutations. Neuromuscul Disord. 2016;26:153-9.
15. Sandweiss AJ, Patel S, Bader MY, Kylat RI. A Truncating Variant of CHRNG as a Cause of Escobar Syndrome: A Multiple Pterygium Syndrome Subtype. J Pediatr Genet. 2020;11(2):144-6.
16. Chen CP. Prenatal diagnosis and genetic analysis of fetal akinesia deformation sequence and multiple pterygium syndrome associated with neuromuscular junction disorders: a review. Taiwan J Obstet Gynecol. 2012;51(1):12-7.
17. Otero-Cruz JD, Báez-Pagán CA, Dorna-Pérez L, Grajales-Reyes GE, Ramírez-Ordoñez RT, Luciano CA, et al. Decoding pathogenesis of slow-channel congenital myasthenic syndromes using recombinant expression and mice models. P R Health Sci J. 2010;29(1):4-17.
18. Palace J, Lashley D, Bailey S, Jayawant S, Carr A, McConville J, et al. Clinical features in a series of fast channel congenital myasthenia syndrome. Neuromuscul Disord. 2012;22(2):112-7.
19. Palace J. DOK7 congenital myasthenic syndrome. Ann N Y Acad Sci. 2012;1275:49-53.
20. Ben Ammar A, Soltanzadeh P, Bauché S, Richard P, Goillot E, Herbst R, et al. A mutation causes MuSK reduced sensitivity to agrin and congenital myasthenia. PLoS One. 2013;8(1):e53826.
21. Han JY, Park J. Novel compound heterozygous mutations in SCN4A as a potential genetic cause contributing to myopathic manifestations: A case report and literature review. Heliyon. 2024;10(7):e28684.
22. Engel AG. The therapy of congenital myasthenic syndromes. Neurotherapeutics. 2007;4(2):252-7.
23. Siddiqui S, Polavarapu K, Bardhan M, Preethish-Kumar V, Joshi A, Nashi S, et al. Distinct and Recognisable Muscle MRI Pattern in a Series of Adults Harbouring an Identical GMPPB Gene Mutation. J Neuromuscul Dis. 2022;9:95-109.
24. Malfatti E, Catchpool T, Nouioua S, Sihem H, Fournier E, Carlier RY, et al. A TOR1AIP1 variant segregating with an early onset limb girdle myasthenia-Support for the role of LAP1 in NMJ function and disease. Neuropathol Appl Neurobiol. 2022;48:e12743.
25. Hoffmann A, Spengler D. Chromatin Remodeler CHD8 in Autism and Brain Development. J Clin Med. 2021;10:366.
26. Reijnders MRF, Janowski R, Alvi M, Self JE, van Essen TJ, Vreeburg M, et al. PURA syndrome: Clinical delineation and genotype-phenotype study in 32 individuals with review of published literature. J Med Genet. 2018;55:104-13.
27. Polavarapu K, Sunitha B, Töpf A, Preethish-Kumar V, Thompson R, Vengalil S, et al. Clinical and genetic characterisation of a large Indian congenital myasthenic syndrome cohort. Brain. 2024;147:281-96.
28. Murtazina A, Borovikov A, Marakhonov A, Sharkov A, Sharkova I, Mirzoyan A, et al. Mild phenotype of CHAT-associated congenital myasthenic syndrome: case series. Front Pediatr. 2024;12:1280394.
29. Lee HE, Kim YH, Kim SM, Shin HY. Clinical Significance of Repetitive Compound Muscle Action Potentials in Patients with Myasthenia Gravis: A Predictor for Cholinergic Side Effects of Acetylcholinesterase Inhibitors. J Clin Neurol. 2016;12(4):482-8.
30. Engel AG, Shen XM, Selcen D, Sine SM. Congenital myasthenic syndromes: pathogenesis, diagnosis, and treatment. Lancet Neurol. 2015;14(4):420-34.

31. McMacken G, Abicht A, Evangelista T, Spendiff S, Lochmuller H. The increasing genetic and phenotypical diversity of congenital myasthenic syndromes. Neuropediatrics. 2017;48:294-308.
32. Thompson R, Bonne G, Missier P, Lochmüller H. Targeted therapies for congenital myasthenic syndromes: systematic review and steps towards a treatabolome. Emerg Top Life Sci. 2019;3(1):19-37.
33. Beeson D. Congenital myasthenic syndromes: recent advances. Curr Opin Neurol. 2016;29:565-71.
34. Farmakidis C, Pasnoor M, Barohn RJ, Dimachkie MM. Congenital Myasthenic Syndromes: a Clinical and Treatment Approach. Curr Treat Options Neurol. 2018;20(9):36.
35. Burke G, Hiscock A, Klein A, Niks EH, Main M, Manzur AY, et al. Salbutamol benefits children with congenital myasthenic syndrome due to DOK7 mutations. Neuromuscul Disord. 2013;23(2):170-5.
36. Rodríguez Cruz PM, Palace J, Ramjattan H, Jayawant S, Robb SA, Beeson D, et al. Salbutamol and ephedrine in the treatment of severe AChR deficiency syndromes. Neurology. 2015;85(12):1043-7.
37. Lorenzoni PJ, Scola RH, Kay CS, Filla L, Miranda AP, Pinheiro JM, et al. Salbutamol therapy in congenital myasthenic syndrome due to DOK7 mutation. J Neurol Sci. 2013;331(1-2):155-7.
38. Schara U, Lochmüller H. Therapeutic strategies in congenital myasthenic syndromes. Neurotherapeutics. 2008;5(4):542-7.

CHAPTER 4

Idiopathic Inflammatory Myopathies and Current Immunology

Sruthi S Nair, Deepti Narasimhaiah

ABSTRACT

Idiopathic inflammatory myopathies (IIMs) comprise a diverse group of autoimmune myopathies which share a common clinical presentation, laboratory markers, and therapeutic response to immunotherapy to varying degrees. Over decades, many classification systems have attempted to reconcile the heterogeneity among IIMs. The widespread acceptance of immunological diagnosis with myositis specific and myositis-associated antibodies have identified relatively homogeneous groups among these entities. Currently, five main clinicoseropathological subgroups are recognized, namely: (1) dermatomyositis (DM), (2) antisynthetase syndrome (ASS), (3) immune-mediated necrotizing myopathy (IMNM), (4) sporadic inclusion body myositis (IBM), and (5) overlap myositis. Newer pathological insights classify DM as a type 1 interferonopathy distinct from its phenocopy, ASS. A relatively newer syndrome, IMNM, is classified as an IIM based on autoimmune pathogenesis though histopathological evidence for inflammation is classically sparse. Sporadic IBM has long been considered an IIM, though the poor response to immunotherapy and demonstrable degenerative processes in the myofibers delegate it to the border-zone of autoimmune myopathies. This review discusses the current classification, immunological phenotypes, and diagnostic and therapeutic approach to IIMs.

Keywords: Idiopathic inflammatory myopathy, Muscle specific antibodies, Dermatomyositis, Immune-mediated necrotizing myopathy, Antisynthetase syndrome.

■ INTRODUCTION AND CLASSIFICATION

Introduction

Idiopathic inflammatory myopathies (IIMs) comprise a heterogeneous group of autoimmune disorders characterized by immune-mediated injury to the muscles. Hallmarks include acute to subacute muscle weakness, elevated muscle enzymes, characteristic histopathology, and variable association with extramuscular disease and cancer. The identification of autoantibodies in IIMs which are closely linked with the pathogenic mechanisms has produced better precision in the subtype classification and therapeutic planning. This chapter will discuss the updates in IIM classification and management with special focus on the immunology.

Epidemiology and Clinical Presentation

The true epidemiology of IIMs is marred by diverse and incomplete classification systems. A recent review estimated the incidence at 0.2–2 per 100,000 person-years and the prevalence at 2–25 per 100,000 people.[1] Most of the studies showed a female preponderance. Adult and juvenile forms exhibit differences in subtype distribution and pathophysiology. Peak incidence is seen between 40 and 50 years of age except sporadic inclusion body myositis (sIBM) which has a later onset.[2]

The onset of illness is acute to subacute in the majority. The classical pattern of weakness is a symmetric limb–girdle pattern with variable neck and/or pharyngeal weakness. The exception is sIBM where the weakness is asymmetric, affecting quadriceps, long finger flexors, and facial muscles. Muscle pain can occur, while ophthalmoplegia is exclusionary. Cutaneous, lung, joint, cardiac, and other system involvement as well as cancer association vary across subtypes.

Evolution of Classification of Idiopathic Inflammatory Myopathies

The traditional classification of the IIMs by Bohan and Peter in 1975 defined inflammatory myopathies by symmetric limb girdle weakness, elevation of skeletal muscle enzymes, muscle biopsy with evidence of myositis, and electromyography (EMG) features of myositis. They were subclassified as polymyositis (PM) and dermatomyositis (DM) based on the absence or presence of cutaneous manifestations, respectively. These criteria had many fallacies, not least being the lack of specificity. sIBM was identified as a separate entity in 1995 and specific clinicopathological criteria were identified subsequently.[3] Immune-mediated necrotizing myopathy (IMNM) was identified as a separate entity based on distinct antibodies and pathology.[4]

The latest European League Against Rheumatism and the American College of Rheumatology (EULAR/ACR) classification of 2017 recognizes adult and juvenile IIMs with high specificity based on clinical, laboratory, and muscle biopsy criteria, but is less stringent on the subtype identification. The juvenile and adult forms of DM, amyopathic DM (ADM), PM, IBM and IMNM are defined in these criteria. The overlapping clinic-laboratory features in the various subtypes, particularly PM and IMNM, and the nonincorporation of serology with the exception of anti Jo-1 are major drawbacks.[5]

A paradigm shift in IIM classification was brought about by the wider acceptance of specific phenotypes linked to muscle-directed autoantibodies. A large-scale study proposed to elucidate a better classification based on immunological profile in addition to numerous clinic-pathological variables using machine learning algorithms. They identified four clinically and pathologically distinct clusters corresponding to DM, IMNM, antisynthetase syndrome (ASS), and sIBM. There were no unidentified clusters, thereby establishing the crucial role of antibodies in the diagnostic classification.[6] The same four classes were recognized by transcriptomic analysis of muscle biopsies by a different group.[7] A fifth subtype, overlap myositis, with less specific autoantibodies is also acknowledged by most of the authors. PM lacks any distinct serological or pathological markers, calling into dispute its very existence as an independent entity. Likewise, sIBM occupies an unusual position in the border zone as it differs from the classical IIM phenotype and exhibits pathology other than immune damage.[8] Some of the newer entities with immune muscle injury remains unclassified such as immune checkpoint inhibitor (ICI)-associated myositis and COVID-19-associated myositis.

This general classification is applicable for childhood-onset or juvenile IIMs as well with similar diagnostic certainty associated with autoantibodies and muscle pathology. However, they differ from adult IIM in terms of clinical phenotype, antibody positivity, and treatment response. Juvenile DM is overwhelmingly the most common subtype, contributing to nearly 85% of juvenile IIMs.[9]

Myositis Specific and Myositis-associated Antibodies

Autoantibodies are detected in about 70% of patients with IIM.[10] Though the earliest antibodies, Mi-2 and Jo-1 were discovered back in 1976 and 1980, respectively, their widespread use in diagnosis occurred only the latter half of 2010s.[11]

The antibodies are broadly classified as myositis-specific antibodies (MSAs) and myositis-associated antibodies (MAAs). MSAs are well-characterized and generally specific for an IIM subtype whereas MAAs are seen in systemic autoimmune diseases which have associated myositis. The MSAs are (1) Mi2, NXP2, TIF1γ, MDA5, and SAE related to DM, (2) anti-synthetase antibodies (Jo-1, PL-7, PL-12, EJ, OJ, Zo, Ha, and KS) related to ASS, (3) signal recognition particle (SRP) and 3-hydroxy-3-methylglutaryl-CoA reductase (HMGCR) related to IMNM, and (4) cN1A related to sIBM. MSAs are usually exclusive and disease specific [with the exception of anti-cytosolic 5' nucleotidase1A (cN1A)].[10] MAAs identify less homogeneous patient populations and coexist with other autoantibodies. **Tables 1 and 2** illustrate the clinical phenotypes in relation to the MSAs and MAAs.

The population positivity of these antibodies is not clearly known; hence, the testing should be appropriate to the clinical setting to avoid false-positives. In addition to patients with suspected IIMs, testing for MSAs may also be indicated in chronic

TABLE 1: Muscle specific antibodies in idiopathic inflammatory myopathies.

Antibody	Frequency within the subtype	Clinical features	Prognosis
Dermatomyositis			
Mi2	2–45% ADM 4–10% JDM	Classic cutaneous symptoms, low risk of ILD and cancer	Good response to therapy
TIF1γ	19% ADM 17–35% JDM	Significant cancer association in adults (>50%), dysphagia common, mild ILD	Poor prognosis, reduced survival with cancer
NXP2	17% ADM 17–35% JDM	Calcinosis cutis in JDM, subcutaneous edema, muscle ischemia, cancer association, fewer skin lesions	Poorer prognosis, remission less likely
MDA5	4–20%	Amyopathic or mild myopathy, rapidly progressive ILD, mucocutaneous ulceration, alopecia, palmar pustules, panniculitis, alopecia, arthritis, constitutional signs	Poorer prognosis in ILD and vasculopathic phenotypes, good prognosis for rheumatoid phenotype
SAE	1–8%	20% have amyopathic presentation, dysphagia common, low ILD risk, cancer risk related to ethnicity (higher in Chinese)	Moderate prognosis, rash could be refractory to treatment

Continued

Continued

Antibody	Frequency within the subtype	Clinical features	Prognosis
Antisynthetase syndrome			
Jo-1	70–75%	Myositis dominant, arthritis, ILD uncommon	Good prognosis
PL-7, PL-12	-	ILD dominant, mild myopathy	Poor prognosis
EJ, OJ, Zo, Ha, KS	-	EJ has myositis, ILD dominant in KS and OJ	Variable prognosis
Immune mediated necrotizing myopathy			
HMGCR	~30–60%	Statin use in 60–70%, low cancer association, rare extramuscular manifestations	Intermediate prognosis, could be treatment resistant
SRP	~18–30%	Severe necrotizing myositis with dysphagia, ILD, risk of severe myocarditis	Poor prognosis, severe disease
Seronegative	~20%	High cancer association	Poorer prognosis
Sporadic inclusion body myositis			
cN1A		Moderate association with IBM, also seen in Sjögren's syndrome, SLE and other IIM	Presence may be associated with more severe dysphagia

(ADM: adult dermatomyositis; sIBM: sporadic inclusion body myositis; IIM: idiopathic inflammatory myopathy; ILD: interstitial lung disease; JDM: juvenile dermatomyositis; SLE: systemic lupus erythematosus)

TABLE 2: Clinical phenotypes related to myositis associated antibodies.

Antibody	Connective tissue disease/autoimmune disease	Clinical phenotype
Pm/Scl	Systemic sclerosis	Myositis with deltoid weakness more than hip flexor weakness, ILD, skin disease
U1-RNP	Systemic sclerosis	ILD, arthralgia, glomerulonephritis, pericarditis, pulmonary hypertension
Ku	Systemic sclerosis, Sjögren's syndrome, SLE, MCTD, RA	More distal weakness, higher risk of steroid resistant-ILD, skin rash is less common
Mitochondrial M2	Primary biliary cholangitis, systemic sclerosis, Sjögren's syndrome, autoimmune hepatitis	Chronic myopathy, cardiac disease

(ILD: interstitial lung disease; MCTD: mixed connective tissue disease; RA: rheumatoid arthritis; SLE: systemic lupus erythematosus)

limb–girdle myopathies with raised muscle enzymes which are genetically unconfirmed (for necrotizing myopathy) and inflammatory arthritis/interstitial lung disease (ILD) of uncertain etiology (ASS and MDA5-DM).[12]

Line blot immunoassay for these antibodies is the most widely available technique in commercial use. The gold standard, immunoprecipitation technique, is highly specific and sensitive, but poorly accessible.[13]

SUBTYPES OF IDIOPATHIC INFLAMMATORY MYOPATHIES

Dermatomyositis

Dermatomyositis is the most common and best characterized IIM subtype. Typically, DM has proximal weakness developing subacutely and one-third of patients having neck weakness and dysphagia. Myalgias have been reported in about 30%. Cutaneous manifestations are the hallmark of the disease and had been the main diagnostic point in many classifications **(Figs. 1A to G)**. Other system disease including ILD, myocarditis, Raynaud's phenomenon, and arthritis are common as is cancer association. Juvenile DM is prevalent and contributes to 85% of childhood IIM. Recently, identification of DM-specific antibodies and amplified type I interferon signature in pathology have redefined DM diagnosis.[14]

Distinct human leukocyte antigen (HLA) associations have been noted for adult and juvenile DM and for specific antibodies. Pathophysiologically, DM, an interferonopathy and the disease mechanisms resulting in myofiber and vascular injury, is linked to an overexpression in the interferon I pathway.[14]

The distinctive skin manifestations of DM include heliotrope rash (periorbital bluish–purplish rash), Gottron's papules (erythematous scaly papules over bony prominences of joints), and Gottron's sign (erythematous rash over the extensor aspect of fingers). Others are erythematous rash over face, sun-exposed regions of chest (V-sign) or shoulders and neck (shawl sign), and lateral aspect of hips (holster sign), erythroderma, and dry itchy skin. Vasculopathic lesions of DM include periungual or gingival telangiectasias, vasculitic ulcers, and livedo

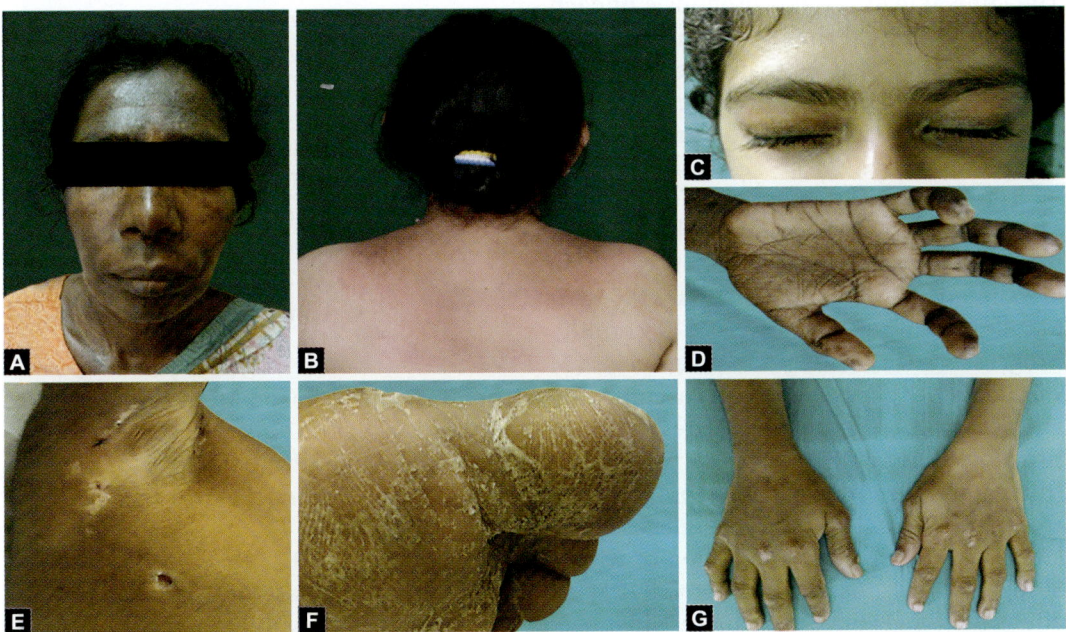

FIGS. 1A TO G: Cutaneous manifestations of idiopathic inflammatory myopathies. (A) Forehead and facial hyperpigmentation, (B) shawl sign, (C) heliotrope rash, (D) hand contractures, (E) vasculitic ulcers, (F) Mechanic's foot, and (G) Gottron's papules.
Courtesy: Seena Venganil, Associate Professor of Neurology, National Institute of Mental Health and Neurosciences, Bengaluru.

reticularis. Thickened and cracked skin over the palmar and lateral surfaces of hands termed as "mechanic's hands" is a feature shared by DM and ASS. Subcutaneous swelling may occur. Chronic lesions show intermixed hyper- and hypopigmented macular lesions referred to as poikiloderma.[14,15] Darker skin tone as in Indians could produce black or brown rashes than erythema.[16] Calcinosis cutis (subcutaneous or intramuscular) occurs more commonly in juvenile DM and is a late, difficult-to-treat complication.[15] Presence of active skin lesions and worsening calcinosis cutis indicates ongoing disease activity.[3] Clinically ADM occurs in nearly 20% with only cutaneous manifestations usually produce diagnostic delay.

The clinical heterogeneity of DM is closely linked to MSAs. Five MSAs have been described in DM—anti-Mi2, anti-SAE, anti MDA, anti TIF1γ, and anti NXP2 and each has specific clinicopathological signature.[11] The clinical features and prognosis of each antibody subtype are noted in **Table 1**. Nearly 25% of DM are autoantibody negative. The most common MSA in adult DM is Mi2 whereas TIF1γ and NXP2 are more frequent in juvenile DM.[9]

The classical DM phenotype is seen with Mi2 positivity which has a good prognosis in general. NXP2 in children is strongly associated with calcinosis cutis. DM with MDA5 have three phenotypes—(1) rapidly progressive ILD with poor prognosis, (2) vasculopathic phenotype (skin vasculopathy with weakness) having intermediate prognosis, and (3) rheumatoid phenotype (more joint disease) with a good prognosis.[11]

Among IIMs, DM has the highest correlation with cancer (at presentation or within 3 years of diagnosis) in 10–20%. TIF1γ in adults is strongly linked to cancer. Older age, male, severe skin rash, and raised acute phase reactants were associated with higher cancer risk.[14]

Antisynthetase Syndrome

Antisynthetase syndrome is defined by the presence of antibodies against aminoacyl-transfer ribonucleic acid (tRNA) synthetases of which eight have been identified, namely, antibodies to Jo-1, PL-7, PL-12, EJ, OJ, Zo, Ha, and KS. The clinical triad of ASS comprises myositis, ILD, and inflammatory arthritis which is seen in 20% at onset and 50% along the disease course.[12] Fever, Raynaud phenomenon, and mechanic's hand are other classical features. A rash mimicking DM may be seen in ASS, but they are pathologically distinct as ASS does not display prominent interferon I signatures. In contrast, activation of type 2 interferon pathway is more common in ASS. Cancer association and juvenile forms are quite rare.[11]

Generally, ASS is a severe syndrome though the phenotype and prognosis are variable with the specific MSA **(Table 1)**. Jo-1 antibody was one of the earliest MSAs identified and occurs in 70–75% of ASS. Anti Jo-1 has severe myositis whereas PL-7 and PL-12 antibodies more commonly present as ILD. The prognosis is poorer with coexistent ILD. Ro52 antibodies are seen concurrently with Jo-1 in 58–70% and this portends a more severe phenotype with arthritis and myositis.[12]

Immune-mediated Necrotizing Myopathy

The IIM entity associated with anti-SRP antibodies was initially classified as PM, but was later pathologically classified as necrotizing autoimmune myopathy (current terminology being IMNM). Later, a second antibody anti-HMGCR was described in IMNM. Antigen targets of both the antibodies are ubiquitously expressed in cells, but are found to translocate to muscle fiber surface in patients. IMNM presents as acute to subacute sever myopathy and often has very high levels of creatine kinase (CK) to the tune of >100 times. The antibodies are pathogenic and correlate with serum CK levels. However, both of them can present as a slowly progressive myopathy mimicking muscular dystrophy.[4,17] Pediatric involvement is more common with anti-HMGCR than anti-SRP IMNM. IMNMs represent nearly 30–35% of IIMs.[18]

Anti-SRP IMNM typically has onset after 30s and predominantly affects females. Weakness is severe and lower limb predominant with frequent dysphagia. Anti-SRP is associated with a higher risk of lung disease and rarely severe myocarditis. There is no cancer association. There is a higher risk of atrophy, fat replacement, disability, and longer duration of disease than other IIMs. Recovery is often suboptimal.[17]

Association of statin use with anti-HMGCR has been definitively proven and the drug could be the trigger for autoimmunity. Nearly two-thirds have history of statin exposure. Younger patients, those with higher CK and Asian race, more commonly do not report prior statin use. There is an increased risk of malignancy and needs follow-up, however, extramuscular involvement is not seen.[17]

A subgroup of IMNM negative for both the antibodies has very strong association with malignancy.[4]

Overlap Syndrome

Myositis occurring in the course of a systemic connective tissue disease is referred to as overlap myositis. The diagnosis requires the independent diagnosis of a connective tissue disease with specific criteria, the most important ones being systemic sclerosis (SSc), Sjögren's syndrome (SS), and systemic lupus erythematosus (SLE). Overlap syndromes in myositis may also be defined by less specific MAAs rather than MSAs.[11] Antibodies and associated clinical syndromes are noted in **Table 2**.

Sporadic Inclusion Body Myositis

Sporadic IBM has characteristic clinicopathological features and treatment response compared to other IIMs. Concurrent inflammatory and degenerative processes in this disease have been shown. The disease occurs in people aged over 40 years affecting males more often. Weakness evolves chronically over months to years. The pattern of weakness is distinct from other IIMs. Weakness is asymmetric affecting quadriceps or forearm finger flexors (particularly ulnar flexor digitorum profundi) initially. Marked muscle wasting is noted. Pharyngeal weakness leading to dysphagia and facial weakness are common.[3] There is no extramuscular involvement or malignancy.[19]

Criteria for sIBM were first proposed by Griggs et al. in 1995 and relied heavily on muscle biopsy findings for definite or possible diagnostic certainty. The more recent 2011 European Neuromuscular Centre diagnostic criteria defined clinicopathologically defined, clinically defined, and probable IBM classes allowing the diagnosis to be made with classical clinical features even when biopsy is not pathognomonic.[20]

Serum CK elevation is mild-to-moderate (usually <10 times). Anti-cN1A antibody has moderate specificity for sIBM and is positive in 37–76% patients. However, this antibody has also been reported in connective tissue disorders and motor neuron disease.[21]

Pathology reveals a combination of CD8+ lymphocyte infiltrate in addition to pathological features of degeneration like rimmed vacuoles with granular inclusions, protein aggregates staining with special stains such as amyloid, TDP43 and p62, and mitochondrial abnormalities.

Other IIM Phenotypes

Immune Checkpoint Inhibitor Associated IIM

Immune checkpoints are proteins which inhibit overactivity of T-cell and other immune responses. These include cytotoxic T-lymphocyte-associate protein 4 (CTLA-4), programmed cell death 1 (PD-1) and PD-1 ligand (PDL-1). ICIs such as pembrolizumab, nivolumab, and ipilimumab enhance T-cell activity and could induce immune-related adverse events. ICI-related myositis is a rare complication (<0.5%), but could be fatal due to myocarditis and respiratory failure. Oculomotor weakness could suggest coexisting myasthenia and has a poorer prognosis. Acute or subacute weakness occurs after a median duration of 4 weeks after ICI initiation. Limb–girdle and axial weakness with myalgia and raised serum CK comprise the phenotypes. A good response is seen with prompt ICI withdrawal and immunotherapy.[22,23]

Polymyositis

The existence of PM as an independent entity is uncertain. There are no specific clinical, serological, or pathological markers for PM, relegating it as a diagnosis by exclusion. A seminal follow-up study showed that among 165 patients initially diagnosed as PM, all except four could be assigned an alternate diagnosis with reevaluation.[24] In reality, PM may represent the forme fruste of the traditional IIMs where a definite subtype classification is not yet made.

■ DIAGNOSIS

Muscle Enzymes

Serum levels of muscle enzymes [CK, lactate dehydrogenase (LDH), aldolase, aspartate aminotransferase (AST), and alanine aminotransferase (ALT)] are typically elevated. Serum CK is the most sensitive and is elevated nearly 5–50 times the normal range. Extremely high levels of up to 100 times can be seen in IMNM whereas nearly 20% of DM could have normal CK levels. CK elevation is mild to moderate in sIBM, usually <10 times of upper limit of normal. Serial monitoring of CK levels does not always help with disease monitoring. Serum aldolase levels are reported to be elevated in DM patients with normal CK levels.[25]

Electromyography

Electromyography is generally nonspecific shows increased irritability evidenced by fibrillations, positive sharp waves, and repetitive discharges in addition to myopathic motor unit potentials. In sIBM, nerve conduction study may rarely show polyneuropathy and neurogenic potentials in EMG in chronic stages.[21,25]

Muscle Imaging

Magnetic resonance imaging (MRI) of the muscles is widely used in IIM. Main sequences of interest are T1-weighted images for fat replacement and T2 short tau inversion recovery (STIR) for muscle edema. MRI has high sensitivity for muscle edema in active and early stages. Even in active stages, fatty changes may be appreciated.[26] DM has symmetric muscle edema of proximal muscles which may be associated subcutaneous edema while ASS may show hyperintense and thickened fasciae. IMNM shows more severe edema and early fatty changes and muscle atrophy compared to DM.[27] Muscle MRI in IBM follows clinical pattern with involvement of quadriceps (with relative sparing of rectus femoris), finger flexors, and medial gastrocnemius, often in an asymmetric fashion. Fatty infiltration is predominant over muscle edema.[19] Wavy fascia between affected vasti is called the undulating fascia sign and indicates severe disease.[26] Although the specificity of MRI in

IIM is limited, it is useful to confirm myositis, exclude mimics, for specific pattern identification, for localization for biopsy and as an outcome measure in longitudinal studies.[27]

The utility of muscle ultrasound is limited, but rapid availability and pediatric-friendliness are advantageous in specific situations for screening. Fluorine 18-fluorodeoxyglucose positron emission tomography (FDG-PET) is a good marker of inflammatory activity and is gaining acceptance as a useful tool for early detection.[26]

Muscle Biopsy

Assessment of muscle pathology is still considered the gold standard for diagnosis of IIMs. Routine enzyme histochemistry and immunohistochemistry (IHC) are the two major tools used by the pathologist for diagnosis of IIM. The histological and immunohistochemical features associated with IIMs are summarized in **Table 3**.

Dermatomyositis

Hematoxylin and eosin (H&E) staining shows patchy involvement of myofibers, fiber size variation, perifascicular atrophy **(Figs. 1A and B)**, myonecrosis and myophagocytosis, regenerating fibers, some cuffing necrotic fibers[28] and microinfarction.[29] Capillaries are thickened and reduced in number. Inflammatory cells seen are lymphocytes (predominant), dendritic cells, and macrophages with perimysial, endomysial, and perivascular localization **(Figs. 1C and D)**. Connective tissue may be increased **(Figs. 2A to D)**. A caveat is that muscle biopsy may be entirely normal with absent inflammatory cells. The histological features specific to MSAs are summarized in **Table 1**.

Enzyme histochemistry does not show any diagnostic hallmarks, though the following features may be seen, namely, moth-eaten fibers or core-like areas in nicotinamide adenine dinucleotide-tetrazolium reductase (NADH-TR), cytochrome c oxidase (COX) deficient fibers, increased acid phosphatase activity in muscle fibers, and increased alkaline phosphatase in perimysium.[8,28]

Immunohistochemistry plays an important role in diagnosis. The diagnostically useful markers include sarcolemmal and focal sarcoplasmic expression of major histocompatibility complex I (MHC-I) (in normal muscle MHC-I is expressed only on blood vessels).[8] However, sarcolemmal MHC-I expression can also be seen in muscular dystrophies and acid maltase deficiency. Membrane attack complex (MAC, C5b-9) is expressed on capillaries and sarcolemma.[30] Human myxovirus resistance protein A (MxA) is expressed capillaries and sarcoplasm with perifascicular, diffuse, and scattered patterns. It is useful in differentiating DM (MxA-positive) from ASS (mostly MxA-negative).[31,32] Inflammatory cells are CD4+ T-cells and dendritic cells and ultrastructural studies may show tubuloreticular inclusions in endothelial cells.

Antisynthetase Syndrome

The H&E show perifascicular necrosis of myofibers rather than atrophy which is seen in DM. There is paucity of capillaries, inflammatory infiltrates with lymphocytes and macrophages, and fragmentation of connective tissue.[8]

Enzyme histochemistry shows perimysial connective tissue staining with alkaline phosphatase. IHC reveals sarcolemmal expression and focal sarcoplasmic expression of MHC-I, and sarcolemmal expression (perifascicular distribution) of MHC-II.[8] MAC is sometimes expressed on sarcolemma[30] and MxA is generally negative, but can be rarely positive.[31]

Immune-mediated Necrotizing Myopathy

Predominant muscle fiber necrosis in the absence of significant inflammation characterizes the syndrome. Scattered necrotic

TABLE 3: Histological and immunohistochemical features in idiopathic inflammatory myopathies.

Auto-antibody	Significant histopathology	MHC Class I	MHC Class II	MAC (C5b-9) deposition	MxA
Anti-Mi-2 DM	• Prominent muscle fiber damage • Inflammatory cell infiltration • Perifascicular atrophy and necrosis • Increased perimysial alkaline phosphatase activity	+ sarcolemma and sarcoplasm	−	+ sarcolemma > capillaries	+ sarcoplasmic, perifascicular area
Anti-MDA5 DM	Less muscle pathology and inflammatory features	+ sarcolemma and sarcoplasm	−	+ capillaries > sarcolemma	+ sarcoplasmic, scattered/diffuse
Anti-TIF-1γ DM	Vacuolated/punched out fibers	+ sarcolemma and sarcoplasm	−	+ capillaries > sarcolemma	+ sarcoplasmic, perifascicular area
Anti-NXP-2 DM	Microinfarction	+ sarcolemma and sarcoplasm	−	+ capillaries > sarcolemma	+ sarcoplasmic, perifascicular area
Anti-SAE DM	Perifascicular atrophy	+ sarcolemma and sarcoplasm	−	+ capillaries	+ sarcoplasmic, perifascicular area
Anti-SRP IMNM	• Scattered necrotic and regenerating fibers • Macrophages ++ • Paucity of lymphocytes • p62: Tiny sarcoplasmic dots	+ sarcolemma and sarcoplasm	−	+ sarcolemma	−
Anti-HMGCR IMNM	Same as for anti-SRP IMNM	+ sarcolemma and sarcoplasm	−	+ sarcolemma	−

Continued

Continued

Auto-antibody	Significant histopathology	MHC Class I	MHC Class II	MAC (C5b-9) deposition	MxA
Anti-Jo-1 ASS	• Perifascicular necrosis • Perimysial connective tissue fragmentation • Perifascicular atrophy +/-	+ sarcolemma and sarcoplasm	+ perifascicular	+ sarcolemma	–
Anti-PL-7 ASS	Same as for anti-Jo-1 ASS	+ sarcolemma and sarcoplasm	+ perifascicular	+ sarcolemma	–
Anti-OJ ASS	Same as for anti-Jo-1 ASS	+ sarcolemma and sarcoplasm	+ perifascicular	+ sarcolemma	–
Anti-PL-12 ASS	Not characterized	+ sarcolemma and sarcoplasm	+ perifascicular	+ sarcolemma	–
Sporadic IBM	• Endomysial (CD8+ KLRG1+) lymphocytic invasion surrounding or invading non-necrotic fibers • MGT: Rimmed vacuoles • COX-SDH: COX-deficient fibers • p62: Coarse aggregates in myofibers	+ sarcolemma and sarcoplasm	+ sarcolemma	+ sarcolemma	–

(DM: dermatomyositis; IMNM: immune-mediated necrotizing myopathy; ASS: anti-synthetase syndrome; IBM: inclusion body myositis; MHC: major histocompatibility complex; MAC: membrane attack complex; MxA: myxovirus resistance protein A)

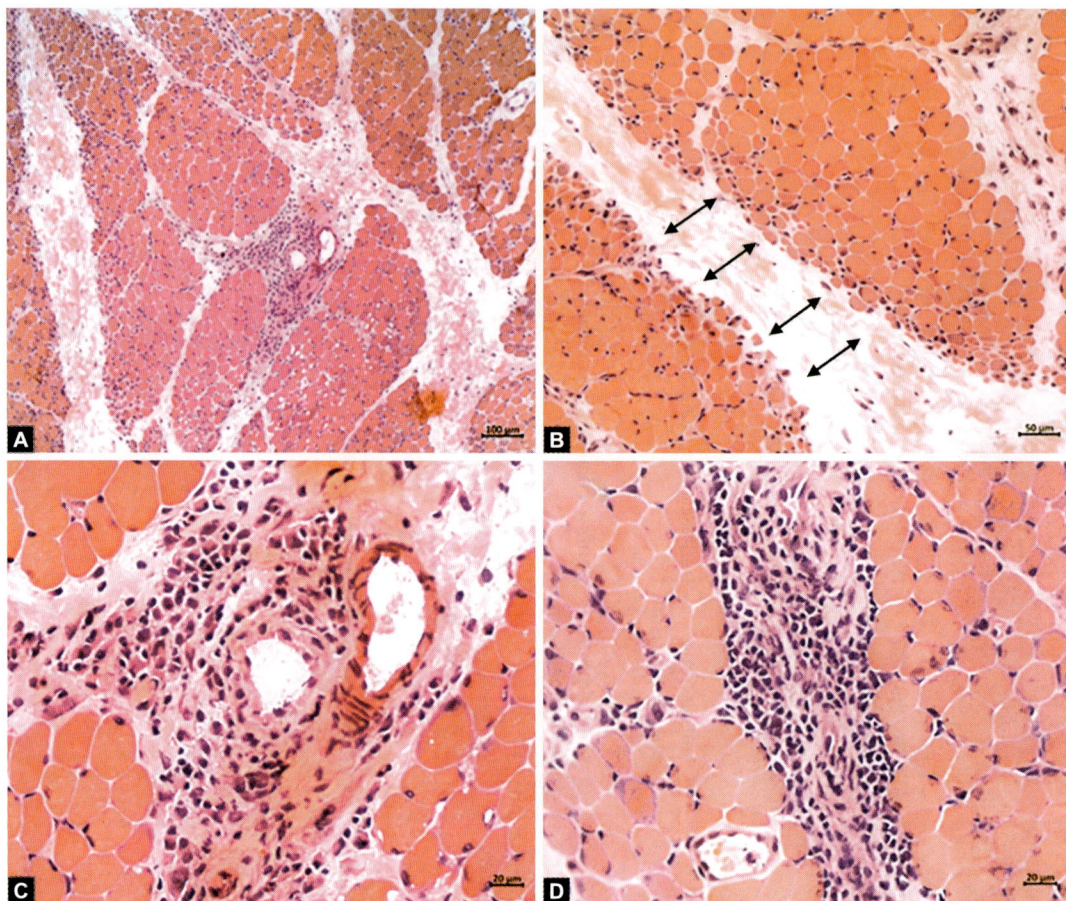

FIGS. 2A TO D: Dermatomyositis. Muscle biopsy with preserved architecture, (A) interstitial edema, (B) perifascicular atrophy (black arrows), and (C and D) perivascular epimysial and perimysial inflammation (A to D) hematoxylin and eosin.

fibers, several regenerating fibers, and inflammatory cells composed mainly of macrophages, but with paucity of lymphocytes is noted in H&E.[28] MHC-I may show sarcolemmal and focal sarcoplasmic expression and MAC is expressed in the in the sarcolemma of non-necrotic fibers.[30] Staining for p62/SQSTM1 appears as tiny dots in sarcoplasm.[33]

Sporadic Inclusion Body Myositis

Myofibers show fiber size variation (atrophy and hypertrophy), and internalized nuclei and may show myonecrosis and myophagocytosis and regenerating fibers. Vacuoles rimmed by granular basophilic material is classically seen.[28] Inflammatory cells are lymphocytes (predominant) and macrophages. Endomysial connective tissue can be increased.

Modified Gomori trichrome (MGT) highlights vacuoles rimmed by reddish granular material. COX-deficient fibers may be noted and the inclusions within the vacuoles are congophilic and show birefringence **(Figs. 3A to D)**.[28]

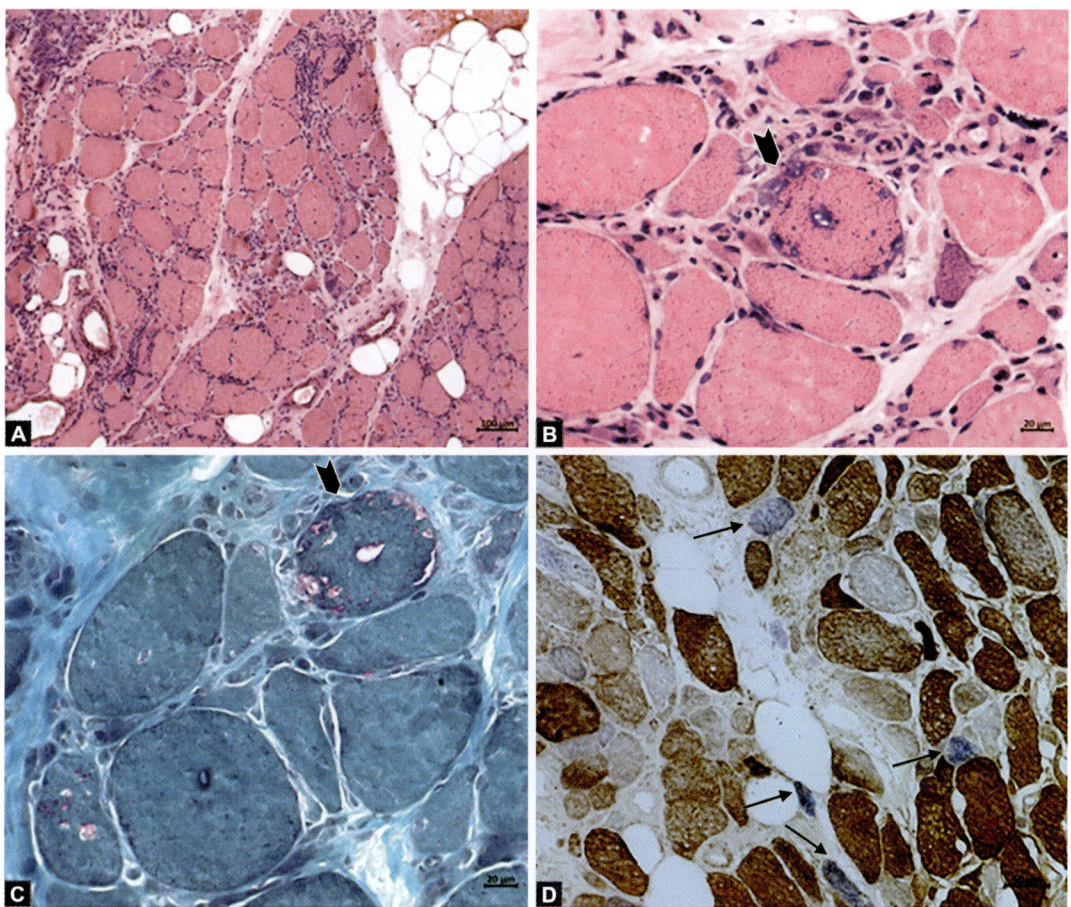

FIGS. 3A TO D: Inclusion body myositis. Muscle biopsy with partially effaced architecture with endomysial inflammation (1A), myofibers with rimmed vacuoles (B and C, black arrowheads) and COX-deficient fibers (D, black arrows) (A and B: Hematoxylin and eosin, C: Modified Gomori trichrome, and D: COX-SDH)
(COX: cytochrome c oxidase; SDH: succinate dehydrogenase)

Sarcolemmal and focal sarcoplasmic expression of MHC-I and sarcolemmal expression of MHC-II are noted.[34] There are coarse aggregates positive for p62/SQSTM1 within vacuoles, perinuclear and subsarcolemmal localization,[35] and predominantly CD8+ KLRG1+ (killer cell lectin-like receptor G1) lymphocytes.[36] Ultrastructural studies show filamentous inclusions in nuclei and/or cytoplasm and myelin-like whorls and cytoplasmic bodies.[28]

TREATMENT OF IDIOPATHIC INFLAMMATORY MYOPATHIES

Treatment of IIMs aim at restoration of muscle strength, maintain long-term remission, and management of multisystem and cancer complications.

Immunotherapy

Immunotherapy is the cornerstone of IIM management. However, there are few randomized controlled trials to substantiate the choices. Treatment is guided by the disease subtype, severity and risk of cancer, and severe systemic involvement.[3] Doses and indications are summarized in **Table 4**. sIBM has poor response to immunotherapy and is discussed separately.

In mild-to-moderate DM, IMNM, and ASS, therapy is initiated with high-dose oral corticosteroid along with simultaneous

TABLE 4: Immunotherapy for idiopathic inflammatory myopathies.

Therapeutic agent	Dose	Indication	Prophylaxis and monitoring
Oral prednisolone	1–1.5 mg/kg at initiation, maintained for 4–6 weeks (or till stable). Taper at a dose of 10 mg every 2 weeks till 30 mg, 5 mg every 2 weeks till 20 mg/day, 2.5 mg every 2 weeks to final dose	First line agent in all	Prophylaxis for gastritis and osteoporosis and monitor for hyperglycemia, hypertension, osteoporosis, sleep and mood disturbances, glaucoma, cataract
Oral pulse dexamethasone	Monthly dose of 40 mg × 4 days	Alternative to oral prednisolone, shown to be equally effective with fewer side effects	Same as above
Intravenous methylprednisolone	500–1,000 mg for 3–5 days	Induction in severe or refractory disease	Acute gastritis, hypokalemia, behavioral problems, hyperglycemia, hypertension
Methotrexate	Initiated orally as a single weekly dose of 5 mg/week and increased to 25 mg/week in increments of 2.5 mg weekly. Subcutaneous can be used in suboptimal response	Steroid sparing agent with maximum evidence, particularly in juvenile IIM. Risk of ILD makes it unattractive	• Supplementation of folic acid 1 mg/day (6 days a week) or folinic acid 5 mg/week is required. Stomatitis, gastroenteritis, alopecia, teratogenicity likely. Bone marrow suppression, hepatic dysfunction to be monitored • Cumulative risk of hepatic fibrosis and lung toxicity
Azathioprine	Started as a dose of 25–50 mg daily and increased by 25 mg every week to a maximum dose of 2–3 mg/kg of ideal body weight per day (in two divided doses)	First line steroid sparing immunotherapy	• Thiopurine methyltransferase (TPMT) genotype status prior to initiation • Gastritis, flu like syndromes, marrow suppression, hepatic dysfunction, long-term oncogenicity

Continued

Continued

Therapeutic agent	Dose	Indication	Prophylaxis and monitoring
Mycophenolate mofetil	Initiated at a dose of 500 mg/day and slowly increased to 2–3 g/day in two divided doses	Optional first line steroid sparing immunotherapy, less preferred in children	Gastrointestinal side effects, cytopenia, hepatic dysfunction, infections, teratogenicity
Cyclosporine A	6 mg/kg/day	Optional agent, limited use	Hypertension, renal dysfunction, neurotoxicity, metabolic side effects, oncogenicity
Tacrolimus	0.2 mg/kg/day	Optional agent, limited use	Gastrointestinal and hepatic dysfunction, nephrotoxicity, tremors, confusion, headache, dermatological problems
Intravenous immunoglobulin	2 g/kg infusion over 5 days	Refractory patients and severe relapses	Headache, thrombotic side effects, allergy
Rituximab	1,000 mg infusion 2 weeks apart, repeated 6–9 monthly	Refractory IIM, especially antibody positive	Infusion reactions, infections, hypogammaglobulinemia
Cyclophosphamide	0.6–1 g/m² weekly for 6–12 months	Refractory IIM	Hemorrhagic cystitis (mitigated by hydration and mesna), bone marrow suppression, infections, ovarian failure

addition of a steroid-sparing immunotherapy. Oral methotrexate, azathioprine, or mycophenolate mofetil is the preferred agents, though the propensity of the former to produce ILD makes it less attractive. Steroid taper is initiated when the weakness plateaus.[26]

In severe or refractory situations, treatment may be initiated with pulse intravenous methyl prednisolone with or without intravenous immunoglobulin (IVIg). Rituximab is particularly useful as a second-line agent in antibody positive patients, juvenile IIM and those with moderate deficits.[37] Cyclophosphamide pulse therapy can also be used in refractory patients.

Table 5 summarizes the newer and emerging biological agents for refractory IIM.[2,38-40]

Precision therapy includes early use of IVIG for HMGCR IMNM and rituximab for IIM with SRP, Jo-1, or Mi antibodies. Tacrolimus is effective for pulmonary improvement with anti Jo-1 and ani SRP positive IIMs and early cyclophosphamide for all ILD.[3,25]

Response to immunotherapy has been disappointing in sIBM. Corticosteroids may have temporary benefits for muscle power. IVIG showed partial benefit for dysphagia in one study. Multiple therapeutic trials have been attempted, notably, alemtuzumab, bimagrumab, and arimoclomol, but results

TABLE 5: Emerging and experimental therapies in refractory idiopathic inflammatory myopathies.

Agent	Mechanism of action	Evidence
Tocilizumab	IL-6 inhibitor	Case reports of positive effects in refractory ASS, OM and DM with rapidly progressive ILD and skin disease. Phase 2B study in refractory DM/PM failed to meet the efficacy endpoints
Abatacept	CTLA-4 fusion protein	Case reports and series showed effectiveness in JDM and OM. A phase 2b delayed start trial showed efficacy in 42% refractory DM/PM, phase 3 study is ongoing
Tofacitinib	JAK 1/3 inhibitor	Small series and pilot study showed moderate benefit, particularly in DM with rapidly progressive ILD
Baricitinib	JAK 1/2 inhibitor	Clinical improvement reported in individual cases and small series. Phase 2 study is ongoing
Ruxolitinib	JAK 1/2 inhibitor	Case report of efficacy in DM-myelofibrosis overlap
Etanercept	Anti-TNF-α agent	Conflicting evidence in refractory DM and PM, improvement and worsening of myositis reported in different case series. Not recommended for therapy
Infliximab	Anti-TNF-α agent	Conflicting results in case reports and series. Not recommended for therapy
Anakinra	IL-1 inhibitor	Nearly half of patients with refractory DM/PM responded to therapy in case series and reports
Sifalimumab	Anti-interferon-α antibody	Phase 1B study showed suppression of interferon signatures with clinical correlate. Phase 2 study in SLE with myositis showed a high rate of adverse effects
Belimumab	BAFF antagonist	Phase 2 RCT failed to show significant benefit
Eculizumab	Complement inhibitor	Effective in case report, phase 2 trial is ongoing
Apremilast	Phosphodiesterase-4 inhibitor	Positive impact on refractory DM in case reports, particularly for cutaneous manifestations
Lenabasum	Type 2 cannabinoid receptor agonist	Phase 2/3 studies are ongoing. Tolerance and positive benefit demonstrated for refractory cutaneous disease in a phase 2 study
ACTH gel/ corticotropin	Stimulates adrenal gland	Effective in refractory DM/PM in small series

(ACTH: adrenocorticotropic hormone; ASS: anti-synthetase syndrome; BAFF: B cell activating factor; CTLA: cytotoxic T-lymphocyte associated protein; DM: dermatomyositis; IL: interleukin; ILD: interstitial lung disease; JAK: Janus kinase; OM: overlap myositis; PM: polymyositis; RCT: randomized controlled trial; TNF: tumour necrosis factor)

were negative or inconclusive. Two of the promising drugs under investigation are sirolimus and anti-KLRG1 antibody **(Table 6)**.[21]

Treatment of juvenile IIM follows a similar pattern. Prednisolone may be initiated at a higher dose of 2 mg/kg. Methotrexate escalated to 15 mg/m^2 is the immunotherapy of choice whereas mycophenolate mofetil is not generally used. IVIg and rituximab are preferred for refractory cases.[37]

Symptomatic and Supportive Management

Management of cutaneous manifestations and calcinosis cutis are important in DM therapy.[41] Use of sunscreens and avoidance of sun exposure are essential and hydroxychloroquine at doses of 200–400 mg/day is helpful for skin rashes of DM.[42] Early detection and aggressive management of pulmonary

TABLE 6: Treatment trials (selected) in sporadic inclusion body myositis.

Agent	Mechanism of action	Evidence and current status
Sirolimus	mTOR pathway inhibitor	Phase 2b study did not show efficacy in primary outcome, but secondary measures were favorable. Phase 3 trial is ongoing
ABC008	Anti-KLRG1 monoclonal antibody	Phase 2/3 trial is ongoing
Arimoclomol	Heat shock protein amplification	Phase 2/3 randomized controlled trial did not show efficacy against placebo
Bimagrumab	Myostatin inhibitor	Phase 2b study showed good safety profile, failed to demonstrate efficacy
Lithium	Glycogen synthase kinase 3 inhibitor	No benefit in a case series
Oxandrolone	Myotrophic property	Pilot study showed borderline benefits
Follistatin gene therapy	Myostatin inhibitor	Moderate benefits in a pilot trial
Alemtuzumab	Anti CD52 monoclonal antibody	Pilot study showed promising results
Prednisone and other immunosuppressants	Immunosuppression by multiple mechanisms	Mixed results in case series and small studies including exacerbation of weakness with therapy
IV immunoglobulin	Immunomodulation by multiple mechanisms	Short term and minor effects on dysphagia and weakness

(CD: cluster of differentiation; IV: intravenous; KLRG1: killer cell lectin-like receptor G1; mTOR: mammalian target of rapamycin)

and cardiac complications and dysphagia can be lifesaving. Physical therapy and assistive devices are essential for all patients with disability, particularly in sIBM.[3,20]

Risk of Cancer and Screening

Idiopathic inflammatory myopathies are associated with an increased risk of cancer within 3 years of diagnosis. All adult patients should be screened for cancer, but particular vigilance is required in high-risk situations, namely, older age of onset, rapid worsening and poor response to therapy, presence of dysphagia or cutaneous ulcers, and specific serostatus (positive anti-TIF1-γ or anti-NXP2 antibodies or seronegative). The risk stratification and recommendation for screening for cancers have been defined in a recent guideline.[42] Children and adults with sIBM do not need routine cancer screening.

■ CONCLUSION

Focus on immunological signatures in serum and tissue has been successful in recognizing homogeneous groups among IIMs. Five main subtypes have emerged—(1) DM, (2) IMNM, (3) ASS, (4) sIBM, and (5) overlap myositis. The key paradigm shift in clinical medicine has been the wide application of MSAs for diagnosis, precision therapy, and prognostication of IIMs. Further understanding of the pathomechanisms of each subtype in the future will aid in identification of specific and efficacious therapies.

REFERENCES

1. Khoo T, Lilleker JB, Thong BY, Leclair V, Lamb JA, Chinoy H. Epidemiology of the idiopathic inflammatory myopathies. Nat Rev Rheumatol. 2023;19(11):695-712.
2. Selva-O'Callaghan A, Pinal-Fernandez I, Trallero-Araguás E, Milisenda JC, Grau-Junyent JM, Mammen AL. Classification and management of adult inflammatory myopathies. Lancet Neurol. 2018;17(9):816-28.
3. Malik A, Hayat G, Kalia JS, Guzman MA. Idiopathic inflammatory myopathies: Clinical approach and management. Front Neurol. 2016;7:64.
4. Allenbach Y, Mammen AL, Benveniste O, Stenzel W; Immune-Mediated Necrotizing Myopathies Working Group. 224th ENMC International Workshop: Clinico-sero-pathological classification of immune-mediated necrotizing myopathies Zandvoort, The Netherlands, 14-16 October 2016. Neuromuscul Disord. 2018;28(1):87-99.
5. Lundberg IE, Tjärnlund A, Bottai M, et al. 2017 European League Against Rheumatism/American College of Rheumatology classification criteria for adult and juvenile idiopathic inflammatory myopathies and their major subgroups Ann Rheum Dis. 2017;76(12):1955-64.
6. Mariampillai K, Granger B, Amelin D, Guiguet M, Hachulla E, Maurier F, et al. Development of a new classification system for idiopathic inflammatory myopathies based on clinical manifestations and myositis-specific autoantibodies. JAMA Neurol. 2018;75(12):1528-37.
7. Pinal-Fernandez I, Casal-Dominguez M, Derfoul A, Pak K, Miller FW, Milisenda JC, et al. Machine learning algorithms reveal unique gene expression profiles in muscle biopsies from patients with different types of myositis. Ann Rheum Dis. 2020;79(9):1234-42.
8. Tanboon J, Nishino I. Classification of idiopathic inflammatory myopathies: Pathology perspectives. Curr Opin Neurol. 2019;32(5):704-14.
9. Papadopoulou C, Chew C, Wilkinson MGL, McCann L, Wedderburn LR. Juvenile idiopathic inflammatory myositis: An update on pathophysiology and clinical care. Nat Rev Rheumatol. 2023;19(6):343-62.
10. Damoiseaux J, Vulsteke JB, Tseng CW, et al. Autoantibodies in idiopathic inflammatory myopathies: Clinical associations and laboratory evaluation by mono- and multispecific immunoassays. Autoimmun Rev. 2019;18(3):293-305.
11. Tanboon J, Uruha A, Stenzel W, Nishino I. Where are we moving in the classification of idiopathic inflammatory myopathies?. Curr Opin Neurol. 2020;33(5):590-603.
12. Damoiseaux J, Mammen AL, Piette Y, Benveniste O, Allenbach Y; ENMC 256th Workshop Study Group. 256th ENMC international workshop: Myositis specific and associated autoantibodies (MSA-ab): Amsterdam, The Netherlands, 8-10 October 2021. Neuromuscul Disord. 2022;32(7):594-608.
13. Rietveld A, Lim J, de Visser M, van Engelen B, Pruijn G, Benveniste O, et al. Autoantibody testing in idiopathic inflammatory myopathies. Pract Neurol. 2019;19(4):284-94.
14. Mammen AL, Allenbach Y, Stenzel W, Benveniste O; ENMC 239th Workshop Study Group. 239th ENMC International Workshop: Classification of dermatomyositis, Amsterdam, the Netherlands, 14-16 December 2018. Neuromuscul Disord. 2020;30(1):70-92.
15. Marvi U, Chung L, Fiorentino DF. Clinical presentation and evaluation of dermatomyositis. Indian J Dermatol. 2012;57(5):375-81.
16. Ghosh R, Dubey S, Benito-León J. Black rash in dark-skinned people: Do not forget dermatomyositis. Neuromuscul Disord. 2023;33(10):788-9.
17. Allenbach Y, Benveniste O, Stenzel W, Boyer O. Immune-mediated necrotizing myopathy: clinical features and pathogenesis. Nat Rev Rheumatol. 2020;16(12):689-701.
18. Merlonghi G, Antonini G, Garibaldi M. Immune-mediated necrotizing myopathy (IMNM): A myopathological challenge. Autoimmun Rev. 2022;21(2):102993.
19. Naddaf E. Inclusion body myositis: Update on the diagnostic and therapeutic landscape. Front Neurol. 2022;13:1020113.
20. Machado P, Brady S, Hanna MG. Update in inclusion body myositis. Curr Opin Rheumatol. 2013;25(6):763-71.
21. Goyal NA. Inclusion Body Myositis. Continuum (Minneap Minn). 2022;28(6):1663-77.
22. Hamada N, Maeda A, Takase-Minegishi K, Kirino Y, Sugiyama Y, Namkoong H, et al. Incidence and distinct features of immune checkpoint inhibitor-related myositis from idiopathic inflammatory myositis: A single-center experience with systematic literature review and meta-analysis. Front Immunol. 2021;12:803410.

23. Touat M, Maisonobe T, Knauss S, Ben Hadj Salem O, Hervier B, Auré K, et al. Immune checkpoint inhibitor-related myositis and myocarditis in patients with cancer. Neurology. 2018;91(10):e985-94.
24. van der Meulen MF, Bronner IM, Hoogendijk JE, Burger H, van Venrooij WJ, Voskuyl AE, et al. Polymyositis: An overdiagnosed entity. Neurology. 2003;61(3):316-21.
25. Manousakis G. Inflammatory myopathies. Continuum (Minneap Minn). 2022;28(6):1643-62.
26. Zubair AS, Salam S, Dimachkie MM, Machado PM, Roy B. Imaging biomarkers in the idiopathic inflammatory myopathies. Front Neurol. 2023;14:1146015.
27. Malartre S, Bachasson D, Mercy G, Sarkis E, Anquetil C, Benveniste O, et al. MRI and muscle imaging for idiopathic inflammatory myopathies. Brain Pathol. 2021;31(3):e12954.
28. Dubowitz V, Sewry CA, Oldfors A. Muscle Biopsy, 5th ed. Amsterdam: Elsevier-OHCE; 2020.
29. Tanboon J, Inoue M, Saito Y, Tachimori H, Hayashi S, Noguchi S, et al. Dermatomyositis: Muscle pathology according to antibody subtypes. Neurology. 2022;98(7):e739-49.
30. Honda M, Shimizu F, Sato R, Nakamori M. Contribution of complement, microangiopathy and inflammation in idiopathic inflammatory myopathies. J Neuromuscul Dis. 2024;11(1):5-16.
31. Uruha A, Allenbach Y, Charuel JL, Musset L, Aussy A, Boyer O, et al. Diagnostic potential of sarcoplasmic myxovirus resistance protein A expression in subsets of dermatomyositis. Neuropathol Appl Neurobiol. 2019;45(5):513-22.
32. Uruha A, Nishikawa A, Tsuburaya RS, Hamanaka K, Kuwana M, Watanabe Y, et al. Sarcoplasmic MxA expression: A valuable marker of dermatomyositis. Neurology. 2017;88(5):493-500.
33. Fischer N, Preusse C, Radke J, Pehl D, Allenbach Y, Schneider U, et al. Sequestosome-1 (p62) expression reveals chaperone-assisted selective autophagy in immune-mediated necrotizing myopathies. Brain Pathol. 2020;30(2):261.
34. Uruha A, Goebel HH, Stenzel W. Updates on the immunopathology in idiopathic inflammatory myopathies. Curr Rheumatol Rep. 2021;23(7):56.
35. Nogalska A, Terracciano C, D'Agostino C, King Engel W, Askanas V. p62/SQSTM1 is overexpressed and prominently accumulated in inclusions of sporadic inclusion-body myositis muscle fibers, and can help differentiating it from polymyositis and dermatomyositis. Acta Neuropathol. 2009;118(3):407-13.
36. Greenberg SA, Pinkus JL, Kong SW, Baecher-Allan C, Amato AA, Dorfman DM. Highly differentiated cytotoxic T cells in inclusion body myositis. Brain. 2019;142(9):2590-604.
37. Oldroyd AGS, Lilleker JB, Amin T, Aragon O, Bechman K, Cuthbert V, et al. British Society for Rheumatology guideline on management of paediatric, adolescent and adult patients with idiopathic inflammatory myopathy. Rheumatology (Oxford). 2022;61(5):1760-8.
38. Grazzini S, Rizzo C, Conticini E, D'Alessandro R, La Barbera L, D'Alessandro M, et al. The role of bDMARDs in idiopathic inflammatory myopathies: A systematic literature review. Autoimmun Rev. 2023;22(2):103264.
39. Zeng R, Glaubitz S, Schmidt J. Antibody therapies in autoimmune inflammatory myopathies: Promising treatment options. Neurotherapeutics. 2022;19(3):911-21.
40. Moghadam-Kia S, Oddis CV, Aggarwal R. Modern therapies for idiopathic inflammatory myopathies (IIMs): Role of biologics. Clin Rev Allergy Immunol. 2017;52(1):81-7.
41. Cobos GA, Femia A, Vleugels RA. Dermatomyositis: An update on diagnosis and treatment. Am J Clin Dermatol. 2020;21(3):339-53.
42. Oldroyd AGS, Callen JP, Chinoy H, Chung L, Fiorentino D, Gordon P, et al. International guideline for idiopathic inflammatory myopathy-associated cancer screening: An International Myositis Assessment and Clinical Studies Group (IMACS) initiative. Nat Rev Rheumatol. 2023;19(12):805-17.

Updates on Limb–girdle Dystrophies and Gene Therapies

Vaibhav Wadwekar, Abhijeet K Kohat, Ragavendar Bhuvaneswaran

ABSTRACT

Limb–girdle muscular dystrophies (LGMDs) represent a diverse group of genetic muscle disorders. These conditions are characterized by proximal muscle weakness, elevated creatine kinase levels, and autosomal inheritance patterns. Genetic diagnosis remains definitive method for diagnosing LGMD and its subtype. Due to various problems in the previous classification and nomenclature of these disorders, the 229th European Neuromuscular Consortium (ENMC) international workshop which was held in Netherlands in 2017 has proposed a new definition, classification, and nomenclature. Currently lot of exciting research in the field of genetic therapies of LGMD is going on, which gives us a hope of a treatment alternative being available in the near future.

Keywords: Limb–girdle muscular dystrophies, Gene therapy, Muscle weakness, Muscle disorders.

■ INTRODUCTION

Limb–girdle muscular dystrophies (LGMDs) represent a diverse group of genetic muscle disorders. Among the muscle weakness caused by genetic disorders these rank fourth most common cause globally. These conditions are characterized by proximal muscle weakness, elevated creatine kinase levels, and autosomal inheritance patterns. Among the Western populations, LGMD affects approximately four to seven individuals per 100,000 population. Their exact prevalence in India is uncertain.[1] References to muscle weakness involving hip and shoulder muscles date back to the early 1800s. Subsequent descriptions by Erb and Leyden-Möbius differentiated these disorders by their specific patterns of muscle weakness, particularly the shoulder and hip girdle weakness while sparing facial muscles. Initially, LGMD served as an umbrella term encompassing various disorders involving these proximal muscles. In 1876, Leyden classified muscular dystrophies into two categories: One affecting children, famously described by Duchenne, and the other causing progressive degeneration in adults. As understanding expanded, additional categories such as facioscapulohumeral and distal muscular dystrophies were incorporated. By the 1950s, Walton identified 18 types of myopathic disorders, refining the classification further. The term "limb–girdle muscular dystrophy" itself emerged in the mid-19th century.[2]

Advances in genetics over the past six decades have revealed that LGMDs stem from mutations in genes that lead to abnormal proteins across various parts of muscle

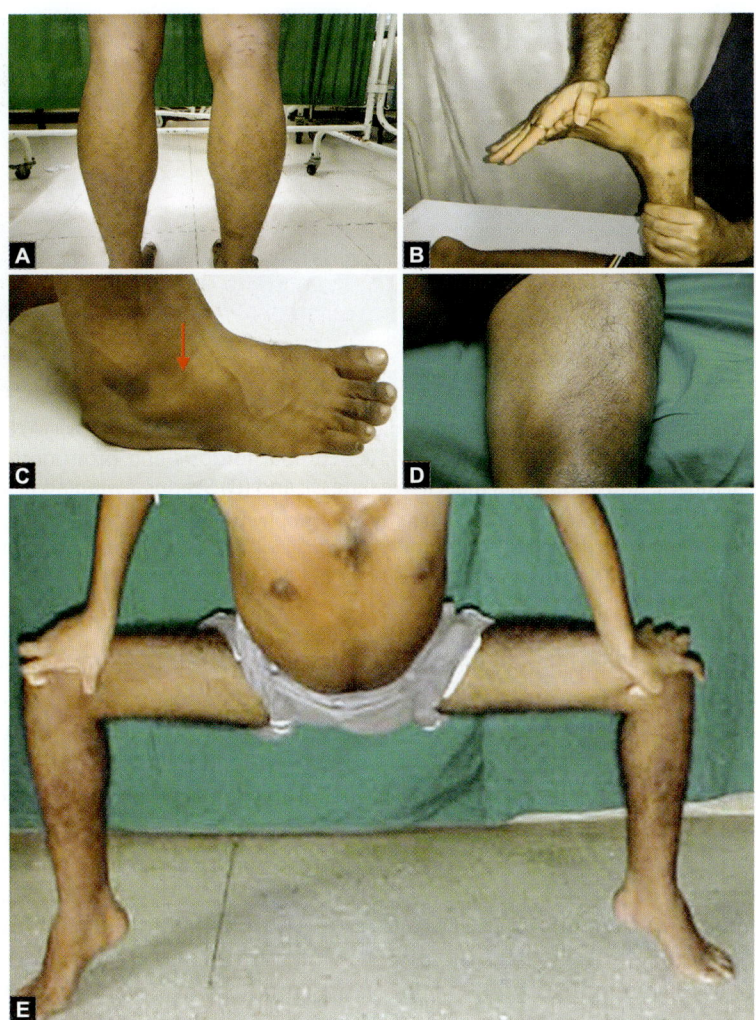

FIGS. 1A TO E: Few clinical signs found in limb–girdle muscular dystrophies (LGMDs). (A) Calf hypertrophy (in sarcoglycanopathies); (B) Ankle contracture (calpainopathy); (C) Extensor digitorum brevis hypertrophy/sparing (nonspecific finding), helpful in differentiating LGMDs from neuropathies where it is wasted; (D) Diamond sign (dysferlinopathy); and (E) Hip splaying or abduction sign due to preferential adductor weakness (sarcoglycanopathies).

Note: Most signs develop as a result of selective atrophy and/or hypertrophy/pseudohypertrophy of muscles. Additionally, it should be noted that although a particular sign indicates a particular LGMD subtype, it may also occur atypically in other subtype and even other disorder (e.g., calf hypertrophy is characteristic of Duchenne/Becker's muscular dystrophy also).

Courtesy (Part D and E): Department of Neurology National Institute of Mental Health and Neurosciences (NIMHANS), Bangalore, Karnataka, India.

cells, including the extracellular matrix, sarcolemma, cytosol, and nuclei. LGMD 2A was the first subtype to be genetically defined.[3] The clinical course and phenotype of each LGMD subtype varies widely and is also based on the specific genetic mutation's severity. Many signs based on the various phenotypic appearances have been described in an attempt to identify the subtypes of LGMD **(Figs. 1 and 2)**. Diagnosis of LGMD relies on

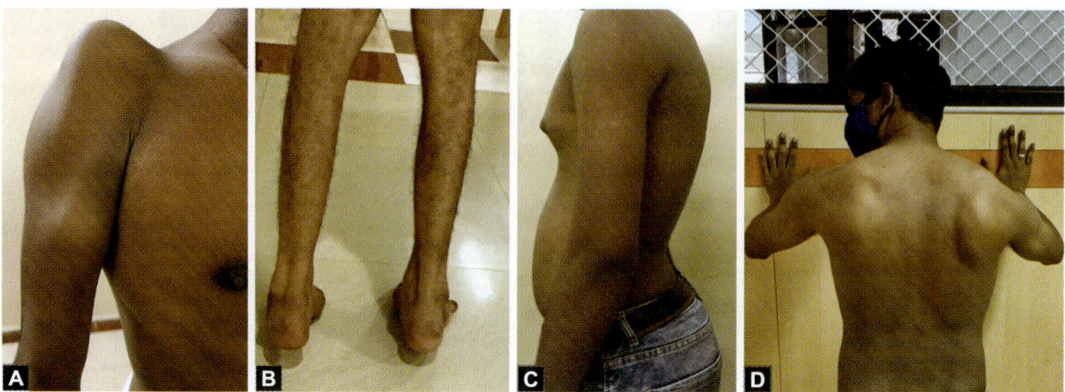

FIGS. 2A TO D: Few clinical signs found in limb–girdle muscular dystrophies (LGMDs). (A) Bicep bulge sign (dysferlinopathy); (B) Calf atrophy (dysferlinopathy); (C) Lumbar lordosis and protrudent abdomen (any LGMD with truncal muscle and abdominal muscle weakness); and (D) Scapular winging (calpainopathy).

Note: Most signs develop as a result of selective atrophy and/or hypertrophy/pseudohypertrophy of muscles. Additionally, it should be noted that although a particular sign indicates a particular LGMD subtype, it may also occur atypically in other subtype and even other disorder (e.g., scapular winging is also found in facioscapulohumeral muscular dystrophy).

a comprehensive medical and family history, physical examination, and various laboratory tests such as creatine kinase levels, muscle histochemistry, immunohistochemistry, muscle magnetic resonance imaging, and electrodiagnostics. However, genetic testing remains the definitive method for diagnosing LGMD and the subtype.

Despite strides in understanding LGMD's genetics and pathophysiology, significant challenges persist in managing and treating these conditions effectively. Addressing these unmet needs remains a crucial focus for ongoing research and clinical care in the field of neuromuscular disorders.

■ LIMB–GIRDLE MUSCULAR DYSTROPHY IN INDIA

In India, LGMDs are increasingly being recognized with the advancements in specifically the immunohistochemistry and genetic tests. Still, the medical literature remains fragmented and is predominantly comprised of case studies and series. The understanding of LGMDs has progressed slowly over recent years, initially highlighted by Srinivas et al. in their report detailing 35 cases.[4] As diagnostic capabilities have evolved in tertiary care centers, immunohistochemistry revealed sarcoglycanopathy to be the most common subtype of LGMD in early 2000s India. Among the sarcoglycanopathies described, the α-sarcoglycanopathy was most notably prevalent, followed by β- and γ-sarcoglycanopathies but this observation was based on isolated case reports and small series.[5] Khadilkar et al. provided further detailed description of multiple sarcoglycan deficiencies in a series of 25 patients, contributing significantly to the understanding of these disorders.[5] Additional common LGMD subtypes in India, identified through immunohistochemistry included dysferlinopathy and calpainopathy.

In the current era of genetics, LGMD subtypes are increasingly being documented in higher institutional and corporate sectors in India, revealing variable phenotypes and expanding the spectrum of these recognized conditions. However, due to limited diagnostic availability and cost issues, the exact prevalence of genetically confirmed LGMDs across India remains challenging to estimate.

One notable factor influencing the prevalence of LGMDs in India worth mentioning is the tradition of consanguineous marriages, particularly within specific caste, subcaste, or *gotra* (clan) communities. The practice of endogamy can lead to an increased incidence of autosomal recessive diseases, including LGMDs, due to the genetic homogeneity within these communities. In some regions and communities, consanguineous marriages, including unions between first cousins, are culturally accepted, further contributing to the concentration of recessive genetic traits.

Overall, while progress is being made in understanding and diagnosing LGMDs in India, continued efforts are necessary to improve diagnostic accessibility and expand epidemiological knowledge, particularly due to genetic and cultural diversity.

LIMB-GIRDLE MUSCULAR DYSTROPHY NEW CLASSIFICATION AND NOMENCLATURE

Understanding the nomenclature of disease classification is crucial for clinicians and patients alike. Changes to accepted terminology should be approached cautiously and should involve consultation with leading clinical experts and patient advocacy groups.

The previous classification system, which is still quite popular, came into existence in 1990 and was based on the defective protein and responsible genetic mutation.[6] Subtypes were classified by a number that indicates whether the disorder was autosomal dominant (LGMD1) or recessive (LGMD2). An alphabet followed the numeric which denoted the specific gene.[6] For example, LGMD1A denoted its autosomal dominant inheritance, and "A" specified the mutation in the *MYOT* gene which is responsible for myotilin which controls the sarcomere assembly. To date over 50 genetic loci have been identified. Dominantly inherited LGMD is less common and reported to be only 5-10% of all LGMD.[7] This classification system had certain limitations:

- The alphabet had no more letters to designate in case a newer form of autosomal recessive LGMD was to be discovered. The latest autosomal recessive condition that has been suggested to be an LGMD has been classified as LGMD 2Z.[8]
- With more than 30 LGMDs it is difficult to remember what a number and letter exactly signifies.
- Several conditions that resemble LGMD phenotypes are not listed in this classification system.
- Some classified LGMD phenotypes overlap with other classification systems.
- Some listed LGMD subtypes do not appear to be a classical LGMD phenotype.

With the evolving genetic shreds of evidence, it was clear that single genetic mutation can give rise to a variety of phenotypes or very similar phenotypes can be caused by various mutations in different genes. For example, the mutation in the *LMNA* gene which is responsible for congenital muscular dystrophy can also result in a LGMD phenotype. Also, some conditions that were classified as LGMD had a prominent distal weakness. In addition, Pompe disease which is a glycogen storage disease was classified as LGMD 2V. With advancing genomic sequencing techniques the multiple newer genetic variants of LGMD are continuously being discovered.

There is currently no consensus on nomenclature beyond LGMD 2Z within the previous classification system. The Online Mendelian Inheritance in Man (OMIM) catalog defaults to assigning the name LGMD 2AA to the next identified autosomal recessive form of LGMD. However, this classification system lacks support from the clinical community.

Observing all the earlier-mentioned problems, 229th European Neuromuscular Consortium (ENMC) international workshop which was held in Netherlands in 2017 for LGMDs, a new definition and classification of LGMD was proposed.[9] According to the proposed definition:
- LGMD is a genetically inherited condition that primarily affects skeletal muscle leading to progressive, predominantly proximal muscle weakness at presentation caused by a loss of muscle fibers.
- To be considered a form of LGMD the condition:
  - Must be described in at least two unrelated families with affected individuals achieving independent walking.
  - Must have an elevated serum creatine kinase activity.
  - Must demonstrate degenerative changes on muscle imaging throughout the disease.
  - Have dystrophic changes on muscle histology, ultimately leading to end-stage pathology for the most affected muscles.

In the same meeting, Straub et al. proposed a new classification system for LGMDs. The new nomenclature included the mode of inheritance: "D" for dominant or "R" for recessive, with "X" representing an X-linked LGMD, if discovered. It is to be noted that Duchenne/Becker's muscular dystrophies which are X-linked are not considered LGMDs. The proposed scheme includes LGMD, inheritance (R or D), order of discovery (number), and affected protein. Congenital muscular dystrophies were excluded as these patients did not achieve independent walking.[9] It is suggested that if a patient fulfils the earlier-proposed definition of LGMD with no known pathogenic gene identified until diagnosis is confirmed they should be referred to as "LGMD unclassified". The proposed LGMD classification by Straub et al. can therefore only serve as a guideline to assign a specific diagnosis to a patient.

Table 1 shows the current and previous classification systems. LGMD 1A, LGMD 1B,

TABLE 1: Comparison of old and new classification/nomenclature of limb–girdle muscular dystrophies (LGMDs).

Old nomenclature	New nomenclature	Gene involved	Protein involved
LGMD type 1 or 2 Alphabet	• LGMD type D or R • Numeric to be followed by affected protein name		
Dominant forms of LGMD (now called as LGMD D)			
LGMD 1D	LGMD D1 DNAJB6 related	DNAJB6	DNAJB6
LGMD 1F	LGMD D2 TNPO3 related	TNPO3	Transportin 3
LGMD 1G	LGMD D3 HNRNPDL related	HNRNPDL	Heterogeneous nuclear ribonucleoprotein D-like
LGMD 1I	LGMD D4 calpain 3 related	CAPN3	Calpain 3
LGMD 1H	LGMD D5 collagen 6 related	COL6A1	Collagen 6α1
		COL6A2	Collagen 6α2
		COL6A3	Collagen 6α3
"LGMD 1 has been renamed to LGMD-D (for dominant)"			
"LGMD A, B, C, E are no longer considered as LGMDs"			

Continued

Continued

Old nomenclature	New nomenclature	Gene involved	Protein involved
Recessive forms of LGMD (now called as LGMD R)			
LGMD 2A	LGMD R1 calpain 3 related	CAPN3	Calpain 3
LGMD 2B	LGMD R2 dysferlin-related	DYSF	Dysferlin
LGMD 2D	LGMD R3 α-sarcoglycan related	SGC α	α-sarcoglycan
LGMD 2E	LGMD R4 β-sarcoglycan related	SGC β	β-sarcoglycan
LGMD 2C	LGMD R5 γ-sarcoglycan related	SGC γ	γ-sarcoglycan
LGMD 2F	LGMD R6 δ-sarcoglycan related	SGC δ	δ-sarcoglycan
LGMD 2G	LGMD R7 telethonin related	TCAP	Telethonin
LGMD 2H	LGMD R8 TRIM 32 related	TRIM32	Tripartite motif containing protein 32
LGMD 2I	LGMD R9 FKRP related	FKRP	Fukutin-related protein
LGMD 2J	LGMD R10 titin related	TTN	Titin
LGMD 2K	LGMD R11 POMT1 related	POMT1	Protein O-mannosyltransferase 1
LGMD 2L	LGMD R12 anoctamin 5 related	ANO5	Anoctamin5
LGMD 2M	LGMD R13 fukutin related	FKTN	Fukutin
LGMD 2N	LGMD R14 POMT2 related	POMT2	Protein O-mannosyltransferase 2
LGMD 2O	LGMD R15 POMGnT1 related	POMGnT1	Protein O-linked mannose N-acetylglucosaminyltransferase 1
LGMD 2P	LGMD R16 α-dystroglycan related	DAG1	Dystroglycan 1
LGMD 2Q	LGMD R17 plectin related	PLEC	Plectin
LGMD 2S	LGMD R18 TRAPPC11 related	TRAPPC11	Trafficking protein particle complex 11
LGMD 2T	LGMD R19 GMPPB related	GMPPB	GDP-mannose pyrophosphorylase B
LGMD 2U	LGMD R20 ISPD related	ISPD/ CRPPA	CDL-L-ribitol pyrophosphorylase A
LGMD 2Z	LGMD R21 POGLUT1 related	POGLUT1	Protein O-glucosyltransferase 1
NONE	LGMD R22 collagen 6 related	COL6A1	Collagen 6α1
		COL6A2	Collagen 6α2
		COL6A3	Collagen 6α3
NONE	LGMD R23 laminin α2 related	LAMA2	Laminin α2
NONE	LGMD R24 POMGNT2 related	POMGnT2	Protein O-linked mannose N-acetylglucosaminyltransferase 2
2X	LGMD R25 BVES related	BVES	Blood vessel epicardial substance
None	R pending	PYROXD1	Pyridine nucleotide-disulfide oxidoreductase domain-containing protein1

"LGMD 2 has been renamed to LGMD R (for recessive)"

"LGMD R, V, W are no longer considered as LGMDs"

"LGMDs α (alpha), β (beta), γ (gamma), and δ (delta) (sarcoglycanopathies) have been reordered for ease"

LGMD 1C, LGMD 1E, LGMD 2R, LGMD 2V, LGMD 2W, and LGMD 2Y are not included in the current classification as LGMDs due to various reasons which include predominant distal weakness, higher incidences of cardiomyopathy, myopathy related to metabolic derangements, and their rarity. It was decided that these conditions instead be considered by either their more commonly used names or as stand-alone entities (e.g., "myofibrillar myopathy" for LGMD 1E) rather than being classified as LGMD.

GENE THERAPY IN LIMB–GIRDLE MUSCULAR DYSTROPHY

Principles of Gene Therapy

The term "gene therapy" primarily refers to the addition, removal, or alteration of genetic material in human cells through viral transduction. Wayback in 1972 Friedmann and Roblin hypothesized genetic modification as the cure for hereditary diseases.[10] Following many years of scientific and technical development today, gene therapies have evolved as potential treatment options for various inherited and acquired diseases including primary myopathies, neurodegenerative disorders, immune-mediated diseases, hemoglobinopathies, etc. The monogenic nature of primary myopathies facilitates mutation-specific therapeutic interventions, notably viral vector-mediated gene therapy.[11] Gene therapy follows certain basic principles which include gene addition, gene suppression, and genome editing. Genes with "loss-of-function" defects are treated with gene addition while genes with "gain-of-functions" defects are treated with gene suppression. Gene editing is a newer tool that can repair genetic defects in situ. Gene editing mostly relies on the site-specific introduction of a double-strand break into deoxyribonucleic acid (DNA).[12] Exon skipping is a type of gene editing that involves using ribonucleic acid (RNA) splicing to skip over faulty sections of genetic code. The notable techniques used in the treatment of limb–girdle dystrophies are given in **Flowchart 1**.

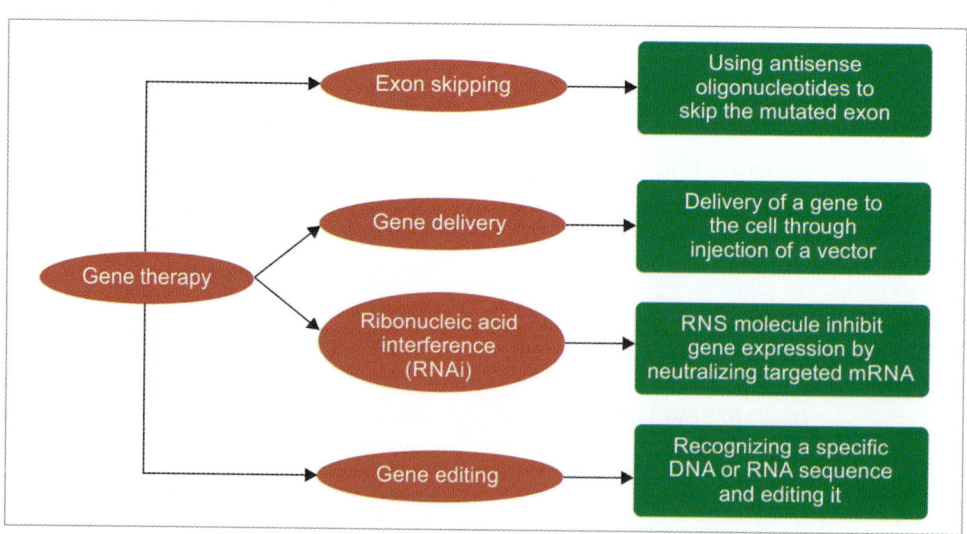

FLOWCHART 1: Various genetic techniques used in the treatment of LGMD.
(DNA: deoxyribonucleic acid; LGMD: limb–girdle muscular dystrophy; mRNA: messenger ribonucleic acid; RNA: ribonucleic acid)

GENE THERAPY FOR LIMB–GIRDLE MUSCLE DYSTROPHIES

Limb–girdle Muscle Dystrophy R1/2A (Calpainopathy)

Limb–girdle muscle dystrophy R1/2A is due to recessive mutations in the *CAPN3* gene encoding calpain-3, which is a sarcomeric protein, a calcium-dependent cysteine protease whose function in the muscle is not completely known. Symptom onset is in early adolescence and is characterized by the predominant involvement of posterior thigh muscles. Ambulation loss is noted around 10–20 years. Bartoli et al. (2006) evaluated the safety and efficacy of adeno-associated virus (AAV)-mediated calpain 3 gene transfer in a mouse model[13] and reported efficient and stable transgene expression in muscle with restoration of the proteolytic activity. However, dose-dependent cardiac toxicity and death were reported when the therapy was given intravenously. In subsequent studies, this problem of cardiac toxicity was overcome by adding a target sequence from the heart-specific microRNA-208a in the promoter region. This prevented cardiac toxicity while enabling proper transgene expression in skeletal muscle. This approach also reversed the signs of calpain 3 deficiency. These findings were reproduced by another group who demonstrated that employing muscle-specific promoters can prevent cardiac toxicity even in a primate model of the disease.[14] So far there is no clinical trial has been initiated to test gene therapy in LGMD R1/2A human patients.

Limb–girdle Muscle Dystrophy R2/2B (Dysferlinopathies)

Dysferlinopathies have proximal and distal phenotypes. Defects in the *DYSF* gene that maps to chromosome 2p13 is responsible for the defect. Hip girdle muscles are mainly involved and the disease later progresses to calf muscles. The dysferlin gene plays a role in the calcium-mediated repair of the muscle membrane, vesicle trafficking, and calcium homeostasis, as well as the expression of nonselective calcium-permeable channels that contribute to the inflammatory process. Muscle biopsy of the dysferlinopathy patients mimics with inflammatory myopathies mainly because of the presence of marked inflammation.[15] The dysferlin transcript is 6.9 kb of size, exceeding the AAV vectors load carrying capacity. To overcome this, a dual vector strategy utilizing two recombinant AAV (rAAV) vectors, each carrying a segment of the dysferlin complementary DNA (cDNA) was tested by intramuscular injection in mutated mice. This resulted in 27% of normal protein expression while restoring muscle force.[16] Another study demonstrated the benefit of intravenous injection of dual rAAV vectors leading to full-length dysferlin production without toxicity and with improvement in muscle pathology and strength.[17] Preliminary human studies also validated dual vector intramuscular delivery to small forearm muscles in two LGMD R2/2B subjects without significant safety concerns.[14] An open-label, phase I, single dose, systemic gene transfer study to evaluate the safety, tolerability, and efficacy of SRP6004 in ambulatory subjects with LGMD R2/2B is ongoing using a rAAVrh74.MHCK7.DYSF.DV vector (NCT05906251, Sarepta Therapeutics) and results are awaited.

Sarcoglycanopathies

The sarcoglycan complex, including the α-, β-, γ-, and δ-sarcoglycans (LGMDR3/2D, LGMDR4/2E, LGMDR5/2C, and LGMDR6/2F, respectively) is a subcomplex of the dystrophin-glycoprotein complex composed of four transmembrane glycoproteins. These proteins have a special role in the mechanical stabilization of the sarcolemma. Clinically, sarcoglycanopathies are autosomal recessive LGMDs with variable disease severity and phenotypes usually onset in early childhood to young adulthood. The later age of onset has milder severity of the disease.[17] Respiratory and cardiac involvement are not that uncommon, especially in some subtypes of the disease[18] (LGMDR4/2E and LGMDR5/2C).

Limb–girdle Muscle Dystrophy R3/2D (α-sarcoglycanopathy, SGCA)

The preclinical studies on mice models demonstrated positive outcomes. Intramuscular (into the tibialis anterior muscle) delivery of full-length human SGCA cDNA using an rAAV and its expression driven by muscle-specific creatine kinase promoter (tMCK) did not generate any toxicity.[19,20] The use of the tMCK promoter to package the full-length SGCA into an AAVrh74 vector for both intramuscular delivery and isolated limb infusion demonstrated improved local muscle function and lasting SGCA protein expression on muscle membranes for up to 180 days after injection.[21]

In humans, a phase I/II, double-blind randomized controlled trial (NCT00494195) using gene transfer with AAV1 was completed on six subjects. This trial demonstrated *SGCA* gene expression accompanied by full restoration of the sarcoglycan complex under the control of the tMCK promoter (rAAV1.tMCK.hSGCA) after injection into the extensor digitorum brevis muscles. One patient in this trial failed to express α-sarcoglycan protein because of pre-exposure to AAV.[22]

Limb–girdle Muscle Dystrophy R4/2E (β-sarcoglycanopathy, SGCB)

Preclinical studies in mouse models showed efficacy and safety of gene transfer using a rAAVrh74 vector carrying a human *SGCB* gene by intramuscular injection, enhancing gene expression by 88.4 ± 4.2% after 6 weeks post-procedure. Furthermore, vascular delivery by isolated limb perfusion showed better restoration of the *SGCB* gene.[23] Systemic delivery using the MHCK7 promoter was successfully performed and the results showed 98.1% transgene expression across all muscles with improvement in histopathology, 85% reductions in the serum CK level, and overall ambulation was increased by 57%. No cardiac toxicity was reported. These findings have established a path for clinically beneficial AAV-mediated gene therapy for LGMD2E. In humans, a phase I, multicenter, open-label, single-dose, systemic gene transfer study to evaluate the safety, tolerability, and efficacy of SRP-9003 (NCT05876780, Sarepta Therapeutics, rAAVrh74.MHCK7.hSGCB) is ongoing.

Limb–girdle Muscle Dystrophy R5/2C (γ-sarcoglycan, SGCG)

Intramuscular administration of rAAV *SGCG* gene therapy showed enhanced expression of γ-sarcoglycan in muscles if injected before the development of muscle fibrosis.[24] In a phase 1 human trial, intramuscular injection of AAV1.des.hγ-SGC vector was given in extensor carpi radialis muscles of nine patients in escalating doses. The highest dose-receiving group showed the maximum γ-sarcoglycan expressions.[25]

One phase I clinical trial aiming at testing ATA-200 (AAV8) in six children between 6 and 12 years of age is open (NCT05973630, Atamyo Therapeutics).

Limb–girdle Muscle Dystrophy R9/2I

The missense mutation p.(Leu276Ile) is the most commonly responsible for the LGMD 2I.[26] FKRP deficiency results in α-dystroglycan hypoglycosylation in the muscle and heart, leading to a variety of phenotypes that range from severe congenital muscular dystrophies with central nervous system involvement, exertional myalgia, and asymptomatic hyperCKemia. Systemic delivery of the human *FKRP* gene by AAV9 vector in the *L276IKI* mice, at either neonatal age or at the age of 9 months, rendered body-wide FKRP expression and restored glycosylation of α-dystroglycan in both skeletal and cardiac muscles within 3 months.[27] Treatment of mice with a different mutation (Pro488Leu) showed similar positive results in terms of restoring alpha-dystroglycan glycosylation and improving dystrophic symptoms in heart and skeletal muscles.[28] At present two clinical trials are ongoing. The first, from Asklepios Biopharmaceutical, Inc. (NCT05230459), to evaluate the safety of AB-1003 (previously LION-101) in subjects with genetic confirmation of LGMD R9/2I (part 1). It is a two-part multicenter study. Part one is a randomized, double-blind, and placebo-controlled dose-escalation safety phase followed by a double-blind, placebo-controlled, adaptive phase (part 2) in adult ambulatory patients with LGMD R9/2I.

The second study is by Atamyo Therapeutics multicenter, phase 1–2 study evaluating safety, pharmacodynamic, efficacy, and immunogenicity of GNT0006 (rAAV9 mediated). This study will consist of two phases: An open-label dose escalation phase (Stage 1) and a double-blind placebo-controlled, randomized phase (Stage 2), both with long-term follow-up period NCT05224505).

■ CONCLUSION

Limb–girdle muscular dystrophies represent a group of diverse genetic muscle disorders characterized by progressive proximal muscle weakness. Over the years, significant progress has been made in understanding their genetic basis, classification, and potential therapeutic strategies, particularly in the realm of gene therapy.

The classification of LGMDs has evolved from protein-based nomenclature to include more precise genetic and clinical criteria, reflecting advancements in genetic testing and diagnostic capabilities. However, challenges remain, including the classification of overlapping phenotypes and the need for standardized diagnostic criteria across diverse populations.

Gene therapy has emerged as a promising treatment approach for LGMDs, targeting specific genetic defects to potentially restore muscle function. Encouraging preclinical and early clinical trial results have demonstrated feasibility and safety in various subtypes such as calpainopathy (LGMD 2A/R1), dysferlinopathies (LGMD 2B/R2), and sarcoglycanopathies (LGMDs R3, R4, and R5). Ongoing research continues to refine delivery methods, enhance efficacy, and address safety concerns, particularly in systemic administration.

The landscape of LGMD research in India, though in nascent phase, is rapidly expanding with increasing recognition and characterization of different subtypes through advanced diagnostic tools. Challenges such as limited accessibility to genetic testing and variability in disease presentation due to ethnic and regional differences underscore the need for concerted efforts in diagnosis and management.

Looking forward, collaborative efforts among researchers, clinicians, and patient advocacy groups are essential to further delineate the genetic underpinnings, refine diagnostic criteria, and advance therapeutic options for individuals affected by LGMDs worldwide. Continued investment in research and clinical trials hold promise for improving outcomes and quality of life for patients with these challenging neuromuscular disorders.

REFERENCES

1. Norwood FL, Harling C, Chinnery PF, Eagle M, Bushby K, Straub V, et al. Prevalence of genetic muscle disease in Northern England: in-depth analysis of a muscle clinic population. Brain. 2009;132:3175-86.
2. Walton JN, Nattrass FJ. On the classification, natural history and treatment of the myopathies. Brain. 1954;77:169-231.
3. Richard I, Broux O, Allaman V, Fougerousse F, Chiannilkulchai N, Bourg N, et al. Mutations in the proteolytic enzyme, calpain 3, cause limb-girdle muscular dystrophy type 2A. Cell. 1995;81:27-40.
4. Srinivas K. The myopathies (19501975). Proc Inst Neurol. 1975;5:102-12.
5. Khadilkar SV, Faldu HD, Patil SB, Singh R. Limb-girdle muscular dystrophies in India: A review. Ann Indian Acad Neurol. 2017;20:87-95.
6. Bushby KM. Diagnostic criteria of the limb-girdle muscular dystrophies: Report of the ENMC consortium on limb-girdle dystrophies. Neuromuscul Disord. 1995;5:71-4.
7. van der Kooi AJ, Barth PG, Busch HFM, de Haan R, Ginjaar HB, van Essen AJ, et al. The clinical spectrum of limb girdle muscular dystrophy. A survey in the Netherlands. Brain. 1996;119(5):1471-80.
8. Servián-Morilla E, Takeuchi H, Lee TV, Clarimon J, Mavillard F, Area-Gómez E, et al. A POGLUT1 mutation causes a muscular dystrophy with reduced Notch signaling and satellite cell loss. EMBO Mol Med. 2016;8:1289-309.
9. Straub V, Murphy A, Udd B, Corrado A, Aymé S, Bönneman C, et al. 229th ENMC international workshop: Limb girdle muscular dystrophies–Nomenclature and reformed classification Naarden, the Netherlands, 17–19 March 2017. Neuromuscul Disord. 2018;28:702-10.
10. Friedmann T, Roblin R. Gene therapy for human genetic disease? Science. 1972;175(4025):949-55.
11. Gomez Limia C, Baird M, Schwartz M, Saxena S, Meyer K, Wein N. Emerging Perspectives on Gene Therapy Delivery for Neurodegenerative and Neuromuscular Disorders. J Pers Med. 2022;12(12):1979.
12. Anguela XM, High KA. Entering the modern era of gene therapy. Annu Rev Med. 2019;70:273-88.
13. Bartoli M, Roudaut C, Martin S, Fougerousse F, Suel L, Poupiot J, et al. Safety and efficacy of AAV-mediated calpain 3 gene transfer in a mouse model of limb-girdle muscular dystrophy type 2A. Mol Ther. 2006;13(2):250-9.
14. Pozsgai E, Griffin D, Potter R, Sahenk Z, Lehman K, Rodino-Klapac LR, et al. Unmet needs and evolving treatment for limb girdle muscular dystrophies. Neurodegener Dis Manag. 2021;11(5):411-29.
15. McNally EM, Ly CT, Rosenmann H, Mitrani Rosenbaum S, Jiang W, Anderson LV, et al. Splicing mutation in dysferlin produces limb-girdle muscular dystrophy with inflammation. Am J Med Genet. 2000;91(4):305-12.
16. Lostal W, Bartoli M, Bourg N, Roudaut C, Bentaïb A, Miyake K, et al. Efficient recovery of dysferlin deficiency by dual adeno-associated vector-mediated gene transfer. Hum Mol Genet. 2010;19(10):1897-907.
17. Potter RA, Griffin DA, Sondergaard PC, Johnson RW, Pozsgai ER, Heller KN, et al. Systemic Delivery of Dysferlin Overlap Vectors Provides Long-Term Gene Expression and Functional Improvement for Dysferlinopathy. Hum Gene Ther. 2018;29(7):749-62.
18. Guimarães-Costa R, Fernández-Eulate G, Wahbi K, Leturcq F, Malfatti E, Behin A, et al. Clinical correlations and long-term follow-up in 100 patients with sarcoglycanopathies. Eur J Neurol. 2021;28(2):660-9.
19. Skopenkova VV, Egorova TV, Bardina MV. Muscle-Specific Promoters for Gene Therapy. Acta Naturae. 2021;13(1):47-58.
20. Rodino-Klapac LR, Lee JS, Mulligan RC, Clark KR, Mendell JR. Lack of toxicity of alpha-sarcoglycan overexpression supports clinical gene transfer trial in LGMD2D. Neurology. 2008;71(4):240-7.
21. Mendell JR, Chicoine LG, Al-Zaidy SA, Sahenk Z, Lehman K, Lowes L, et al. Gene Delivery for Limb-Girdle Muscular Dystrophy Type 2D by Isolated Limb Infusion. Hum Gene Ther. 2019;30(7):794-801.
22. Dressman D, Araishi K, Imamura M, Sasaoka T, Liu LA, Engvall E, et al. Delivery of alpha- and beta-sarcoglycan by recombinant adeno-associated virus: efficient rescue of muscle, but differential toxicity. Hum Gene Ther. 2002;13(13):1631-46.
23. Pozsgai ER, Griffin DA, Heller KN, Mendell JR, Rodino-Klapac LR. β-Sarcoglycan gene transfer decreases fibrosis and restores force in LGMD2E mice. Gene Ther. 2016;23(1):57-66.
24. Cordier L, Hack AA, Scott MO, Barton-Davis ER, Gao G, Wilson JM, et al. Rescue of skeletal muscles of gamma-sarcoglycan-deficient mice with adeno-associated virus-mediated gene transfer. Mol Ther. 2000;1(2):119-29.

25. Herson S, Hentati F, Rigolet A, Behin A, Romero NB, Leturcq F, et al. A phase I trial of adeno-associated virus serotype 1-γ-sarcoglycan gene therapy for limb girdle muscular dystrophy type 2C. Brain. 2012;135(Pt 2):483-92.
26. Bolano-Diaz C, Diaz-Manera J. Therapeutic Options for the Management of Pompe Disease: Current Challenges and Clinical Evidence in Therapeutics and Clinical Risk Management. Ther Clin Risk Manag. 2022;18:1099-115.
27. Qiao C, Wang CH, Zhao C, Lu P, Awano H, Xiao B, et al. Muscle and heart function restoration in a limb girdle muscular dystrophy 2I (LGMD2I) mouse model by systemic *FKRP* gene delivery. Mol Ther. 2014;22(11):1890-9.
28. Xu L, Lu PJ, Wang CH, Keramaris E, Qiao C, Xiao B, et al. Adeno-associated Virus 9 Mediated *FKRP* Gene Therapy Restores Functional Glycosylation of α-dystroglycan and Improves Muscle Functions. Mol Ther. 2013;21(10):1832-40.

Clinical Utility and Interpretation of Genetic Testing in Neuromuscular Disorders

Ajith Sivadasan, Karthik Muthusamy, Aditya Nair

ABSTRACT

The diagnosis of inherited neuromuscular disorders requires careful phenotyping, understanding mutational mechanisms, and selecting appropriate genetic tests. Detecting genetic variants with therapeutic options is crucial. Despite advances, many patients still have negative tests. A systematic approach involves rephenotyping, ancillary tests, and judicious interpretation of uncertain variants.

Keywords: Variants, Next-generation sequencing (NGS), Pathogenic, Repeat disorders.

■ INTRODUCTION

The emergence and accessibility of genetic testing have revolutionized the care of patients with neuromuscular disorders, especially considering the sizeable proportion of inherited diseases in clinical practice. Having a definite diagnosis by genetic testing aids in the optimal management by (1) guiding specific treatment when available, (2) avoiding unnecessary and often invasive tests such as muscle and nerve biopsies, (3) predicting prognosis, (4) restricting empiric use of immunotherapy and other interventions such as thymectomy, (5) optimizing monitoring strategies for systemic involvement such as cardiomyopathy and arrhythmogenic risk in certain muscular dystrophies, (6) enabling patient recruitment in clinical trials and gene therapies, and (7) prospective genetic counseling and family planning.[1]

As practicing neuromuscular neurologists, a sound knowledge on the genetic basis of various inherited neuromuscular disorders, available genetic tests, and their clinical applications as well as understanding the limitations is desirable in the current era of precision medicine.[2] This chapter provides a summary of the genetic basis of neuromuscular disorders, currently available genetic tests, their interpretations, and the optimal genetic testing strategies in diseases such as inherited myopathies, congenital myasthenic syndromes (CMSs), neuropathies, and amyotrophic lateral sclerosis (ALS).

■ BASIC CONCEPTS IN GENETICS

Genes are considered the basic unit of inheritance. They comprise segments of deoxyribonucleic acid (DNA) that encode information for making a ribonucleic acid

CHAPTER 6: Clinical Utility and Interpretation of Genetic Testing in Neuromuscular Disorders

(RNA) molecule by transcription, subsequent translation results in the formation of protein. Exons are regions of the DNA that are transcribed to RNAs and remain after the splicing of the introns. Introns are the intervening/noncoding segments of a RNA transcript (or DNA coding it), that are spliced out before the RNA is translated into a protein. An allele is used to denote the DNA sequence at a specific chromosomal position, presenting as a variant or alternate form of a gene. Alleles can vary according to the nucleotide base present at a particular genome location. The term "variant" is being increasingly used in place of "mutation". A variant refers to the alteration in DNA nucleotide sequence, which can be benign, pathogenic, or of unknown significance.

Mendelian (monogenic) disorders are ones in which defects in a single gene can cause disease; their inheritance following certain rules. Autosomal dominant disorders occur when there is the presence of one pathogenic allele in the heterozygous state. However, autosomal recessive disorders require pathogenic variants in both alleles to manifest a disease (either as homozygous or compound heterozygous state). The term "anticipation" is used when the clinical manifestations tend to occur at an earlier age and/or are more severe as the disease is passed from one generation to the next. Penetrance refers to the proportion of individuals with the pathogenic variant who manifest the disease, whereas expressivity refers to the severity of clinical manifestations that can vary even within the same family. Sporadic disorders (without any apparent family member being affected) can occur when a pathogenic variant occurs "de novo" (for the first time) in an individual with the variant being absent in the unaffected parents. Seemingly sporadic occurrence can also happen due to reduced penetrance when parents test positive for the pathogenic variant that is detected in the proband. Wide age range at first symptom often leads to age-related changes in penetrance of the specific condition.

An individual's unique sequence of DNA is termed the "genotype". "Phenotype" refers to the clinical presentation, i.e., the observed expression of this genotype. The phenomenon of different and variable clinical presentations associated with a specific genetic defect is known as "phenotypic pleiotropy" (e.g., variants in SCN4A are known to cause both hypokalemic periodic paralysis and paramyotonia congenita). Clinically similar phenotypes can be caused by variants in different genes, this denotes the concept of "genetic heterogeneity" (e.g., hypokalemic periodic paralysis is described with variants in both *CACNA1* and *SCN4A* genes).

Single nucleotide substitutions leading to the exchange of an amino acid are known as missense variants, and they comprise the most common type of genetic variation. Insertion of a stop codon resulting in premature translation termination is known as nonsense mutation. Insertion–deletion (indel) refers to the insertion or deletion of bases in the gene. The indels of length >50 bases are termed structural variants, typically >1 kbp of DNA. A change of the reading frame due to small insertions/deletions of nucleotides occurs in frameshift mutations (the number of indels being not divisible by 3). These variants can cause severe reduction or a completely absent protein product (loss-of-function mutations). Copy number variants (CNVs) are structural variants, deletions, or duplications of segments of DNA leading to variations in the number of copies of a particular sequence of DNAs.

Apart from the known reduced penetrance and variable expressivity, the type and location of the variants and their effect on protein translation could also correlate with the clinical severity. These "genotype-phenotype" correlations are being extensively analyzed in several inherited neuromuscular disorders. Different diseases differ in their candidate genes as well as the underlying mechanisms of mutation (genetic variations). Type of mutation also has theranostic implications as specific variants are targetable by various gene therapies and related treatments. The molecular mechanism of the common inherited myopathies, neuropathies, and neuromuscular junction disorders have been provided in **Tables 1 and 2**.[3]

TABLE 1: Disease mechanisms in the common inherited myopathies.

Disease	Molecular mechanism	Genetic testing strategy
• Dystrophinopathies • Duchenne muscular dystrophy (DMD) • Becker muscular dystrophy (BMD)	• X-linked recessive • Deletions (65%), duplications (10%) or nonsense point mutations (20%) affecting reading frame of *DMD* gene (out-of-frame mutations) • In-frame mutation with preserved reading frame, dystrophin protein shorter but partly functional	• Multiple ligation dependent probe amplification (MLPA) or targeted comparative genomic hybridization assay (CGH) for deletion/duplication followed by sequence analysis for point mutations • Next-generation sequencing (NGS) panels capable of detecting deletion, duplications in addition to point mutations • Ribonucleic acid (RNA) sequencing from muscle tissue
• Myotonic dystrophy type 1 • Myotonic dystrophy type 2	• Autosomal dominant, CTG repeats in *DMPK* gene (noncoding region >34 repeats) • CCTG repeat expansion in first intron of *CCTG* gene (>75 repeats)	• Fragment analysis • Repeat primed polymerase chain reaction (PCR) • Southern blot • No correlations between length of repeat expansion and phenotype in DM2
Facioscapulohumeral dystrophy (FSHD)	• Autosomal dominant/digenic • Contraction of D4Z4 repeats (<11) in chromosome 4 with a permissive haplotype 4q35A (FSHD1) or hypomethylation of D4Z4 repeat assay due to heterozygous variant in SMCHD1 in chromosome 18 or rarely in DNMT3B, LRIF1 (FSHD2)	• Southern blot to determine D4Z4 repeats (1–10 with typical phenotype, confirmed). 4q35 (A) haplotyping for confirmation in atypical presentations • In > 11 D4Z4 repeats with typical phenotype, proceed with D4Z4 methylation, 4q35 haplotyping and SMCHD1 sequencing • Hypomethylation and SMCHD1 variant confirms FSHD2 • Optical genome mapping
Limb–girdle muscular dystrophy (LGMD)	• Autosomal dominant or recessive forms • Sarcoglycan, calpain, dysferlin, and other genes	• NGS-based testing • Whole exome sequencing • RNA-seq or whole genome testing if inconclusive and compatible phenotype

Continued

Continued

Disease	Molecular mechanism	Genetic testing strategy
Distal myopathies	• Autosomal dominant or recessive forms • Testing for GNE (quadriceps sparing myopathy), VCP, TTN, and others	• NGS-based testing • WES • Of note, add on MLPA/deletion/duplication testing may be needed in heterozygous variants in recessive disorders
• Oculopharyngeal muscular dystrophy (OPMD) • Oculopharyngeal distal myopathy (OPDM)	• Autosomal dominant > recessive. GCN repeat expansion in *PABPN1* gene (>12 repeats) • Triplet repeats in LRP12, GIPC1, and NOTCH2NLC	Fragment analysis for triplet repeats, rarely add-on sequencing of *PABPN1* gene
• Metabolic myopathies • Pompe disease • Multiple acyl-CoA dehydrogenase deficiency • McArdle disease	• Sequencing of *GAA* gene (including known intronic variants) • Variants in EDFHD (*flavoprotein genes*) • Variants in *PYGM* gene	• NGS-based panels for sequencing, WES • Complementary tests include muscle biopsy, dried blood spot for acid maltase deficiency, carnitine, plasma acylcarnitine, and urinary organic acids
Muscle channelopathies including nondystrophic myotonias	Autosomal dominant and recessive forms due to variants in SCN4A or CLCN1	NGS-based panels, WES
Congenital myopathies and congenital muscular dystrophies	• Congenital myopathies (RYR1, NEB, and ACTA1) can be autosomal dominant, recessive or X-linked • Majority of congenital muscular dystrophies (LAMA2, COL6A1, and SEPN1) are autosomal recessive	• NGS-based panels, WES • *NEB* gene associated with nemaline myopathy, long gene difficult to sequence
Congenital myasthenic syndromes (CMSs)	Autosomal dominant and recessive forms. Variants in CHRNE, COLQ, DOK7, and others	NGS-based panels. Therapeutic options available

TABLE 2: Disease mechanisms of the common neurogenic disorders.

Disease	Molecular mechanism	Genetic testing strategy
Spinal muscular atrophy (SMA)	• Autosomal recessive • Homozygous deletion of *SMN1* gene, 5q13 • Non 5qSMAs are rare, can have varied phenotypes and genetically heterogeneous, variants in BICD2, ATP7A, CHCHD10, DYNC1H1, and TRPV4	• Classical form may be missed by next-generation sequencing (NGS) technique because of pseudogene SMN2, MLPA may help • Non-5q SMAs by NGS

Continued

Continued

Disease	Molecular mechanism	Genetic testing strategy
Spinal bulbar muscular atrophy (SBMA-Kennedy disease)	• X-linked recessive • CAG repeat expansion (>38) in androgen receptor (*AR* gene)	Fragment analysis
Amyotrophic lateral sclerosis (ALS), familial	C9orf72 (G4C2) intronic hexanucleotide repeats, other variants FUS, SOD1, and TARDBP	Fragment analysis, repeat primed PCR for C9orf72 expansions. Rest by NGS-based panels
Charcot–Marie–Tooth (CMT) disease	• *Demyelinating*: Autosomal dominant: PMP22 duplication, MPZ, EGR2, LITAF. Autosomal recessive: PRX, GDAP1 • *X-linked recessive*: GJB1 • *Axonal*: Autosomal dominant: MFN 2, MPZ, GARS, RAB7, NEFL, HSPB1. Autosomal recessive: GDAP1. X-linked recessive: GJB1	• CMT 1A, PMP 22 duplication analysis • NGS-based assays for the remaining CMTs
Hereditary neuropathy with liability to pressure palsies (HNPP)	• Autosomal dominant, • Deletions in *PMP22* gene	MLPA and NGS may detect
Familial amyloid polyneuropathy (FAP)	• Autosomal dominant • Heterozygous pathogenic variants in *TTR* gene	NGS-based assays. Availability of newer therapies such as TTR stabilizers, gene therapies

■ GENETIC TESTING STRATEGIES

Multiplex Ligation-dependent Probe Amplification Assay

Multiplex ligation-dependent probe amplification (MLPA) assay utilizes multiple probes, each being specific for different exons of interest **(Figs. 1A to C)**. The DNA isolated from the subject is denatured and hybridized with the probes. Each probe consists of half-probes that identify target-specific sequences and can be ligated and then amplified [polymerase chain reaction (PCR)]. The amplification is performed using a PCR primer pair, one of which is fluorescently labeled. Only the ligated probes are amplified, which are then separated by capillary electrophoresis. The height of the PCR-derived fluorescent peaks is compared with those from the control DNA sample, the date being analyzed by different software programs.[4] Homozygous deletions are evident, however, the demonstration of heterozygous deletions, duplications, and CNVs can be challenging. MLPA is an excellent test in the diagnosis of inherited neuromuscular disorders due to gene deletions and duplications such as dystrophinopathies (Duchenne and Becker muscular dystrophy), spinal muscular atrophy (SMA), Charcot–Marie–Tooth disease type 1A (CMT-1A) and hereditary neuropathy with pressure palsies (HNPP).[4,5] Other diseases of note with pathogenesis related to deletions include NEB and titin, these also being large genes.

Comparative genomic hybridization (CGH) arrays, quantitative PCRs, fluorescence

CHAPTER 6: Clinical Utility and Interpretation of Genetic Testing in Neuromuscular Disorders

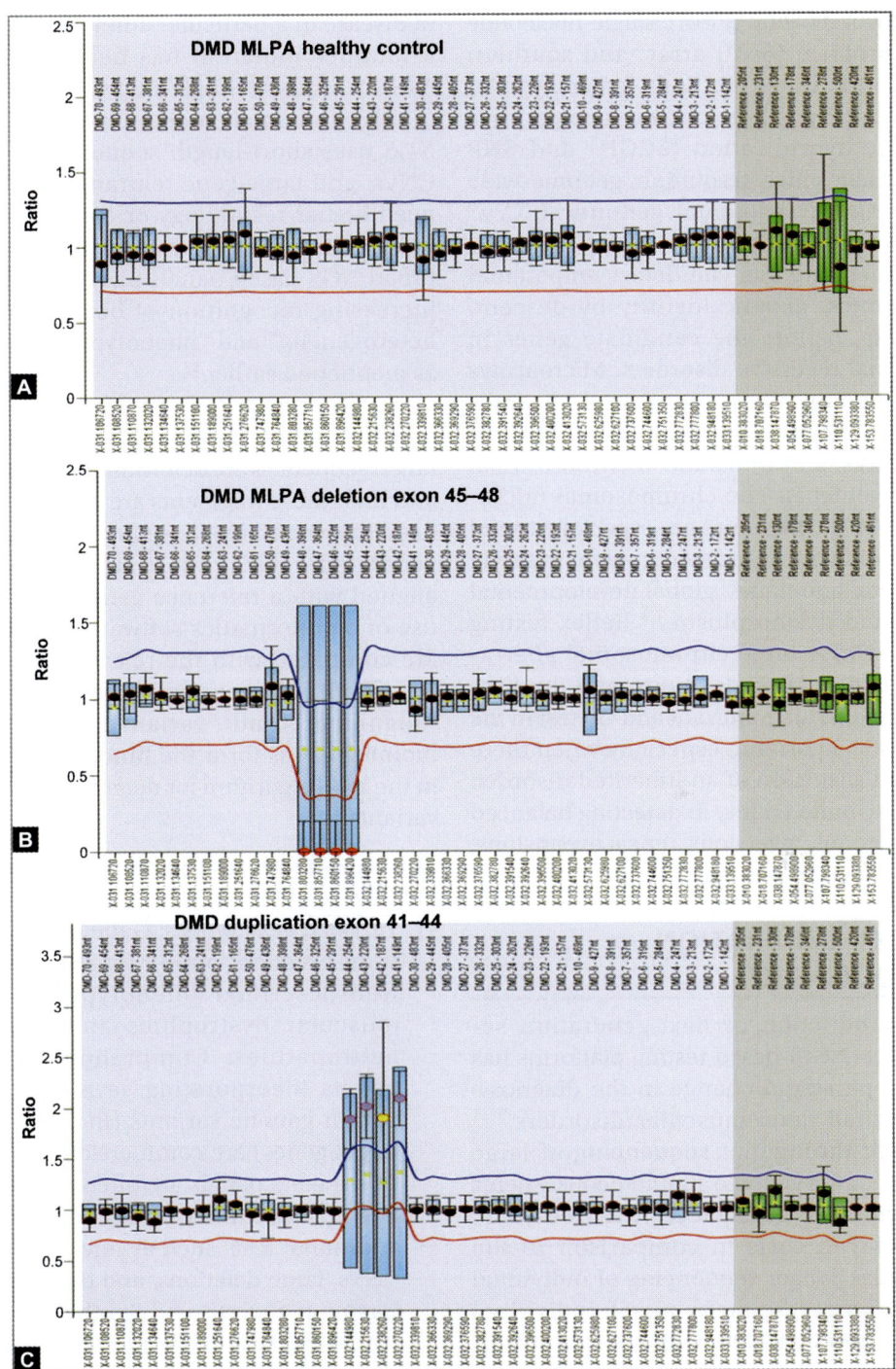

FIGS. 1A TO C: Multiplex ligation-dependent probe amplification (MLPA) analysis of the duchenne muscular dystrophy (DMD) gene in (A) healthy control, (B) patient with exon 45–48 deletion as shown by ratio on the Y-axis, < 0.75, and (C) patient with duplication of exons 41–44 with ratio > 1.3.

in situ hybridization (FISH), single-nucleotide polymorphism (SNP) array, and southern blot are the other methods for analysis of deletions/duplications. Array comparative genomic hybridization (aCGH) and SNP array enables high-resolution, genome-wide screening for segmental genomic CNVs.[6] SNP arrays additionally allow homozygosity mapping that can detect uniparental isodisomies, genetic identity by descent, and help explore the candidate genes in autosomal recessive disorders. Microarrays detect aneuploidies, recognized chromosomal microdeletion/duplication syndromes, CNVs, and unbalanced chromosomal rearrangements. The chromosomal microarray (CMA) techniques are especially useful in children with associated autism, multiple congenital anomalies, global developmental delay, and dysmorphism.[7,8] Reflex testing with CMA for large chromosomal aberrations such as large deletions, and duplications remains an important add-on test in the diagnostic algorithm, especially when there is a high suspicion of an inherited disorder. CMA has limited utility in detecting balanced translocations, inversions, repeat expansions, and low-level mosaicisms.

■ NEXT-GENERATION SEQUENCING

The introduction of next-generation sequencing (NGS)-based testing platforms has made a paradigm change in the diagnosis of inherited neuromuscular disorders.[9-11] The high-throughput sequencing of large portions of the genome simultaneously helps with improved efficiency, increased yield, and reduced costs in comparison to the sequential Sanger sequencing of individual genes. Sanger sequencing of individual genes is now considered only in specific circumstances such as the presence of a very characteristic phenotype, the presence of a known familial variant, or the manifestation of disease in a particular ethnic group where a founder mutation has been identified. NGS can detect single nucleotide variants (SNVs) and small indels. As conventional NGS uses short-length sequencing, exonic CNVs, and large gene rearrangements may need higher technology or complementary testing strategies. The implementation of broad NGS based panels has resulted in an increasing recognition of both "genotypic heterogeneity" and "phenotypic pleiotropy" as mentioned earlier.[12]

In NGS, the DNA isolated from the subject is broken down into short fragments. The target sequences are determined ("captured") and then these fragments are clonally amplified. Subsequently, the sequencing machine generated several short reads which are aligned with a reference genome. With the use of bioinformatics software, the variants are compared with the reference genome, identified, and reported. Hence, "capturing", "alignment", and "variant calling" using bioinformatics form the fundamental steps in the NGS algorithm for determining genetic variants.[13]

The NGS-based testing platforms available include:
- *Targeted gene panels*: Gene panel testing is an excellent option for diseases with well-described phenotypes such as muscular dystrophies and inherited neuropathies. Comprehensive gene panels incorporating several possible culprit genetic variants (including >100 target genes) are commercially available. These gene panels are often customized, and in addition to NGS, also include additional tests such as microarrays (for CNVs, large deletions, and duplications), fragment analysis and Southern blot (for repeat expansion disorders), and Sanger sequencing of certain genes to improve coverage.[14] For example, including microarray or MLPA of dystrophin/*SMN*

gene in a targeted panel for muscular dystrophy (and proximal myopathy) may help diagnose DMD/SMA where the pathology (large deletion/duplication) could be missed by using NGS alone. The whole exome may be sequenced; however, the analysis could be restricted to the target genes that were previously defined in the panel.

The yield of genetic testing has been historically mentioned to be around 30%, but this is a conservative estimate that can improved by carefully identifying the phenotype, population prevalence of the disease and customizing/tailoring the targeted gene panel.[15] The costs are lower, and more importantly, less number variants of uncertain significance (VUSs) are reported with targeted panels; hence the interpretation is easier compared to whole exome sequencing (WES). Of note, one major limitation of targeted gene panels is that atypical phenotypes and novel disease-related genes may not be reported if only targeted gene panels are used.

- WES: It utilizes NGS of the coding regions (exons), comprising 1–2% of the genome. WES has become less costly, extensively available, and is one of the most used genetic testing strategies. The extensive phenotypic overlap noted with inherited neuromuscular disorders justifies the simultaneous sequencing of multiple genes that may be associated with a particular disorder. A typical instance will be the phenotype of proximal myopathy not being confined to limb–girdle muscular dystrophy (LGMD) alone and seen with variants in genes associated with congenital myopathy, congenital muscular dystrophy, and CMS. Diagnostic yields of up to 60% have been reported with WES.[16] WES may be more advantageous over a target gene panel in patients with complex diseases, multiple organ system involvement and when dual or multiple genetic diagnoses are suspected.[17] Moreover, novel genes causing disease can be identified and the data is available for reanalysis.[18,19] Availability of parental DNA (trio sequencing) helps in better analysis of the identified variants and improved yield and should be strongly recommended and implemented.[16,20]

Newer technologies have resulted in better coverage of exon-intron boundaries, intronic splice site variants, and CNVs involving the coding regions. Deep intronic variants, inversions, and transpositions may not be detected.[21] It is very important to note that WES may not detect repeat expansions and some structural variations such as large deletions/duplications. Certain regions that are GC-rich and where repetitive sequences can be found (such as *TTN* and *NEB* genes) may not be covered completely with WES.[22]

Moreover, many VUS in genes both related and unrelated to the disease phenotype may be identified, the proper interpretation of which will need more expertise. Predictors that have been identified for attaining a definite molecular diagnosis using WES include consanguinity, positive family history, onset in childhood, and abnormalities in laboratory findings (such as elevations in creatine kinase, abnormal nerve conduction studies, needle electromyogram, muscle MRI, and muscle biopsy findings).[19,23,24]

Despite the availability of WES, the causative variant may not be identified in a sizeable proportion (up to 50–75%) of cases.[25,26] These deep intronic variants are causative in certain dystrophinopathies and collagenopathies (COL6A1-related muscle disease). These variants can alter RNA splicing by inducing pseudo exons, introducing premature stop codons which lead to functional defects in the proteins.[27] Their detection needs complementary testing strategies that are mentioned here.

- *Whole genome sequencing*: The use of whole genome sequencing was till recently mainly limited to research settings given the prohibitive costs. Compared to WES, genome sequencing is more extensive, and uniform coverage of the coding regions can be achieved, however, the depth of coverage may be less. CNVs are better detected and delineated in comparison with WES.[2] Deep intronic variants may be detected; however, their interpretation may need the use of "add-on"/complementary techniques such as transcriptome sequencing (RNA-seq, which is mentioned later). Similarly, large data sets and VUSs (up to 5 million variants) are identified. These data sets may need judicious interpretation and data storage space. Like WES, genome sequencing offers the advantages of novel disease-related gene identification and future reanalysis.
- *Transcriptome sequencing*: The majority of the deep intronic and intergenic variants may cause disease by affecting splicing. Sequencing of the affected tissue is useful for the interpretation of these genetic variants. RNA-seq provides information regarding the transcriptional disturbances caused by genetic changes and has been used to observe the effect of pathogenic changes.[21,26] Here, RNA obtained from affected tissues such as muscle is compared with controls [from large transcriptome data sets such as Genotype-Tissue Expression (GTEx) Consortium Project] to detect transcriptional aberrations and to determine aberrant splicing, allele imbalance, and abnormal variants. This technique can provide interpretation of coding and noncoding, splice-altering, and splice-disrupting variants. Transcriptome analysis was shown to have an additional diagnostic yield of 35% in a cohort of 50 patients with genetically undiagnosed muscle diseases.[21] Importantly, novel genes can also be identified.

Long-read sequencing such as that used in Oxford Nanopore Technology can have better yields compared to conventional short-read NGS.[28] Here, the DNA sequences are determined by recording the changes in electric current, depending on each passing nucleotide. Optical genome mapping is a newer technology that is commercially available for facioscapulohumeral dystrophy (FSHD) and other inherited diseases and has an excellent resolution of up to 50 bps.[29] The turnaround times are also shorter.

■ THIRD-GENERATION SEQUENCING

Third-generation sequencing is currently used extensively in research might soon find its clinical utility. The technology involves single molecule sequencing and utilizes long-reads with no amplification, detect epigenetic modifications such as methylation and histone acetylation, explore complex structural rearrangements, and provide uniform coverage of the genome that are inaccessible by short-read sequencing.

■ INTERPRETATION OF VARIANTS OF UNCERTAIN SIGNIFICANCE

The American College of Medical Genetics and Genomics (ACMG) has set guidelines for the classification of genetic variants.[30] The five categories into which variants are classified include: (1) pathogenic, (2) likely pathogenic, (3) VUS, (4) likely benign, and (5) benign.

Pathogenic and likely pathogenic variants are considered diagnostic if they are compatible with the expected mode of inheritance.

The important parameters used to establish the pathogenicity of variants include:
- Population prevalence [databases used Genome Aggregation Database (gnomAD), the previous Exome Aggregation Consortium (ExAC)]
- Effect of variant on protein sequence (whether there are any changes in the amino acid sequence)
- Familial genotype data and segregation studies (variant shared with affected family members or occurs de novo)
- Functional studies (if available)
- Allelic data
- In silico prediction algorithms [based on computational tools such as PolyPhen-2, and Combined Annotation Dependent Depletion (CADD) score] which may predict the impact on a protein level, and
- Concordance with the clinical phenotype.

Databases helpful for variants that have been previously reported to manifest disease in other families include the Human Gene Mutation Database (HMGD) and ClinVar.[31,32] No single feature in isolation is sufficient to prove pathogenicity. One should exercise extreme caution not to overinterpret the observations from in-silico prediction algorithms and segregation in small families.

Correlation with disease phenotype and other ancillary tests such as muscle biopsies and muscle MRI are extremely useful in determining the relevance of the variant identified. Muscle biopsies can have characteristic histopathological findings such as central cores, nemaline rods, amyloid deposits, tubular aggregates, and the use of complementary techniques such as immunohistochemistry, immunoblot (dystrophin, sarcoglycan, calpain, and dysferlin), and electron microscopy can help establish a pathological diagnosis.[3] Muscular dystrophies can have selectivity of muscle involvement with sparing of certain muscle groups, which may be identified with muscle MRI and help in disease phenotyping.[33] Moreover, some of the myopathies have characteristic patterns on MRI (COL6-related myopathy with "target" and "sandwich" signs in rectus femoris and vastus lateralis respectively) which can provide important phenotypic clues.[34]

As a general principle, variants not fulfilling the criteria for pathogenicity should remain classified as VUS to avoid overinterpretation which may have future implications, especially concerning prospective genetic counseling. Segregation studies in parents or similarly affected family members can often help in clarifying a VUS. Multidisciplinary discussions involving the clinician, clinical geneticist, and bioinformaticians are warranted to determine the significance of uncertain variants, and the need for "add-on" tests and may aid in reclassification. For example, an "add-on" MLPA test may help confirm disease in a patient with an identified variant in one allele (heterozygous) in a gene known to be associated with an autosomal recessive disease. Periodic reanalysis of the genetic data is also warranted considering the rate at which novel disease-related genes and varying phenotypes that are being reported. Eventually, all the VUSs need to be followed up by the laboratory in the light of newer literature and evolving disease phenotypes in consult with the clinicians, and should ideally be reclassified in the future.

■ REPEAT EXPANSION DISORDERS

Repeat expansion disorders important in neuromuscular disease include myotonic dystrophy types 1 and 2, spinobulbar muscular atrophy (Kennedy disease), oculopharyngeal muscular dystrophy (OPMD), oculopharyngeal distal myopathy, motor

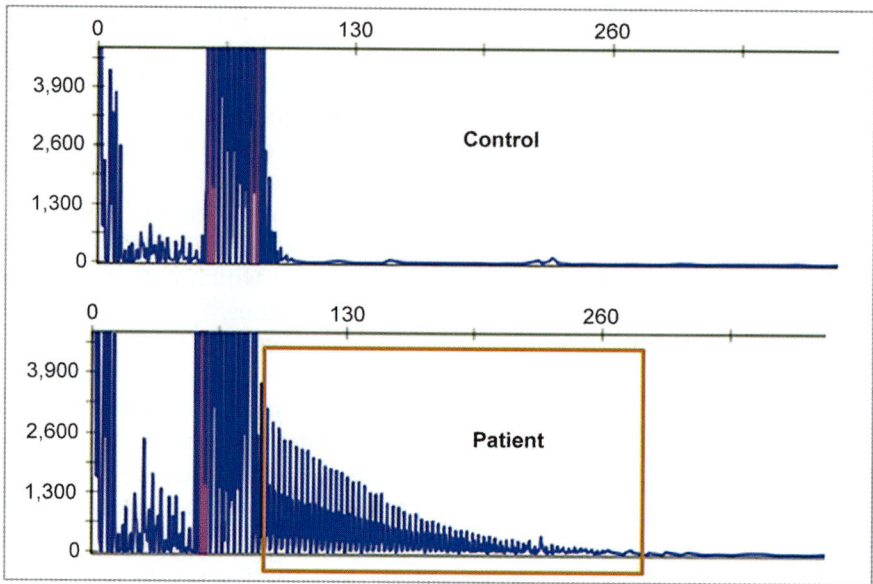

FIG. 2: Triplet-primed reverse transcription-polymerase chain reaction (RT-PCR) in a patient with myotonic dystrophy type 1 showing the "ladder of fragments" from the expanded allele.

neuron disease due to hexanucleotide expansions C9orf72, and NOTCH2NLC-related distal motor neuropathy and myopathy. Each of these diseases differs in terms of the number of repeats and the position of the genetic variant (coding or noncoding region). The triplet repeats as seen in myotonic dystrophy are not stable and can expand when passed on to the next generation, at times exceeding the threshold and manifesting as increasing severity of disease from an earlier age (anticipation).

The repeat disorders are not detected by conventional NGS-based testing strategies. Fragment analysis and triplet repeat-primed PCRs (TP-PCR) are being used for diagnosis.[35] In TP-PCR, a "locus-specific" primer which is "fluorescent-labeled" flanks the repeat along with paired primers that amplify the priming sites from within the repeat sequence. A characteristic "ladder" on the fluorescent trace allows detection of the repeat sequences **(Fig. 2)**.[36] PCR-based techniques are commercially available, less labor intensive have fast turn-around times, and can provide accurate estimation of the number of repeats that has prognostic implications.

When only one allele is detected using PCR-based technique, an alternative method will be required for confirmation and part of reflex testing. Southern blot can be useful in detecting repeats especially for large expansions.[35] It has an advantage in detecting mosaicism, and homozygous alleles, and one could also determine methylation status as an add-on strategy. The limitations of Southern blot include the reduced resolution of small expansions and long turn-around times.

■ PRACTICAL CONSIDERATIONS FOR THE GENETIC DIAGNOSIS OF NEUROMUSCULAR DISORDERS

Muscle Diseases and Congenital Myasthenic Syndromes

A sound basic knowledge regarding the mutational mechanisms **(Table 1)** for the different muscular dystrophies is paramount to choose the appropriate genetic tests. The basic steps in the algorithm include careful determination of the phenotype and targeted genetic testing when possible. Patients with distinct phenotypes such as dystrophinopathies, myotonic dystrophy (type 1 and 2), FSHD, and OPMD may need an individualized choice of genetic tests in contrast to limb–girdle muscular dystrophies, metabolic myopathies, congenital myopathies, congenital muscular dystrophies, and muscle channelopathies. The latter spectrum of myopathies is diagnosed using conventional WES and other NGS-based panels. Optical genome mapping is a commercially available test being used in the diagnosis of FSHD and is lesser time and labor-intensive compared to southern blot.

Congenital myasthenic syndromes are eminently treatable with medicines such as salbutamol, pyridostigmine, and fluoxetine. The spectrum of CMSs includes presynaptic, synaptic, postsynaptic, and glycosylation defects. Delayed diagnosis could occur as they mimic proximal myopathies (limb–girdle myasthenia), distal myopathies (slow channel syndrome), and mitochondrial disorders. CMS could coexist with inherited myopathies. Careful assessment of phenotype and judicious interpretation of electrophysiologic observations such as decrement in repetitive nerve stimulation studies, repetitive compound motor action potentials (CMAPs), and facilitation could help in genotype-phenotype correlations. Considering their varied spectrum and therapeutic implications, testing for genes associated with metabolic myopathies and CMS is an integral part of genetic panels.

Of note, SMA and Kennedy disease also present with proximal muscle weakness and are important differentials to consider in patients with suspected limb–girdle syndromes.

Mitochondrial Cytopathies

Mitochondrial disorders occur from variants in either mitochondrial DNA or nuclear DNA that encoding respiratory chain subunits and mitochondrial maintenance. NGS-based sequencing of the mitochondrial genome is advocated from peripheral blood or urinary epithelial cells. In patients with phenotypes such as external ophthalmoplegia or mitochondrial neurogastrointestinal encephalomyopathy (MNGIE), sequencing of the nuclear DNA (for defects in *POLG* and *TYMP* genes) is also recommended. In patients with multiple mitochondrial DNA deletions and depletions, testing of nuclear genes that are involved in mitochondrial DNA maintenance should always be performed. Of note, in patients with isolated mitochondrial myopathy, the yield of mitochondrial DNA sequencing in peripheral blood is lower compared to the cases with multiple system involvement. Hence, there is an emphasis on the higher diagnostic yield of mitochondrial DNA testing from affected tissues such as a muscle.[37]

Inherited Neuropathies

To date, mutations in over 100 genes have been identified in CMT, highlighting the genetic diversity of this condition. The combination of clinical phenotype, family history, and electrophysiological data (axonal or demyelinating, upper limb conduction velocities in the median, ulnar nerves < 38 m/s) aids in the characterization of the neuropathies and guides genetic testing.[38] CMT 1 is the most common autosomal dominant or seemingly sporadic demyelinating neuropathy. Approximately 90% of CMT 1 cases are due to a 1.5 Mb duplication of the *PMP22* gene on chromosome 17p11.2, which can be detected by MLPA but not by NGS.

Autosomal recessive demyelinating (CMT 4) and both autosomal dominant and recessive axonal sensory motor neuropathies (CMT 2) present a wide spectrum and are generally identified through NGS, common genes implicated include *MFN2*, *SH3TC2*, *GJB1*, and *MPZ*.[38] There could be overlap with diseases such as distal hereditary motor neuropathy (HMN) and hereditary spastic paraplegia (HSP).

An algorithmic approach to genetic testing in suspected inherited neuropathy has been depicted in **Flowchart 1**. Therapeutic options are available/evolving for some neuropathies such as familial amyloid polyneuropathy (FAP), SORD-associated axonal CMT (aldose reductase inhibitors), childhood-onset biotin responsive peripheral motor neuropathy (COMNB), riboflavin transporter deficiencies (SLC52A3, SLC52A2, motor neuropathy with deafness) CMT 1, and HSAN1 (serine). Targeted metabolic workup like blood sorbitol levels (SORD-related neuropathy), and deoxysphingolipids (HSAN1) should be considered when clinically suspected, while interpreting VUSs in these genes, and when genetic testing are not available.

Amyotrophic Lateral Sclerosis

Around 10–15% of ALS are familial, with mutations in genes such as *C9orf72*, *SOD1*, *TARDBP*, and *FUS*. Genetic diversity has been noted across different ethnic groups. Hexanucleotide repeats are more prevalent in Europeans when compared to Asians where SOD1 variants are more. With the emergence of gene therapies such as tofersen for ALS due to SOD1 variant, the indications for genetic testing in ALS has expanded.[39]

An optimal approach for further genetic characterization when confronted with a negative or inconclusive genetic test has been depicted in **Flowchart 2**.

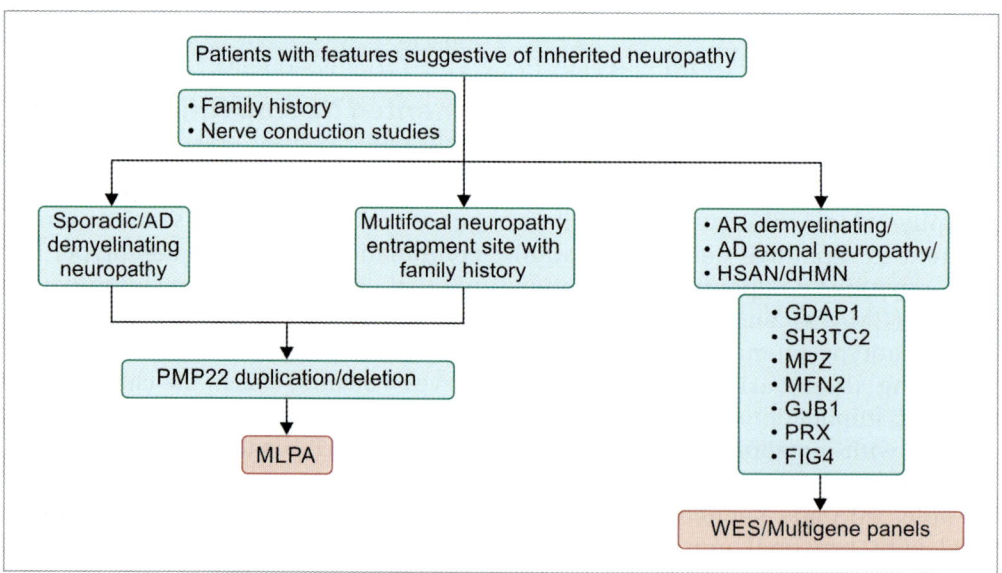

FLOWCHART 1: An algorithm depicting the approach to genetic testing in inherited neuropathies.
(AD: autosomal dominant; AR: autosomal recessive; MLPA: multiplex ligation-dependent probe amplification; WES: whole exome sequencing)

CHAPTER 6: Clinical Utility and Interpretation of Genetic Testing in Neuromuscular Disorders

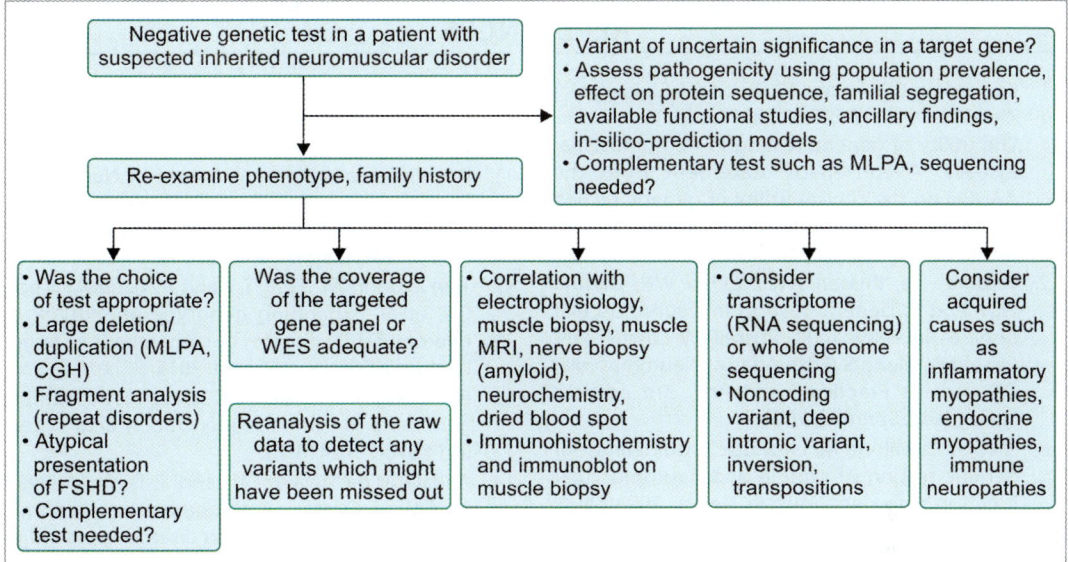

FLOWCHART 2: An algorithm depicting the practical considerations and approach to be taken when confronted with a genetic test which is negative or inconclusive.
(CGH: comparative genomic hybridization; FSHD: facioscapulohumeral dystrophy; MLPA: multiplex ligation-dependent probe amplification; RNA: ribonucleic acid; WES: whole exome sequencing)

■ CONCLUSION

Careful phenotyping, understanding of mutational mechanisms, and appropriate choice of genetic tests are paramount in establishing a definite diagnosis of inherited neuromuscular disorders. In addition to a correct diagnosis, emphasis should also be placed on detecting genetic variants that have therapeutic options such as CMSs, metabolic myopathies (Pompe disease, fatty acid oxidation disorders, and riboflavinopathies), and gene therapies (SMA, DMD amenable to exon skipping, and nonsense mutations). Despite advances in diagnostics, a sizeable proportion of patients may still have negative or inconclusive genetic tests. A systematic approach to this subset involves rephenotyping, the use of ancillary tests, judicious interpretation of uncertain variants, and the potential use of add-on strategies such as genome and RNA sequencing when appropriate. Misinterpretation of VUSs should be avoided considering the potential for misdiagnosis and inappropriate prospective counseling.

■ ACKNOWLEDGMENTS

We acknowledge the contributions of Professor Sumita Danda and Dr Noel Deep Luke from the Department of Clinical Genetics, Christian Medical College, Vellore in preparing this chapter.

REFERENCES

1. Kassardjian CD, Amato AA, Boon AJ, Childers MK, Klein CJ; AANEM Professional Practice Committee. The utility of genetic testing in neuromuscular disease: A consensus statement from the AANEM on the clinical utility of genetic testing in diagnosis of neuromuscular disease. Muscle Nerve. 2016;54(6):1007-9.
2. Feldman EL, Russell JW, Löscher WN, Grisold W, Meng S. Genetic testing in neuromuscular diseases. In: Feldman EL, Russell JW, Löscher WN, Grisold W, Meng S (Eds). Atlas of Neuromuscular Diseases: A Practical Guideline, 3rd edition. Switzerland: Springer; 2021.
3. Nicolau S, Milone M, Liewluck T. Guidelines for genetic testing of muscle and neuromuscular junction disorders. Muscle Nerve. 2021;64(3):255-69.
4. Stuppia L, Antonucci I, Palka G, Gatta V. Use of the MLPA assay in the molecular diagnosis of gene copy number alterations in human genetic diseases. Int J Mol Sci. 2012;13(3):3245-76.
5. Gatta V, Scarciolla O, Gaspari AR, Palka C, De Angelis MV, Di Muzio A, et al. Identification of deletions and duplications of the *DMD* gene in affected males and carrier females by multiple ligation probe amplification (MLPA). Hum Genet. 2005;117(1):92-8.
6. Sagath L, Lehtokari VL, Välipakka S, Udd B, Wallgren-Pettersson C, Pelin K, et al. An Extended Targeted Copy Number Variation Detection Array Including 187 Genes for the Diagnostics of Neuromuscular Disorders. J Neuromuscul Dis. 2018;5(3):307-14.
7. Howell KB, Kornberg AJ, Harvey AS, Ryan MM, Mackay MT, Freeman JL, et al. High resolution chromosomal microarray in undiagnosed neurological disorders. J Paediatr Child Health. 2013;49(9):716-24.
8. Miller DT, Adam MP, Aradhya S, Biesecker LG, Brothman AR, Carter NP, et al. Consensus statement: chromosomal microarray is a first-tier clinical diagnostic test for individuals with developmental disabilities or congenital anomalies. Am J Hum Genet. 2010;86(5):749-64.
9. Ng SB, Turner EH, Robertson PD, Flygare SD, Bigham AW, Lee C, et al. Targeted capture and massively parallel sequencing of 12 human exomes. Nature. 2009;461(7261):272-6.
10. Schofield D, Alam K, Douglas L, Shrestha R, MacArthur DG, Davis M, et al. Cost-effectiveness of massively parallel sequencing for diagnosis of paediatric muscle diseases. NPJ Genom Med. 2017;2:4.
11. Rexach J, Lee H, Martinez-Agosto JA, Németh AH, Fogel BL. Clinical application of next-generation sequencing to the practice of neurology. Lancet Neurol. 2019;18(5):492-503.
12. Tian X, Liang WC, Feng Y, Wang J, Zhang VW, Chou CH, et al. Expanding genotype/phenotype of neuromuscular diseases by comprehensive target capture/NGS. Neurol Genet. 2015;1(2):e14.
13. Biesecker LG, Green RC. Diagnostic clinical genome and exome sequencing. N Engl J Med. 2014;370(25):2418-25.
14. Ankala A, da Silva C, Gualandi F, Ferlini A, Bean LJ, Collins C, et al. A comprehensive genomic approach for neuromuscular diseases gives a high diagnostic yield. Ann Neurol. 2015;77(2):206-14.
15. Beecroft SJ, Yau KS, Allcock RJN, Mina K, Gooding R, Faiz F, et al. Targeted gene panel use in 2249 neuromuscular patients: the Australasian referral center experience. Ann Clin Transl Neurol. 2020;7(3):353-62.
16. Ghaoui R, Cooper ST, Lek M, Jones K, Corbett A, Reddel SW, et al. Use of Whole-Exome Sequencing for Diagnosis of Limb-Girdle Muscular Dystrophy: Outcomes and Lessons Learned. JAMA Neurol. 2015;72(12):1424-32.
17. Haskell GT, Adams MC, Fan Z, Amin K, Guzman Badillo RJ, Zhou L, et al. Diagnostic utility of exome sequencing in the evaluation of neuromuscular disorders. Neurol Genet. 2018;4(1):e212.
18. Salfati EL, Spencer EG, Topol SE, Muse ED, Rueda M, Lucas JR, et al. Re-analysis of whole-exome sequencing data uncovers novel diagnostic variants and improves molecular diagnostic yields for sudden death and idiopathic diseases. Genome Med. 2019;11(1):83.
19. Bugiardini E, Khan AM, Phadke R, Lynch DS, Cortese A, Feng L, et al. Genetic and phenotypic characterisation of inherited myopathies in a tertiary neuromuscular centre. Neuromuscul Disord. 2019;29(10):747-57.
20. Farwell KD, Shahmirzadi L, El-Khechen D, Powis Z, Chao EC, Tippin Davis B, et al. Enhanced utility of family-centered diagnostic exome sequencing with inheritance model-based analysis: results from 500 unselected families with undiagnosed genetic conditions. Genet Med. 2015;17(7):578-86.

21. Cummings BB, Marshall JL, Tukiainen T, Lek M, Donkervoort S, Foley AR, et al. Improving genetic diagnosis in Mendelian disease with transcriptome sequencing. Sci Transl Med. 2017;9(386):eaal5209.
22. Zenagui R, Lacourt D, Pegeot H, Yauy K, Juntas Morales R, Theze C, et al. A Reliable Targeted Next-Generation Sequencing Strategy for Diagnosis of Myopathies and Muscular Dystrophies, Especially for the Giant Titin and Nebulin Genes. J Mol Diagn. 2018;20(4):533-49.
23. Fattahi Z, Kalhor Z, Fadaee M, Vazehan R, Parsimehr E, Abolhassani A, et al. Improved diagnostic yield of neuromuscular disorders applying clinical exome sequencing in patients arising from a consanguineous population. Clin Genet. 2017;91(3):386-402.
24. Thuriot F, Gravel E, Buote C, Doyon M, Lapointe E, Marcoux L, et al. Molecular diagnosis of muscular diseases in outpatient clinics: A Canadian perspective. Neurol Genet. 2020;6(2):e408.
25. Gonorazky H, Liang M, Cummings B, Lek M, Micallef J, Hawkins C, et al. RNAseq analysis for the diagnosis of muscular dystrophy. Ann Clin Transl Neurol. 2015;3(1):55-60.
26. Kremer LS, Bader DM, Mertes C, Kopajtich R, Pichler G, Iuso A, et al. Genetic diagnosis of Mendelian disorders via RNA sequencing. Nat Commun. 2017;8:15824.
27. Grellscheid SN, Smith CW. An apparent pseudo-exon acts both as an alternative exon that leads to nonsense-mediated decay and as a zero-length exon. Mol Cell Biol. 2006;26(6):2237-46.
28. Jain M, Olsen HE, Paten B, Akeson M. The Oxford Nanopore MinION: delivery of nanopore sequencing to the genomics community. Genome Biol. 2016;239:1-17.
29. Guruju NM, Jump V, Lemmers R, Van Der Maarel S, Liu R, et al. Molecular Diagnosis of Facioscapulohumeral Muscular Dystrophy in Patients Clinically Suspected of FSHD Using Optical Genome Mapping. Neurol Genet. 2023;9(6):e200107.
30. Richards S, Aziz N, Bale S, Bick D, Das S, Gastier-Foster J, et al; ACMG Laboratory Quality Assurance Committee. Standards and guidelines for the interpretation of sequence variants: a joint consensus recommendation of the American College of Medical Genetics and Genomics and the Association for Molecular Pathology. Genet Med. 2015;17(5):405-24.
31. Stenson PD, Mort M, Ball EV, Evans K, Hayden M, Heywood S, et al. The Human Gene Mutation Database: towards a comprehensive repository of inherited mutation data for medical research, genetic diagnosis and next-generation sequencing studies. Hum Genet. 2017;136(6):665-77.
32. Landrum MJ, Lee JM, Benson M, Brown GR, Chao C, Chitipiralla S, et al. ClinVar: improving access to variant interpretations and supporting evidence. Nucleic Acids Res. 2018;46(D1):D1062-7.
33. Leung DG. Magnetic resonance imaging patterns of muscle involvement in genetic muscle diseases: a systematic review. J Neurol. 2017;264(7):1320-33.
34. Fu J, Zheng YM, Jin SQ, Yi JF, Liu XJ, Lyn H, et al. "Target" and "Sandwich" Signs in Thigh Muscles have High Diagnostic Values for Collagen VI-related Myopathies. Chin Med J (Engl). 2016;129(15):1811-6.
35. Kamsteeg EJ, Kress W, Catalli C, Hertz JM, Witsch-Baumgartner M, Buckley MF, et al. Best practice guidelines and recommendations on the molecular diagnosis of myotonic dystrophy types 1 and 2. Eur J Hum Genet. 2012;20(12):1203-8.
36. Singh S, Zhang A, Dlouhy S, Bai S. Detection of large expansions in myotonic dystrophy type 1 using triplet primed PCR. Front Genet. 2014;5:94.
37. Parikh S, Goldstein A, Koenig MK, Scaglia F, Enns GM, Saneto R, et al. Diagnosis and management of mitochondrial disease: a consensus statement from the Mitochondrial Medicine Society. Genet Med. 2015;17(9):689-701.
38. Rossor AM, Evans MR, Reilly MM. A practical approach to the genetic neuropathies. Pract Neurol. 2015;15(3):187-98.
39. Roggenbuck J, Eubank BHF, Wright J, Harms MB, Kolb SJ; ALS Genetic Testing and Counseling Guidelines Expert Panel. Evidence-based consensus guidelines for ALS genetic testing and counseling. Ann Clin Transl Neurol. 2023;10(11):2074-91.

Facioscapulohumeral Dystrophy: Update on Treatment

Alisha Reyaz, Vishnu VY

ABSTRACT

Facioscapulohumeral muscular dystrophy (FSHD) is a relatively common muscular dystrophy with a complex pathogenesis. After decades of wait, the FSHD research field has improved dramatically over the last decade ever since the role of DUX4 was identified. Since then, multiple efforts targeting the DUX4 pathways have been initiated and the therapeutic pipeline is exciting for the next decade. With some research molecules reaching phase 3 trials and oligotherapeutic drugs pushing their boundaries in animal studies and will soon knock the doors of human studies, we are hopeful of getting the first approved drug for FSHD in our clinics in this decade.

Keywords: FSHD, DUX4, Losmapimod, of microRNAs, siRNAs, Antisense oligonucleotides.

■ INTRODUCTION

Facioscapulohumeral muscular dystrophy (FSHD) is one of the most common muscular dystrophies which presents as a slowly progressive asymmetric muscle weakness predominantly involving facial, scapular, upper arm, and distal leg muscles. The pathogenetic mechanism in FSHD involves *DUX4* gene's epigenetic derepression in skeletal muscle. A clear understanding of the pathogenesis has paved way opportunities to develop disease modifying therapies in FSHD.

Currently, there is no disease-modifying treatment (DMT) available for treatment of FSHD. The available management strategies involve augmenting daily functioning, reduction of pain and fatigue, and surveillance for extramuscular manifestations.[1] The common assistive devices used are leg braces for foot drop and corset for back support. Low intensity (submaximal and nonfatiguable) aerobic exercises is beneficial for managing chronic fatigue, physical activity, and fitness.[2-4]

The lack of DMTs and other therapies for FSHD represents a high unmet medical need for patients with FSHD. The high burden of disease means patients may have reduced quality of life and report problems with mobility, self-care, daily activities, anxiety, and depression.

■ PATHOGENESIS OF FACIOSCAPULOHUMERAL MUSCULAR DYSTROPHY

The *D4Z4* macrosatellite tandem repeat array occurs in the subtelomeric region of the long arm of chromosome 4 (region 4q35). Normally, *D4Z4* array has 8–100 units which are repressed epigenetically. Mechanism is slightly different in FSHD1 and 2 with a unifying mechanism. In FSHD1, there is contraction of *D4Z4* array in at least one allele to <10 repeats causing opening of chromatin structure and some loss of SMCHD1 which finally leads to *DUX4* transcription. In FSHD2, mutation in SMCHD1 or any other chromatin modifier genes (*DNMT3B* and *LRIF1*) causes derepression of *DUX4*. Though *D4Z4* repeat contraction was necessary for FSHD, it was not sufficient. The repeat contraction results in opening of chromatin structure and, in the setting of a permissive A background, results in the production of stable *DUX4* messenger ribonucleic acid (mRNA) and DUX4 protein from the distal copy of the *D4Z4* repeats. 4qA haplotype displays simple sequence length polymorphisms (SSLPs) in the proximity of the *D4Z4* repeat that allow for distinguishing different 4qA subtypes (4A161, 4A159, and 4A168) **(Fig. 1)**.

■ CURRENT AVAILABLE THERAPIES FOR FACIOSCAPULOHUMERAL MUSCULAR DYSTROPHY

No definite medical therapy is currently available for management of FSHD. Custom made ankle foot orthosis (AFO) for those with foot extensor weakness or knee-ankle-foot-orthosis (KAFO) for those with concomitant knee extensor weakness help in ambulation. Steroids have failed to show any benefit in improving muscle strength. Creatine, methionine, folic acid, and myostatin inhibition (MYO-29) were studied with no benefit in FSHD. Aerobic exercise has utility in improving exercise performance. Retinal vascular and telangiectatic diseases can be treated with photocoagulation to prevent retinal damage or detachment. Keratitis due to facial weakness can be prevented with eye patches and hydrant gels.

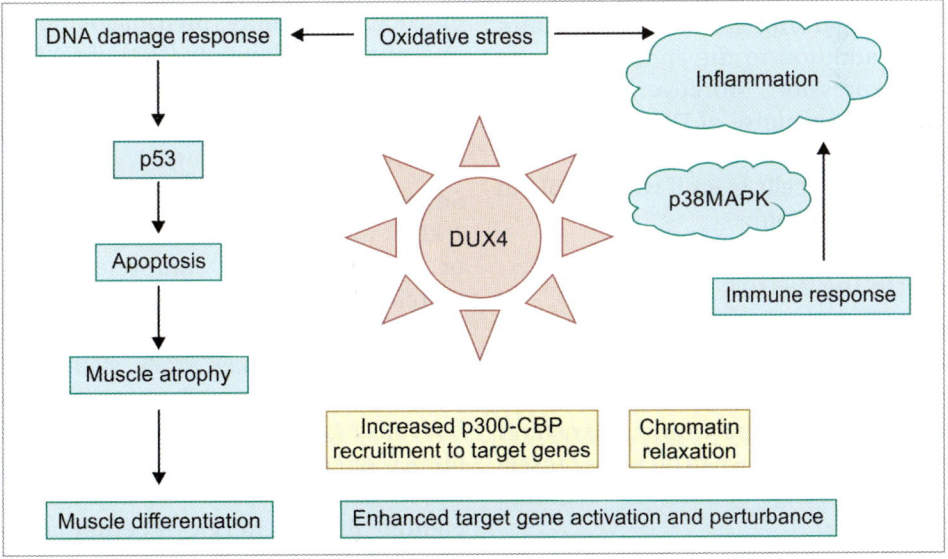

FIG. 1: DUX4 mechanism and pathways in facioscapulohumeral muscular dystrophy (FSHD).[5]

Surgical Options

Scapulothoracic arthrodesis may be tried in FSHD patients with preserved deltoid function and having severe scapular winging, shoulder elevation <90° and marked functional limitation. If there is weakness in deltoid, then surgery is not very useful. The patients should have a detailed discussion with the surgeon regarding their lifestyle and expectations.

Targeted Therapies in Facioscapulohumeral Muscular Dystrophy

Several methods have been tried over the years for developing FSHD-specific, targeted therapies. DUX4 is the primary target and most of the drugs act by affecting directly or indirectly *DUX4*-related transcription, translation, or protein functionality. Most of these promising therapies are in the preclinical stage, except losmapimod, which is currently undergoing a phase 3 clinical trial. Every approach discussed here has challenges regarding safety, delivery, and efficacy in addition to the sporadic nature of *DUX4* expression. Moreover, we do not know the dose response of DUX4 levels and whether we will be able to reverse the already damaged muscle cells even if we are able to stop *DUX4* expression.

Myostatin Inhibitors

Myostatin is a potent negative regulator of muscle growth. It is a growth differentiation factor that inhibits muscle growth and prevents muscular hypertrophy. Myostatin inhibition has been shown to increase muscle mass in a wide range of animals, including humans.[6-9]

GYM329 is an antibody that binds with high specificity to inactive latent myostatin and blocks its conversion to active myostatin. GYM329 was designed to ultimately reduce the levels of myostatin in muscle and blood. It is a recycling and "sweeping" antibody with a high affinity for latent myostatin. GYM329 antibodies are released back into the plasma after eliminating myostatin. This means that the antibody can bind to latent myostatin multiple times and it lasts longer in the body. GYM329 was designed to actively bind FcγRIIb or FcRn receptors and facilitate active uptake of latent myostatin by endocytosis, increasing the rate at which myostatin is degraded and eliminated (or "swept") from plasma. These features are expected to enable lower doses are required for the same level of efficacy, compared to conventional antibodies, subcutaneous administration of the drug with low dosing frequency and more complete blocking of myostatin signaling which could lead to more potent clinical effects. Targeting latent myostatin prevents off-target binding to GDF11. This intervention is hypothesized to lead to increased muscle mass and strength. An ongoing phase 2 trial (MANOEUVRE trial) evaluates safety, efficacy, tolerability, pharmacokinetic (PK) and pharmacodynamic (PD) of GYM329 in ambulant adult patients with FSHD.

Small Molecule Drugs

Small molecule drugs are compounds (0.1–1 kDa) that can easily enter the target cells or any extracellular components.[10] When matched to biologics, small molecules are cheaper, accessible, synthesized much easier, generally taken orally, stable, and not immunogenic. But small molecules can have both off target and on target toxicity. Chemical library screening for these small molecules which can repress *DUX4* expression has yielded β2 adrenergic receptor agonists, bromodomain and extraterminal (BET) inhibitors, p38 inhibitors, and P300 histone acetyltransferase inhibitors **(Table 1)**.

TABLE 1: Small molecule drugs in facioscapulohumeral muscular dystrophy (FSHD) therapeutics.[5]

Agent	Mechanism	Current available findings (preclinical and clinical)
β2 adrenergic receptor agonists	May inhibit transcription of *DUX4* by increasing muscle hypertrophy, partly via cAMP modulation	In FSHD patient-derived muscle cells: • Decreases *DUX4* messenger ribonucleic acid (mRNA) • Decreases DUX4 target gene expression • Increases intracellular cAMP In Randomized controlled trials: • Increases lean muscle mass • Increases grip strength • No change or limited improvement in maximum voluntary isometric strength in some muscles
BRD4 (BET protein) inhibitor	Blocks BRD4-dependent recruitment of transcription regulators to D4Z4 thereby inhibiting *DUX4* transcription	In FSHD patient-derived muscle cells: • Decreases *DUX4* mRNA • Decreases DUX4 target gene expression
Losmapimod (p38 MAPK inhibitor)	Anti-inflammatory effects of p38 MAPK signal inhibition May decrease *DUX4* expression but mechanism is unknown	In FSHD patient-derived muscle cells: • Decreases *DUX4* mRNA • Decreases DUX4 target gene expression In FSHD mouse xenograft model: • Decreases *DUX4* and DUX4 target gene expression In Randomized controlled trials: • Phase 2b RCT (80 patients) with FSHD: No improvement in primary outcome but promising improvement in secondary outcomes. • Phase 3 trial is ongoing
iP300w (P300 histone acetyltransferase inhibitor)	Blocks p300, causing inhibition of recruitment of p300–CBP (mediated by DUX4) to DUX4 target genes	In FSHD myotubes and transgenic mouse model: • Decreases DUX4 target gene expression • Decreases global acetylated histone H3 abundance

β2 Adrenergic Agonists and MAPK Inhibitors (p38MAPK)

Based on the DUX4 repressive action of β2 adrenergic signaling, two trials investigated the role of β2 adrenergic agonists in patients with FSHD.[11,12] Even though they showed some benefits in muscle mass and muscle strength scores, they missed the primary outcome (change in global strength at 52 weeks). Later studies showed that β2 adrenergic signaling activates p38MAPK and some isoforms (p38α and p38β) of MAPK are potent DUX4 inhibitors, probably independent of β2 pathway. Hence, the p38 MAPK inhibitor losmapimod came as a potential candidate drug as it is a small molecule that inhibits p38α MAPK and p38β MAPK. It showed promise in mouse models[13,14] and phase 1 clinical trials with favorable safety and tolerability.[15] The phase 2b trial (ReDUX4) was a randomized double-blind placebo-controlled trial conducted on 80 FSHD participants with Ricci score 2–4.[16] Participants were randomly allocated oral losmapimod 15 mg or similar placebo twice a day in 1:1 ratio for 48 weeks. The change from baseline to either week 16 or 36 in *DUX4*-driven gene expression in muscle biopsy [measured by reverse transcription-polymerase chain reaction (RT-PCR)] was the primary outcome. Though the drug was well tolerated, there was no difference in primary outcome (difference 0.43, SE 0.56; 95% CI 1.04–1.89; $p = 0.56$). But there were potential improvements in prespecified functional outcomes [reachable workspace (RWS)], structural outcomes (muscle fat infiltration), and patient-reported global impression of change (PGIC) compared with placebo. Since losmapimod also has anti-inflammatory properties, the beneficial efforts may be partly because of the anti-inflammatory activity unrelated to DUX4 reduction. The results of this study have paved way to phase 3 trial (REACH, NCT05397470) with primary outcome being absolute change from baseline in RWS. The RWS is a clinical outcome measure that measures the relative surface area that a participant may reach with an outstretched arm. Responses are rated on a scale of 0 (no RWS) to 1.25 (maximal RWS). Higher scores indicate better outcomes. The enrollment of the study was complete in September (260 participants of FSHD 1 or FSHD 2; Ricci score 2–4) and results are expected by early 2026.

Losmapimod targets p38α which is key regulatory role for muscle biology, especially muscle regeneration.[17-19] FSHD treatment will require chronic targeting of p38α which is different from other indications and we do not know the long-term effects of such treatments. Moreover, kinase pathways are very much compensatory, which makes effective long-term inhibition doubtful.[10,20]

Bromodomain and Extraterminal—bromodomain Inhibitors

The BET domain family of proteins comprises of four conserved mammalian members (BRD2, BRD3, BRD4, and BRDT) that modulate the expression of various immunity-related genes and pathways.[21,22] They have BD1 and BD2 bromodomains which attach to acetylated lysines on transcription factors and histones. These BET proteins, which are bound, then stabilize the higher order chromatin structure and thereby offer a platform for transcriptional complexes. BET inhibitors thus cause BET proteins to disentangle from the bound acetylated lysines, and destabilizes chromatin transcriptional complexes, and inhibits transcription.

Small molecule screen studies have shown that BET related, especially BRD4, might influence DUX4 levels. The BET inhibitors can block the activity of BRD4 which in turn suppresses *DUX4* mRNA transcription by reducing the recruitment of transcription regulators and hence abrogating DUX4 activity.

Apabetalone (RVX-208) is a selective BD2 inhibitor which has shown promising results in skeletal muscle cells derived from FSHD patients.[23] Apabetalone inhibited *DUX4* downstream markers expression thereby reversing the hallmarks of FSHD gene expression in differentiated muscle cells. But these results are very early and needs to be confirmed in mouse models and later in human studies.

DUX4 Protein Inhibition

Another therapeutic target is DUX4-mediated recruitment of histone acetyltransferases p300 and CREB-binding protein (CBP) and inducing local H3K27 acetylation which ultimately leads to target gene expression.[24] This DUX4 cascade can be blocked by treatment with the p300-specific inhibitor iP300w which blocks DUX4 target gene induction, inhibiting DUX4 cytotoxicity and reversing the DUX4-induced global accumulation of acetylated histone H3.[25]

The advantages of these small molecule inhibitors are their systemic administration and probably can be taken orally.

Oligonucleotide Therapeutics

The therapeutic potential of microRNAs, small interfering RNAs (siRNAs), and antisense oligonucleotides (AONs) in FSHD is due to the capability to interfere with the *DUX4* mRNA transcription and translation. In healthy human cells, *DUX4* produces a short mRNA isoform which translates to a nontoxic protein. In FSHD myocytes, mRNA splicing generates a full length, pathogenic *DUX4* isoform. Most of the earlier studies in FSHD myotubes showed that siRNAs and ASOs targeting the *DUX4* PAS and mRNA splice sites decreased *DUX4* mRNA and protein.[26,27] When *DUX4* promoter was targeted, siRNAs caused a DICER/AGO-dependent epigenetic transcriptional silencing.[28] Later, PMOs which targeted the *DUX4* PAS decreased *DUX4* levels in FSHD myocytes[29,30] and also in a xenograft model after intramuscular delivery.[30]

There was significant reduction in *DUX4* mRNA levels when siRNAs with identical sequences to D4Z4-derived small siRNAs or miRNAs were used. It also increased H3K9me2 abundance at D4Z4 (indicates transcriptional repression) and enhanced AGO2 recruitment (effector of RNA-mediated epigenetic silencing).[28] Moreover, inhibition of the DICER–AGO2 pathway caused *DUX4* derepression, which shows that the mechanism provides a basal level of suppression also. Human miRNA, miR-675, inhibits *DUX4* expression in vitro and also has shown some protective effects in muscles in FSHD mouse models. Moreover, several molecules such as melatonin and estrogen can increase the endogenous production of miR-675, making miR-675 a promising candidate drug.[31]

Antisense oligonucleotides can cause dysfunction of transcripts by preventing translation or by inducing RNase H1 pathway-mediated degradation. Various in vitro and in vivo studies showed that the AONs are effective in decreasing DUX4 protein, mature *DUX4* mRNA, and also *DUX4* target gene expression.[27,29,30,32,33] Similar results were achieved in transgenic mouse model also using systemic delivery of AONs targeting the *DUX4* transcript. Mice which received *DUX4*-targeted AON showed lesser muscle fibrosis, lesser dysregulation in inflammatory pathways, and improved functional outcome measures related to muscle strength, compared with control mice received a nontargeted AON.[34,35] These results make AONs a feasible therapeutic strategy for FSHD. An AAV vector has been intramuscularly administered in mice cotransduced with AAV-DUX4 to deliver miR-405 (which targets *DUX4* mRNA). It decreased DUX4 protein and also *DUX4*-induced abnormal muscle pathology by guiding the *DUX4* mRNA transcript through RNA interference (RNAi) degradation pathway.[36,37]

An equally promising category of oligonucleotides for *DUX4* inhibition is the altered antisense sequence of the 5′ end of U7 small nuclear RNAs. It is a component of the snRNP complex involved in 3′ end processing of histone pre-mRNAs, which particularly targets *DUX4* pre-mRNA, causing interference with its maturation. Its special advantage is the longevity of the snRNP complex which is relayed to target *DUX4*. This complex guards the small nuclear RNA from degradation and allows intermittent administration of the therapeutic vector (compared to traditional AONs, which need continuous dosing).

Decoy trapping is another method of blocking DUX4 transactivation by utilizing "decoy" DUX4 binding sites, which sequester the endogenous DUX4 and thereby blocking it from the target genes. The DNA aptamers with enhanced DUX4-binding affinity and specificity may enhance this process by increasing "trapping" efficiency.[38]

The advantages of oligonucleotide therapeutic drugs are ability to directly repress DUX4 expression, relatively easier to design, manufacture, and screen and they allow for personalized medicine (sequence-based targeting).[10] Compared with single-dose gene-editing therapies, RNAi-based therapies need lifelong administration, which also allows for dose correction or discontinuation of treatment on occurrence of adverse events. The major disadvantages are off-target effects such as cytotoxicity and immunogenicity. Oligonucleotide therapeutics using RNAi have significant cytotoxicity. miRNAs are less specific than ASOs since they attach using incomplete base-pairing, thereby raising risk of off-target side effects. siRNAs are double-stranded, which might provoke an innate immune response. There is a risk for oligonucleotide therapeutic drugs to oversaturate the natural pathways which they use for their functioning inside the cell. ASOs which use RNase H may develop "ASO tolerance" due to increased premRNA expression. Other major disadvantage is poor uptake to muscle cells and many are developing antibody conjugates to improve the muscle uptake **(Table 2)**.

TABLE 2: Oligotherapeutic drugs in facioscapulohumeral muscular dystrophy (FSHD) therapeutics.[5]

Agent	Mechanism	Current available findings (preclinical and clinical)
PMO ± AON which targets 3'-UTR of *DUX4* pre-mRNA	Affects pre-mRNA processing (polyadenylation or intron splicing) leading to mRNA instability and causing degradation of transcript	In FSHD patient-derived muscle cells and xenograft and/or transgenic FSHD mouse models: • Decreases DUX4 protein • Decreases atrophic myotubes • Increases muscle mass and strength • Decreases myofiber central nucleation and muscle fibrosis
AON which targets exon 1 of *DUX4* transcript	• Inhibition of *DUX4* mRNA translation • Promotes degradation of transcript	In a transgenic FSHD mouse model: • Decreases *DUX4* mRNA • Decreases DUX4 protein • Decreases DUX4 target gene expression • Decreases skeletal muscle pathology • Better treadmill test results • No improvement in strength test results
siRNAs with homologous sequence to *DUX4*	• Targets 5'-UTR of *DUX4* pre-mRNA • Epigenetic silencing via RNA	In FSHD patient-derived muscle cells: • Decreases *DUX4* mRNA • Increases H3K9me2 and recruitment of AGO2
miR-405	• RNA interference • Targets *DUX4* mRNA ORF via RNA interference using artificial miRNA and inhibits transcription	In luciferase assay screen: • Decreases *DUX4* mRNA In AAV-DUX4-transgenic mouse model: • Decreases skeletal muscle pathology • No particular improvement in grip strength • AAV-miDUX4.405 overexpression

Continued

Continued

Agent	Mechanism	Current available findings (preclinical and clinical)
miR-675	RNA interference human miR-675 targets 3′-UTR and *DUX4* mRNA ORF	In HEK293T cells transfected with *DUX4* and in FSHD patient-derived muscle cells: • Decreases *DUX4* mRNA • Decreases DUX4 protein • Decreases DUX4 target gene expression • Decreases DUX4-induced cell death • Decreases transactivation of DUX4-responsive reporter In transgenic (AAV-DUX4 induced) FSHD mouse model: • Decreases skeletal muscle pathology
U7 small nuclear RNA antisense expression cassettes	Alters target specificity of snRNP complex to target *DUX4* pre-mRNA, inhibiting its maturation	In transfected HEK293 cells overexpressing DUX4: • Decreases DUX4-induced cell death • Decreases *DUX4* mRNA • Decreases DUX4 protein In FSHD patient-derived muscle cells: • Decreases *DUX4* mRNA • Decreases DUX4 target gene expression
dsDNA oligonucleotides encoding DUX4 binding sites	Competition of decoy binding sites with real DUX4 target gene-binding sites- Inhibits DUX4 transactivational activity	In FSHD patient-derived muscle cells—Direct electrotransfection of dsDNA: • Decreases DUX4 target gene expression Systemic delivery of AAV-dsDNA decoy in mice overexpressing *DUX4* from transfected plasmid vector: • Decreases DUX4 target gene expression
DNA aptamers	Binds DUX4 protein with enhanced specificity and affinity causing inhibition of DUX4 target binding and activation	Aptamers increase the specificity and affinity of DUX4 "decoy" binding site sequences using recombinant DUX4

Gene Editing

The CRISPR–Cas9 gene-editing system is an encouraging genomic technique for *DUX4* therapy.[39-42] CRISPR modulation of the FSHD locus have been tried with Cas9-mediated gene editing or dCas9-mediated transcriptional inhibition.

The first use of CRISPR system in FSHD was through KRAB transcriptional inhibitor which was fused to inactive Cas9 (dCas9) and attached to the *DUX4* promoter in FSHD myoblasts; thereby successfully repressing *DUX4* and its target genes. It also caused an increase of repressive proteins on D4Z4 even though the levels of H3K9me3 and H3K27me3 did not change significantly.

In FSHD2, CRISPR–Cas9 system target the aberrant splice site created due to the deep intronic mutations in SMCHD1 which restores the wild-type SMCHD1 transcript. This causes reduction in expression of *DUX4* and *DUX4* target genes. Even though this did not restore the DNA methylation on the

D4Z4 locus, it provides a proof of concept for feasibility.[43]

Gene-editing strategies in FSHD have majorly targeted the *DUX4* polyadenylation signal. Targeting of this *DUX4* PAS in FSHD myoblasts using CRISPR and TALEN systems effectively removed the targeted *DUX4* PAS, even though the efficiency of editing was not great.[44] While the *DUX4* transcripts were not completely removed, there was downregulation of the measured *DUX4* target genes (LEUTX, TRIM43, and MDB3L2). The existence of another upstream PAS system was found to be responsible for the persistence of some *DUX4* transcripts. Combining genetic and epigenetic techniques by directly targeting *DUX4* PAS and by utilizing dCas9-KRAB inhibitor to reinstate D4Z4 locus heterochromatin state, led to *DUX4* transcript level reduction and also in DUX4 target gene expression.[45] Another technique targeting PAS is using the adenine base editor system along with Cas9-nickase, creating an AT to CG conversion in the *DUX4* PAS, thereby introducing mutations into the PAS and prevent *DUX4* expression.[46,47]

The major advantage is the potential permanent treatment with a single treatment. The dCas9-mediated transcriptional inhibition may be more suitable and safer in a gain of function disease like FSHD compared to Cas9-mediated gene editing. It is challenging to target the repeat regions because multiple CRISPR–Cas9 binding sites can cause multiple DNA breaks and may create many unwanted effects and give multiple warning signals to the cell and damages the efficiency of editing. The major rate limiting step for gene-editing systems such as CRISPR–Cas9 is their efficient delivery to muscle cells. Other major issues are immunogenicity related to CRISPR components. As of now, recombinant adeno-associated virus (rAAV) vectors are the only realistic way to deliver CRISPR components to skeletal muscles across the body. But we need vectors which more "muscle-tropic" and lesser "liver-tropic" and newer vectors in pipeline such as "AAVMYO" and "MyoAAV" are promising in this aspect.[48,49] The inherent disadvantages of AAV vectors need to be overcome like neutralizing antibodies against capsid which prevents readministration, preexisting immunity, higher doses causing liver toxicity, potential genotoxicity due to genomic integration, and high production cost **(Table 3)**.

TABLE 3: Gene editing in facioscapulohumeral muscular dystrophy (FSHD) therapeutics.[5]

Agent	Mechanism	Current available findings (preclinical and clinical)
Gene editing and CRISPR–dCas9 inhibition		
CRISPR–Cas9	Removes an intronic mutation causing a cryptic splice site and thus restoring *SMCHD1* reading frame	In FSHD2 patient-derived muscle cells: • Increases wild-type SMCHD1 • Decreases *DUX4* mRNA • Decreases DUX4 target gene expression • No effect on D4Z4 DNA methylation
CRISPR–Cas9	CRISPR–Cas9 and TALEN-based removal of *DUX4* PAS (exon 3)	In double-knockout HCT116 (human colorectal cancer cell) model: • Decreases *DUX4* mRNA • Decreases DUX4 target gene expression In FSHD patient-derived muscle cells: • Use of alternative PAS upstream of targeted PAS

Continued

Continued

Agent	Mechanism	Current available findings (preclinical and clinical)
CRISPR–Cas9	CRISPR–Cas9 removal of *DUX4* PAS (exon 3)	In FSHD patient-derived muscle cells and double-knockout HCT116 model: • Decreases *DUX4* mRNA • Decreases DUX4 target gene expression
CRISPR–dCas9 adenine base editor	Causes mutation in *DUX4* PAS (AT → CG conversion)	In FSHD patient-derived muscle cells: • Decreases *DUX4* mRNA • Decreases DUX4 target gene expression
CRISPR–dCas9 transcriptional repression	CRISPR–dCas9 orthologue fused to transcriptional repressors of *DUX4*	In FSHD primary myocytes: • Decreases *DUX4* mRNA • Decreases DUX4 target gene expression In FSHD transgenic mouse model: • Decreases *DUX4* and DUX4 target gene expression
CRISPR–dCas9–KRAB transcriptional repression	KRAB-repressor targeting the *DUX4* gene promoter	In FSHD primary myocytes: • Decreases *DUX4* mRNA • Decreases DUX4 target gene expression • No effect on expression of other genes in the D4Z4 locus (*FRG1* and *FRG2*)
CRISPR–dCas9–KRAB transcriptional repression	KRAB-repressor targeting *DUX4* transcription activators	In FSHD primary myocytes: • Decreases *DUX4* mRNA • Increases H3K9me3 (evidence of altered chromatin) at the targeted D4Z4 locus
CRISPR–dCas9–KRAB transcriptional repression	KRAB-repressor targeting the *DUX4* PAS	In FSHD patient-derived muscle cells: • Decreases *DUX4* mRNA • DUX4 target gene expression • Partial restoration of repressive H3K9me3

■ CONCLUSION

Though FSHD and its pathogenesis is complex, the field has improved dramatically over the last decade ever since the role of *DUX4* was identified. Multiple efforts targeting the DUX4 pathways are ongoing and the therapeutic pipeline is promising. With small molecules reaching phase 3 trial and oligotherapeutic drugs are progressing well in animal studies and poised to human studies, hopefully we will get the first approved drug for FSHD in our clinics in this decade.

REFERENCES

1. Tawil R, Kissel JT, Heatwole C, Pandya S, Gronseth G, Benatar M. Evidence-based guideline summary: Evaluation, diagnosis, and management of facioscapulohumeral muscular dystrophy. Neurology. 2015;85(4):357-64.

2. Voet N, Bleijenberg G, Hendriks J, de Groot I, Padberg G, van Engelen B, et al. Both aerobic exercise and cognitive behavior therapy reduce chronic fatigue in FSHD: an RCT. Neurology. 2014;83(21):1914-22.

3. Andersen G, Prahm KP, Dahlqvist JR, Citirak G, Vissing J. Aerobic training and postexercise protein in facioscapulohumeral muscular dystrophy: RCT study. Neurology. 2015;85(5):396-403.
4. Andersen G, Heje K, Buch AE, Vissing J. High-intensity interval training in facioscapulohumeral muscular dystrophy type 1: a randomized clinical trial. J Neurol. 2017;264(6):1099-106.
5. Tihaya MS, Mul K, Balog J, de Greef JC, Tapscott SJ, Tawil R, et al. Facioscapulohumeral muscular dystrophy: the road to targeted therapies. Nat Rev Neurol. 2023;19(2):91-108.
6. McPherron AC, Lawler AM, Lee SJ. Regulation of skeletal muscle mass in mice by a new TGF-p superfamily member. Nature. 1997;387(6628):83-90.
7. McPherron AC, Lee SJ. Double muscling in cattle due to mutations in the myostatin gene. Proc Natl Acad Sci. 1997;94(23):12457-61.
8. Schuelke M, Wagner KR, Stolz LE, Hübner C, Riebel T, Kömen W, et al. Myostatin Mutation Associated with Gross Muscle Hypertrophy in a Child. N Engl J Med. 2004;350(26):2682-8.
9. Acosta J, Carpio Y, Borroto I, González O, Estrada MP. Myostatin gene silenced by RNAi show a zebrafish giant phenotype. J Biotechnol. 2005;119(4):324-31.
10. Himeda CL, Jones PL. FSHD Therapeutic Strategies: What Will It Take to Get to Clinic? J Pers Med. 2022;12(6):865.
11. Kissel JT, McDermott MP, Mendell JR, King WM, Pandya S, Griggs RC, et al. Randomized, double-blind, placebo-controlled trial of albuterol in facioscapulohumeral dystrophy. Neurology. 2001;57(8):1434-40.
12. van der Kooi EL, Vogels OJM, van Asseldonk RJGP, Lindeman E, Hendriks JCM, Wohlgemuth M, et al. Strength training and albuterol in facioscapulohumeral muscular dystrophy. Neurology. 2004;63(4):702-8.
13. Oliva J, Galasinski S, Richey A, Campbell AE, Meyers MJ, Modi N, et al. Clinically Advanced p38 Inhibitors Suppress DUX4 Expression in Cellular and Animal Models of Facioscapulohumeral Muscular Dystrophy. J Pharmacol Exp Ther. 2019;370(2):219-30.
14. Rojas LA, Valentine E, Accorsi A, Maglio J, Shen N, Robertson A, et al. p38α Regulates Expression of DUX4 in a Model of Facioscapulohumeral Muscular Dystrophy. J Pharmacol Exp Ther. 2020;374(3):489-98.
15. Mellion ML, Ronco L, Berends CL, Pagan L, Brooks S, van Esdonk MJ, et al. Phase 1 clinical trial of losmapimod in facioscapulohumeral dystrophy: Safety, tolerability, pharmacokinetics, and target engagement. Br J Clin Pharmacol. 2021;87(12):4658-69.
16. Tawil R, Wagner KR, Hamel JI, Leung DG, Statland JM, Wang LH, et al. Safety and efficacy of losmapimod in facioscapulohumeral muscular dystrophy (ReDUX4): a randomised, double-blind, placebo-controlled phase 2b trial. Lancet Neurol. 2024;23(5):477-86.
17. Keren A, Tamir Y, Bengal E. The p38 MAPK signaling pathway: A major regulator of skeletal muscle development. Mol Cell Endocrinol. 2006;252(1):224-30.
18. Wissing ER, Boyer JG, Kwong JQ, Sargent MA, Karch J, McNally EM, et al. P38α MAPK underlies muscular dystrophy and myofiber death through a Bax-dependent mechanism. Hum Mol Genet. 2014;23(20):5452-63.
19. Segalés J, Perdiguero E, Muñoz-Cánoves P. Regulation of Muscle Stem Cell Functions: A Focus on the p38 MAPK Signaling Pathway. Front Cell Dev Biol. 2016;4:91.
20. Rask-Andersen M, Zhang J, Fabbro D, Schiöth HB. Advances in kinase targeting: current clinical use and clinical trials. Trends Pharmacol Sci. 2014;35(11):604-20.
21. Wang N, Wu R, Tang D, Kang R. The BET family in immunity and disease. Signal Transduct Target Ther. 2021;6(1):1-22.
22. Campbell AE, Oliva J, Yates MP, Zhong JW, Shadle SC, Snider L, et al. BET bromodomain inhibitors and agonists of the beta-2 adrenergic receptor identified in screens for compounds that inhibit DUX4 expression in FSHD muscle cells. Skelet Muscle. 2017;7(1):16.
23. Sarsons CD, Gilham D, Tsujikawa LM, Wasiak S, Fu L, Rakai BD, et al. Apabetalone, a Clinical-Stage, Selective BET Inhibitor, Opposes DUX4 Target Gene Expression in Primary Human FSHD Muscle Cells. Biomedicines. 2023;11(10):2683.
24. Choi SH, Gearhart MD, Cui Z, Bosnakovski D, Kim M, Schennum N, et al. DUX4 recruits p300/CBP through its C-terminus and induces global H3K27 acetylation changes. Nucleic Acids Res. 2016;44(11):5161-73.
25. Bosnakovski D, da Silva MT, Sunny ST, Ener ET, Toso EA, Yuan C, et al. A novel P300 inhibitor reverses DUX4-mediated global histone H3 hyperacetylation, target gene expression, and cell death. Sci Adv. 2019;5(9):eaaw7781.

26. Vanderplanck C, Ansseau E, Charron S, Stricwant N, Tassin A, Laoudj-Chenivesse D, et al. The FSHD Atrophic Myotube Phenotype Is Caused by DUX4 Expression. PLoS One. 2011;6(10):e26820.
27. Ansseau E, Vanderplanck C, Wauters A, Harper SQ, Coppée F, Belayew A. Antisense Oligonucleotides Used to Target the DUX4 mRNA as Therapeutic Approaches in FaciosScapuloHumeral Muscular Dystrophy (FSHD). Genes (Basel). 2017;8(3):93.
28. Lim JW, Snider L, Yao Z, Tawil R, Van Der Maarel SM, Rigo F, et al. DICER/AGO-dependent epigenetic silencing of D4Z4 repeats enhanced by exogenous siRNA suggests mechanisms and therapies for FSHD. Hum Mol Genet. 2015;24(17):4817-28.
29. Marsollier AC, Ciszewski L, Mariot V, Popplewell L, Voit T, Dickson G, et al. Antisense targeting of 3' end elements involved in DUX4 mRNA processing is an efficient therapeutic strategy for facioscapulohumeral dystrophy: a new gene-silencing approach. Hum Mol Genet. 2016;25(8):1468-78.
30. Chen JC, King OD, Zhang Y, Clayton NP, Spencer C, Wentworth BM, et al. Morpholino-mediated Knockdown of DUX4 Toward Facioscapulohumeral Muscular Dystrophy Therapeutics. Mol Ther. 2016;24(8):1405-11.
31. Saad NY, Al-Kharsan M, Garwick-Coppens SE, Chermahini GA, Harper MA, Palo A, et al. Human miRNA miR-675 inhibits DUX4 expression and may be exploited as a potential treatment for Facioscapulohumeral muscular dystrophy. Nat Commun. 2021;12(1):7128.
32. Lu-Nguyen N, Dickson G, Malerba A, Popplewell L. Long-Term Systemic Treatment of a Mouse Model Displaying Chronic FSHD-like Pathology with Antisense Therapeutics That Inhibit DUX4 Expression. Biomedicines. 2022;10(7):1623.
33. Lu-Nguyen N, Malerba A, Antoni Pineda M, Dickson G, Popplewell L. Improving Molecular and Histopathology in Diaphragm Muscle of the Double Transgenic ACTA1-MCM/FLExDUX4 Mouse Model of FSHD with Systemic Antisense Therapy. Hum Gene Ther. 2022;33(17–18):923-35.
34. Lu-Nguyen N, Malerba A, Herath S, Dickson G, Popplewell L. Systemic antisense therapeutics inhibiting DUX4 expression ameliorates FSHD-like pathology in an FSHD mouse model. Hum Mol Genet. 2021;30(15):1398-412.
35. Bouwman LF, Hamer B den, Heuvel A van den, Franken M, Jackson M, Dwyer CA, et al. Systemic delivery of a DUX4-targeting antisense oligonucleotide to treat facioscapulohumeral muscular dystrophy. Mol Ther Nucleic Acids. 2021;26:813-27.
36. Wallace LM, Liu J, Domire JS, Garwick-Coppens SE, Guckes SM, Mendell JR, et al. RNA Interference Inhibits DUX4-induced Muscle Toxicity In Vivo: Implications for a Targeted FSHD Therapy. Mol Ther. 2012;20(7):1417-23.
37. Wallace LM, Saad NY, Pyne NK, Fowler AM, Eidahl JO, Domire JS, et al. Pre-clinical Safety and Off-Target Studies to Support Translation of AAV-Mediated RNAi Therapy for FSHD. Mol Ther Methods Clin Dev. 2018;8:121-30.
38. Klingler C, Ashley J, Shi K, Stiefvater A, Kyba M, Sinnreich M, et al. DNA aptamers against the DUX4 protein reveal novel therapeutic implications for FSHD. FASEB J. 2020;34(3):4573-90.
39. Ran FA, Hsu PD, Wright J, Agarwala V, Scott DA, Zhang F. Genome engineering using the CRISPR-Cas9 system. Nat Protoc. 2013;8(11):2281-308.
40. Cong L, Ran FA, Cox D, Lin S, Barretto R, Habib N, et al. Multiplex Genome Engineering Using CRISPR/Cas Systems. Science. 2013;339(6121):819-23.
41. Richardson CD, Ray GJ, DeWitt MA, Curie GL, Corn JE. Enhancing homology-directed genome editing by catalytically active and inactive CRISPR-Cas9 using asymmetric donor DNA. Nat Biotechnol. 2016;34(3):339-44.
42. Larson MH, Gilbert LA, Wang X, Lim WA, Weissman JS, Qi LS. CRISPR interference (CRISPRi) for sequence-specific control of gene expression. Nat Protoc. 2013;8(11):2180-96.
43. Goossens R, van den Boogaard ML, Lemmers RJLF, Balog J, van der Vliet PJ, Willemsen IM, et al. Intronic SMCHD1 variants in FSHD: testing the potential for CRISPR-Cas9 genome editing. J Med Genet. 2019;56(12):828-37.
44. Joubert R, Mariot V, Charpentier M, Concordet JP, Dumonceaux J. Gene Editing Targeting the DUX4 Polyadenylation Signal: A Therapy for FSHD? J Pers Med. 2021;11(1):7.
45. Das S, Chadwick BP. CRISPR mediated targeting of DUX4 distal regulatory element represses DUX4 target genes dysregulated in Facioscapulohumeral muscular dystrophy. Sci Rep. 2021;11(1):12598.
46. Gaudelli NM, Komor AC, Rees HA, Packer MS, Badran AH, Bryson DI, et al. Programmable base editing of A•T to G•C in genomic DNA without DNA cleavage. Nature. 2017;551(7681):464-71.
47. Komor AC, Kim YB, Packer MS, Zuris JA, Liu DR. Programmable editing of a target base in genomic DNA without double-stranded DNA cleavage. Nature. 2016;533(7603):420-4.

48. Weinmann J, Weis S, Sippel J, Tulalamba W, Remes A, El Andari J, et al. Identification of a myotropic AAV by massively parallel in vivo evaluation of barcoded capsid variants. Nat Commun. 2020;11(1):5432.

49. Tabebordbar M, Lagerborg KA, Stanton A, King EM, Ye S, Tellez L, et al. Directed evolution of a family of AAV capsid variants enabling potent muscle-directed gene delivery across species. Cell. 2021;184(19):4919-38.e22.

CHAPTER 8

Riboflavinopathies: Potentially Treatable Disorders

Saraswati Nashi, Seena Vengalil, Dipti Baskar, Deepak Menon, Atchayaram Nalini

ABSTRACT

Riboflavinopathies are genetically mediated neurological disorders characterized by motor, sensory, and cranial deficits often associated with respiratory insufficiency in the later stages of disease. The genes implicated are SLC52A2 and SLC52A3, which are riboflavin transporter genes. Onset is typically early in life, however, there are reports with later onset. The disease is relentlessly progressive unless treated with riboflavin at a high dose. Hence, the need to ensure timely identification by genetic testing as also the need to screen siblings and at-risk individuals related to the index patient. Early treatment is a must and is known to be lifesaving.

Keywords: SLC52A2, SLC52A3.

■ INTRODUCTION

Riboflavinopathies are rare neurological disorders characterized by motor, sensory, cranial neuropathies frequently accompanied by ataxia, and respiratory insufficiency. They include the Brown–Vialetto–Van-Laere (BVVL) syndrome and Fazio–Londe syndrome. They are essentially the same except that conventionally Fazio–Londe syndrome lacks deafness. BVVL was first described by Brown in 1894 and subsequently by others. Variants in the genes *SLC52A2* and *SLC52A3* are causative **(Figs. 1 and 2)**. Previously this gene was known as *C20orf54* gene. The role of *SLC52A1*, another riboflavin transporter, is debated, however, an anecdotal report describes its role in this disease.[1] Early treatment is vital and hence the need for knowledge of this rare entity.

Riboflavin is absorbed in the small intestine by the human riboflavin transporters RFVT1 and RFVT3. Another transporter RFVT2 is expressed in the brain.[2] Riboflavin is a precursor for flavin mononucleotide (FMN) and flavin adenine dinucleotide (FAD), these function in the redox reactions in electron transport chain. However, riboflavin cannot be synthesized de novo and hence, riboflavin transporters are crucial in humans. Despite several advances in the understanding of riboflavin transporters, the precise mechanisms underlying disease still remain unclear. The pathophysiology is mediated by mitochondrial dysfunction as riboflavin is an important component of the electron transport chain. Previous studies in Drosophila model and patients' fibroblast cultures have given significant insights into the pathogenesis of this disorder. Drosophila

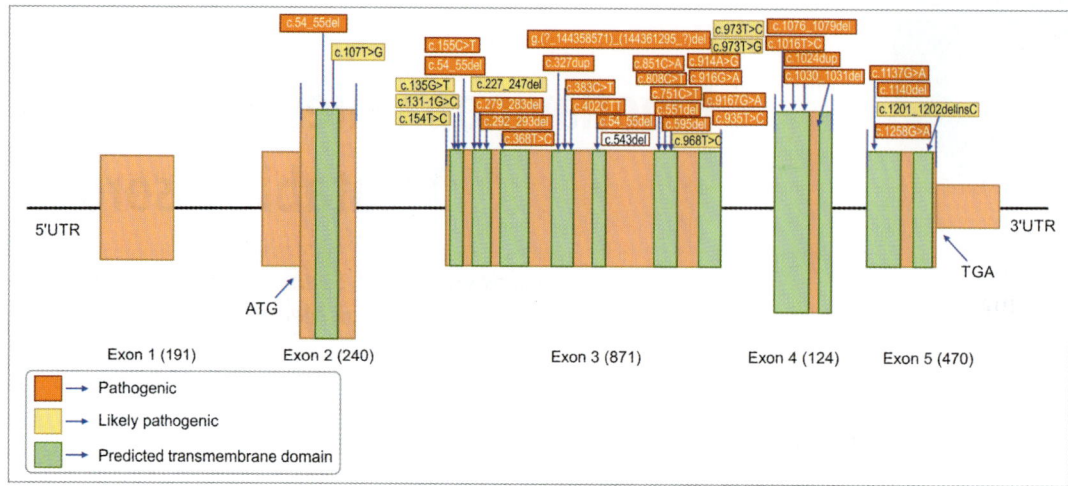

FIG. 1: Gene diagram of the reported variants in *SLC52A2* gene (pathogenic/likely pathogenic).[3]

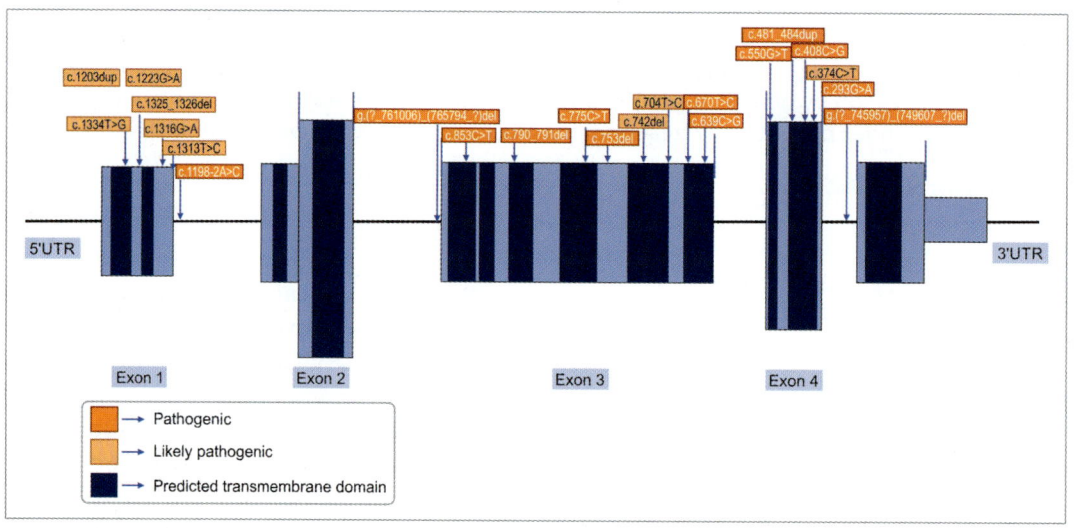

FIG. 2: Gene diagram of the reported variants in *SLC52A3* gene (pathogenic/likely pathogenic).[4]

models with knockout of riboflavin transporter had reduced lifespan which was partly ameliorated with supplementation of riboflavin. In induced pluripotent stem cells (iPSCs)-derived motor neurons from patients' cell lines, reduced axonal growth, and transcriptional alterations in cytoskeletal factors were noted.[5]

■ CASE SCENARIO

Patient: A 12-year-old girl born to consanguineous parents was evaluated during 2014. She presented with progressive hearing impairment for 3 years, repeated falls, difficulty rising from squatting position, and climbing stairs for 3 months. There was difficulty in gripping footwear and a change in gait for 1.5 months. She also reported decreased volume of voice and nasal regurgitation for 15 days. There were no sensory, cerebellar, or extrapyramidal symptoms. Family history was noncontributory. Her brother was diagnosed with thalassemia and died at 18 years of age. Neurological examination revealed mild scapular winging and wasting of intrinsic muscles of the hands with minipolymyoclonus, bilateral 7th to12th nerve involvement **(Figs. 3A to D)** and hypophonia. Muscle strength was significantly decreased in ankle dorsiflexors (grade 2), small muscles of the hand (grade 2), and toe dorsiflexors (grade 1). Babinski sign was positive. All tendon reflexes were elicited. Joint position sense and vibration were predominantly affected in the lower limbs (LLs). Romberg's sign was positive. Coordination tests were impaired, including tandem gait, finger nose, and heel-knee-shin test. A high-stepping ataxic gait was present.

Routine blood investigations were within normal range. Vitamins B12 and E levels were normal. Nerve conduction study (NCS) showed normal sensory conductions, low compound muscle action potential (CMAP) amplitudes from the median and ulnar nerves, and absent CMAP from common peroneal and posterior tibial nerves **(Table 1)**. Visual evoked potentials (VEP) showed prolonged P100 latency (left eye = 121.2 ms; right eye = 124.5 ms), and somatosensory evoked potential (SSEP) from the tibial nerve of left LL showed increased latency of N45 potential of 49.8 ms. Brainstem auditory evoked response (BAER) showed absent waveforms along with audiometry revealing bilateral profound sensorineural hearing loss. Magnetic resonance imaging (MRI) brain done in 2014 showed patchy fluid-attenuated inversion recovery (FLAIR) hyperintense areas in bilateral periventricular and deep white matter without diffusion restriction of lesions. MRI spine screening shows an expansion of the cervical spinal cord with long segment patchy intramedullary T2 hyperintensity in the dorsal aspect.

■ NEUROPATHOLOGY

Nerve biopsies in isolated reports showed signs of chronic axonal neuropathy without signs of inflammation or demyelination; while most muscle biopsies were nonspecific and showed only neurogenic muscle atrophy with some lipid accumulation.[7]

Studies in postmortem samples of brain and spinal cord have shown neuronal loss of the lower cranial nerve nuclei, anterior horn cells, cerebellar nuclei with gliosis, microglial activation, and axonal death. Abnormalities were also reported in the substantia nigra, locus coeruleus, olives, ambiguous nucleus, dorsal nucleus of Clarke, fastigial nucleus, lateral lemnisci, medial longitudinal fasciculus, trapezoid body, optic pathways, cochlear nucleus, inferior colliculi, and solitary tract.[8] Gliosis was

TABLE 1: Differences between BVVL and MMND.[6]

Clinical feature	BVVL	MMND
Gender preponderance	M:F = 1:5	M ≥ F
Cranial nerve involvement	Third or sixth cranial nerve is never noted to be affected	Affected
Lower motor neuron signs	Infrequent	Frequently seen
Upper motor neuron signs	Infrequent	Frequently seen
	50% familial	15% familial

(BVVL: Brown–Vialetto–Van-Laere; MMND: Madras motor neuron disease)

noticed in several tracts of the spinal cord, namely spinothalamic, spinocerebellar, gracile fasciculus, along with loss of anterior horn cells. These findings are in keeping with the clinical features. It was noticed that many patients displayed remarkable recovery despite advanced deficits. Hence, it was postulated that microglia and macrophage-induced inflammation plays a significant role; these changes may be reversible and explain good recovery with treatment.

In Vitro and In Vivo Models of Disease

In fibroblasts derived from patients, there is disruption of mitochondrial activity due to impaired riboflavin transport. In the Drosophila melanogaster studies, knock out of riboflavin transport showed similar changes in mitochondria. This led to reduced life span and impaired locomotion. These changes mirror the findings seen in patients. Interestingly, these changes in Drosophila too were partly reversed with riboflavin supplements.[1] The mitochondrial changes lead to oxidative stress causing impairment in the functioning of motor neurons.

■ CLINICAL SYMPTOMS

Symptoms may occur in early childhood or less frequently in adulthood. Age at presentation ranges from 0.25 to 27.0 years. Rare reports describe onset at a much older age. There is no gender predilection but some reports suggest that females are more commonly affected while males are more severely affected. The most common symptoms are weakness and cranial nerve deficits, usually a relentlessly progressive hearing loss. These children have poor speech discrimination and do not benefit from the conventional hearing aids. Patients manifest clinically with sensorimotor neuropathy in the form of proximal and distal weakness with wasting of upper more than LLs. Upper limb distal wasting may be prominent. Swallowing and speech difficulties in the form flaccid dysarthria and nasal regurgitation, sensorineural deafness, optic atrophy, nystagmus due to visual impairment, tongue fasciculations, tongue atrophy and weakness, development of pyramidal signs, sluggish reflexes, and sensory ataxia may occur later. Few patients may develop early ptosis and facial weakness too. Occasionally, stridor may be noted. Isolated case reports describe central hypoventilation as presenting features.[9] **Figures 3A to O** depict the clinical and imaging findings in patients with BVVL from the authors cohort.

Some reports describe a rapidly progressive weakness mimicking Guillain-Barré syndrome or other autoimmune disorders while others describe a subacute to chronic course of illness.[9,10] Hence, it is very important to have a high index of suspicion; presence of hearing loss prior to the onset of illness gives clue to the diagnosis. However, the history of hearing impairment may be missed in an acute setting. Interestingly, deafness occurs as an initial symptom, is severe, progressive, and may precede other symptoms by a few months to many years. It often responds poorly to treatment too. Axial weakness develops later. Respiratory difficulty occurs later in the course requiring ventilatory assistance and is often the cause of death. Bulbar symptoms need nasogastric feeds and gastrostomy. Higher mental functions are generally preserved. Marked intra- and inter-familial variability is known.[11]

In a review by Zhao et al. (n = 61), the most common initial symptom was ataxia (44.3%). This was followed by hearing loss in 11 cases (18.0%), nystagmus in nine cases (14.8%), muscle weakness in four cases (6.6%), and vision loss in four cases (6.6%). In the course of the disease, 83.9% of patients developed hearing loss, 80.6% developed muscle weakness, 64.5% developed visual

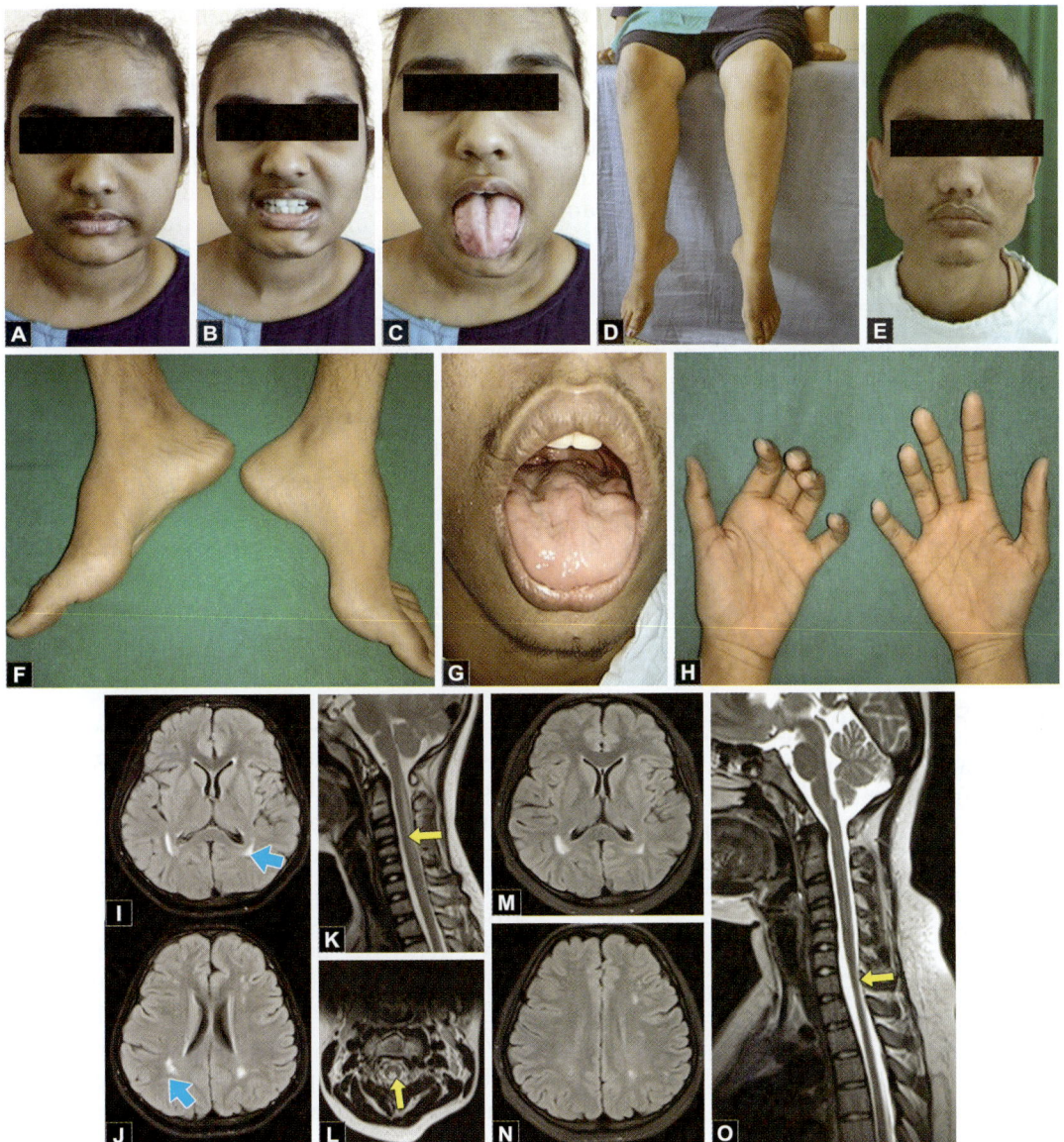

FIGS. 3A TO O: Clinical images of the patients. Patient 1: (A and B) Severe bifacial weakness; (C) Atrophy of tongue; (D) Bilateral foot drop (patient carried *SLC52A3*, p.Asn21Ser, and homozygous pathogenic variant). Patient 3: (E) Severe bifacial weakness with low set ears, broad nose, and depressed nasal bridge; (F) Severe wasting of foot muscles; (G) Severe tongue atrophy and fasciculations; (H) Severe wasting of small muscles of hands (patient carried *SLC52A3*, p.Thr125Ile, and homozygous likely pathogenic variant). Magnetic resonance imaging (MRI) brain and spine of patient 1: (I and J) MRI brain fluid-attenuated inversion recovery (FLAIR) axial section at initial presentation shows patchy hyperintense areas in bilateral periventricular and deep white matter (blue arrow); MRI spine sagittal (K) and axial views (L) show an expansion of the cervical spinal cord (yellow arrow) with long-segment patchy intramedullary T2 hyperintensity in the dorsal aspect. MRI brain FLAIR (M and N) axial section at follow-up after 8 years of initial presentation shows similar changes in the brain parenchyma. However, MRI spine (O) shows cord shows atrophy of the lower cervical and thoracic cord (yellow arrow).

impairment, 59.7% developed optic atrophy, and 21% developed nystagmus. In total, 61.3% had ataxia, 37.1% had respiratory insufficiency, of which 30.4% required mechanical ventilation, bulbar dysfunction occurred in 40.3% of patients, intellectual disability in 11.3%, epilepsy in 3.2%, and breath-holding spells in 4.8% of patients.[7]

Course of Illness

In a study by Bosch et al., 35 publications were reviewed which consisted of 74 patients with onset before age 18 years. Of 61 untreated patients, 28 died. Patients with age of onset before four had poor survival without treatment. The treated group survived.[12] Average age at death was 11.6 years (median 9.3, range 0.9–42 years). The average time between presentation and death was 5.0 years (median 1.3, range 0–32).[12]

■ DIFFERENTIAL DIAGNOSIS

In India, Madras motor neuron disease (MMND) is characterized by limb weakness, lower cranial nerve palsies, and sensorineural hearing loss. However, extensive genetic testing in patients with MMND has been done and no causative gene has been identified so far.[13,14] Patients with MMND develop optic atrophy, pyramidal signs, and cerebellar ataxia however, sensory ataxia is not reported. The differences are listed in **Table 1**.[6,15,16]

Nathalie syndrome is another differential which is accompanied by cataract, cardiac conduction defects, and hypogonadism in addition to lower motor neuron signs and symptoms.

Boltshauser syndrome: Distal muscular atrophy with vocal cord paralysis and sensorineural hearing loss. Unlike BVVL, the brainstem signs are restricted to vocal cord paralysis, and the inheritance is likely to be autosomal dominant.[17]

Amyotrophic lateral sclerosis is a differential; however, it lacks the characteristic features of BVVL, namely sensorineural hearing loss, optic atrophy, and ataxia.

X-linked spinobulbar muscular atrophy: Adult onset, bulbar onset, perioral fasciculations, features of androgen resistance such as gynecomastia, associated sensory neuropathy, tremors, and high 10-year survival rates. CK levels are elevated. Elevated CAG trinucleotide repeats are diagnostic.[17]

Sometimes, BVVL may be mistakenly diagnosed as autoimmune because several patients test positive for antibodies and respond to some extent to intravenous immunoglobulin. They may be misdiagnosed as chronic inflammatory demyelinating polyradiculoneuropathy or multifocal motor neuropathy especially when hearing loss is not on the forefront.[18]

■ LABORATORY FEATURES

Short and medium chain acylcarnitines accumulate in blood in about 50% of patients. Acylcarnitine profile mimics that seen in multiple acyl-coenzyme A (CoA) dehydrogenase deficiency. Some infants develop hyperammonemia. The acylcarnitine profile normalizes with riboflavin supplementation. Amino acid profile may show abnormalities. Riboflavin levels have been demonstrated to improve in blood after supplementation in a previous study by Foley et al., however, the authors do not routinely measure flavin levels.[19]

Electrophysiology/Imaging

Sensorimotor axonal neuropathy is noted on nerve conduction studies. Electromyograms show chronic denervation changes. Evoked potentials including both VEP and auditory show abnormalities. VEPs may reveal reduced amplitudes and prolonged latencies, patterned VEPs are absent in patients with severe visual loss.

Otoacoustic emissions are present, suggesting normal outer hair cell function. Auditory brainstem reflexes are impaired with large ringing cochlear microphonic.[20]

Magnetic resonance imaging of brain may occasionally show cerebellar atrophy, otherwise usually unremarkable. Thinning of optic nerves and tracts, signal changes in dorsal column of spinal cord, T2 hyperintensities in the brainstem, and cerebellum have been described in some patients. Some series report abnormalities in close to 20% of cases with remaining being normal.[7]

■ GENETICS

Biallelic variants in SLC52A2 and SLC52A3 are known with the latter being more commonly reported in previous cohorts.[1] They encode the human riboflavin transporters RFVT3 and RFVT2, respectively. The *SLC52A2* gene (NM_001253815.2) is located at 8q24.3 and contains five exons.[7] *SLC52A2* gene encodes for a transmembrane protein (hRFVT2) containing 445 amino acids and 11 transmembrane helices.[21] Clinical or whole exome sequencing is essential. Several mutations including missense, nonsense, and splice site are known to be causative. To the best of knowledge, large deletions or duplications have not been reported. However, there is no correlation between the genotype and phenotype. Genetic testing is required in this disorder because siblings must be screened for the mutation present in index patients with riboflavinopathies. Sibling screen ensures early identification and treatment with riboflavin in susceptible individuals. Carrier testing and prenatal screening of subsequent pregnancies in the mother may be advised for early diagnosis of this condition. In a rare case report, the proband was diagnosed with BVVL, caused by a homozygous variant of *SLC52A2* with uniparental disomy on chromosome 8.[7]

In patients with variants of uncertain significance, several functional studies are required for confirmation of diagnosis. Riboflavin uptake studies, live cell confocal imaging have been used to test functional consequences cell lines transfected with mutant hRFVT-2 and hRFVT-3 constructs.[22]

Genotype-phenotype Correlation

In a recent review, a total of 62 patients from 43 different families with SLC52A2 variants were described. Of these, there were 40 patients had homozygous and 22 had compound heterozygous variants. A total of 32 variants were found on 124 *SLC52A2* alleles. The most common variant was a missense variant (94.4%), followed by nonsense (2.4%), splice-site (0.8%), deletion (1.6%, including 1 case of an in-frame deletion of 3 amino acids), and insertion (0.8%). Pathogenic variants in *SLC52A2* were distributed throughout the gene including the transmembrane domains and intracellular and extracellular loops. A total of 40.3% of the variants were located in the transmembrane domain, 4.8% in the intracellular loop, and 54.0% were located in the extracellular loop. A total of 10.5% of patients had variants in the C-terminal region, 89.5% were in the intermediate region, and no variant was found in the N-terminal. Exon 3 had the most variants (74.2%), followed by exon 5 (15.3%), and exon 4 (8.9%). The most frequent variants were G306R (41.9%) and C443R (10.5%), accounting for 52.4% of all variants with most detected in the homozygous state, followed by L339P (7.3%), R169C (4.8%), and C325G (4.8%). The G306R (c.916G > A) mutation was most common in Lebanese, followed by Scots, possibly due to a founder effect.[23]

Zhao et al. reported that in patients with homozygous missense variants, ataxia was the most common initial symptom while patients with compound heterozygous missense variants more commonly showed visual impairment and respiratory insufficiency.[7] Visual impairment and hearing impairment were more common in patients with variants in transmembrane domain.[7]

While >30 mutations have been reported in *SLC52A3* gene **(Fig. 2)**, detailed phenotype-genotype correlations are not reported. In India, the variant c.A62G in SLC52A3 is described in five published reports.[22,24]

■ MANAGEMENT

Riboflavin supplementation at a high oral dose of 10–50 mg/kg/day, usually in an escalating dose schedule is advised. Though intravenous supplements are available, commonly oral formulations are used. Riboflavin is very rapidly eliminated; 6 hours after taking oral riboflavin, a situation as in three doses a day, plasma levels are practically back to baseline.[25] Hence, the rationale for frequent dosing. It improves clinical features and some electrophysiological parameters (evoked potentials and nerve conduction studies). Rarely, gastrointestinal symptoms and urine discoloration at high doses have been reported as adverse effects.[2] Early identification and treatment remain crucial. In a previous series, 60% improved and 40% stabilized after treatment. Clinical improvement may take days to months, sometimes as long as 12 months. Dramatic recoveries have been reported even when there were severe deficits and treatment was initiated late into the course of illness.[26] Treatment should be initiated right after suspicion even while genetic report is awaited. While deaths were reported in untreated patients, there were no deaths in previous cohorts of treated patients. Due to limited data on this disorder, it is not known whether treatment would prevent the occurrence of symptoms or delay them.[2] Improvements have been documented in motor symptoms, vision, hearing as well as in diaphragmatic functions. Patients on ventilatory assistance have been taken off the device following riboflavin.[12] However, several patients are quite advanced in their presentation. Hence, supportive care measures employing physiotherapy, occupational therapy, use of orthotics, and speech and swallowing therapy are pivotal. Riboflavin should be continued lifelong.

Hearing loss in BVVL is classified under auditory neuropathy spectrum disorder. Several case reports have detailed the use of cochlear implantation (CI) in patients with BVVL. While some report benefit in isolated cases with a follow-up of 2–3 years postsurgery, others suggest lack of benefit. The decision for implantation is complex as these children additionally also have speech disturbances due to lower cranial nerve involvement and are frequently on tracheostomy for ventilation. In their series of four children, Anderson et al. reported improvement in both sound and speech perception following CI. All these children were treated with riboflavin for a minimum of 1 year before the surgery. Sinnathuray et al. have suggested that the retrocochlear site of the lesion and probable central auditory pathway involvement negatively impacted CI outcomes. In another report of two siblings with BVVL who underwent CI at around 40 years of age, no improvement was noted following CI. It was presumed that since the duration of illness was too long, there may have been irreversible damage and hence lack of improvement following CI. At present, hearing rehabilitation in these patients remains a challenge.

■ FOLLOW-UP

Patients may be followed up once every 3–6 months, measurement of riboflavin/FMN/FAD levels and acylcarnitine profile may be done if feasible, however, there are no recommendations currently on follow-up biochemical testing.

■ GENETIC ANALYSIS OF THE CASE SCENARIO

Genetic analysis in the patient discussed in our case scenario revealed a previously reported pathogenic variant NM_033409.4:c.62A>G in homozygous state in exon 2 of the *SLC52A3* gene. On segregation analysis, the variant was observed in heterozygous state in asymptomatic parents. Further, the clinical phenotype of the proband matches with that of the disorder caused by pathogenic variants in the gene SLC52A3, confirming the diagnosis of BVVL syndrome.

Patient reported significant improvement in bulbar symptoms, mild improvement in hearing ability, increased muscle strength in hands and feet, and improved ability to walk independently after 6 months of riboflavin therapy (600 mg/day).

■ CONCLUSION

Riboflavinopathies clinically present with a wide spectrum of abnormalities including weakness, cranial nerve deficits, sensory ataxia, and respiratory impairment. Despite several advances, pathophysiology still remains elusive. Early identification is crucial as it is a potentially treatable disorder. Current dose of riboflavin is 10–60 mg/kg/day. Treatment is known to stabilize disease and improve symptoms. Untreated, the disease is fatal with a rapid downhill course. It is important to screen at-risk family members of patients diagnosed with riboflavinopathies to ensure early detection and treatment.

REFERENCES

1. Manole A, Jaunmuktane Z, Hargreaves I, Ludtmann MHR, Salpietro V, Bello OD, et al. Clinical, pathological and functional characterization of riboflavin-responsive neuropathy. Brain. 2017;140(11):2820.
2. Jaeger B, Bosch AM. Clinical presentation and outcome of riboflavin transporter deficiency: mini review after five years of experience. J Inherit Metab Dis. 2016;39:559-64.
3. ClinVar—NCBI. SLC52A2 [gene]. [online] Available from https://ncbi.nlm.nih.gov/clinvar/?term=SLC52A2%5Bgene%5D [Last accessed August, 2024].
4. ClinVar—NCBI. SLC52A3[gene]. [online] Available from https://ncbi.nlm.nih.gov/clinvar/?term=SLC52A3%5Bgene%5D&redir=gene [Last accessed August, 2024].
5. Rizzo F, Ramirez A, Compagnucci C, Salani S, Melzi V, Bordoni A, et al. Genome-wide RNA-seq of iPSC-derived motor neurons indicates selective cytoskeletal perturbation in Brown-Vialetto disease that is partially rescued by riboflavin. Sci Rep. 2017;7:46271.
6. Nalini A, Pandraud A, Mok K, Houlden H. Madras motor neuron disease (MMND) is distinct from the riboflavin transporter genetic defects that cause Brown–Vialetto–Van Laere syndrome. J Neurol Sci. 2013;334(1–2):119.
7. Zhao S, Che F, Yang L, Zheng Y, Wang D, Yang Y, et al. First report of paternal uniparental disomy of chromosome 8 with SLC52A2 mutation in Brown-vialetto-van laere syndrome type 2 and an analysis of genotype-phenotype correlations. Front Genet. 2022;13:977914.
8. Sathasivam S. Brown-Vialetto-Van Laere syndrome. Orphanet J Rare Dis. 2008;3:9.
9. Woodcock IR, Menezes MP, Coleman L, Yaplito-Lee J, Peters H, White SM, et al. Genetic, Radiologic, and Clinical Variability in Brown-Vialetto-van Laere Syndrome. Semin Pediatr Neurol. 2018;26:2-9.
10. Anand G, Hasan N, Jayapal S, Huma Z, Ali T, Hull J, et al. Early use of high-dose riboflavin in a case of Brown-Vialetto-Van Laere syndrome. Dev Med Child Neurol. 2012;54(2):187-9.
11. Dipti S, Childs AM, Livingston JH, Aggarwal AK, Miller M, Williams C, et al. Brown–Vialetto–Van Laere syndrome; variability in age at onset and disease progression highlighting the phenotypic overlap with Fazio-Londe disease. Brain Dev. 2005;27(6):443-6.

12. Bosch AM, Stroek K, Abeling NG, Waterham HR, IJlst L, Wanders RJ. The Brown-Vialetto-Van Laere and Fazio Londe syndrome revisited: Natural history, genetics, treatment and future perspectives. Orphanet J Rare Dis. 2012;7(1):83.
13. Govindaraj P, Nalini A, Krishna N, Sharath A, Khan NA, Tamang R, et al. Mitochondrial DNA variations in Madras motor neuron disease. Mitochondrion. 2013;13(6):721-8.
14. Nalini A, Yamini BK, Gayatri N, Thennarasu K, Gope R. Familial Madras motor neuron disease (FMMND): study of 15 families from southern India. J Neurol Sci. 2006;250(1–2):140-6.
15. Nalini A, Thennarasu K, Yamini BK, Shivashankar D, Krishna N. Madras motor neuron disease (MMND): clinical description and survival pattern of 116 patients from Southern India seen over 36 years (1971-2007). J Neurol Sci. 2008;269(1–2):65-73.
16. Gourie-Devi M, Nalini A. Madras motor neuron disease variant, clinical features of seven patients. J Neurol Sci. 2003;209(1–2):13-7.
17. Khadilkar SV, Yadav RS, Patel BA. Brown–Vialetto–Van Laere [BVVL] Syndrome. In: Khadilkar SV, Yadav RS, Patel BA (Eds). Neuromuscular Disorders: A Comprehensive Review with Illustrative Cases. Singapore: Springer; 2018 pp. 231-5.
18. Allison T, Roncero I, Forsyth R, Coffman K, Pichon JBL. Brown-Vialetto-Van Laere Syndrome as a Mimic of Neuroimmune Disorders: 3 Cases From the Clinic and Review of the Literature. J Child Neurol. 2017;32(6):528-32.
19. Foley AR, Menezes MP, Pandraud A, Gonzalez MA, Al-Odaib A, Abrams AJ, et al. Treatable childhood neuronopathy caused by mutations in riboflavin transporter RFVT2. Brain. 2014;137(1):44-56.
20. Menezes MP, O'Brien K, Hill M, Webster R, Antony J, Ouvrier R, et al. Auditory neuropathy in Brown–Vialetto–Van Laere syndrome due to riboflavin transporter RFVT2 deficiency. Dev Med Child Neurol. 2016;58(8):848-54.
21. O'Callaghan B, Bosch AM, Houlden H. An update on the genetics, clinical presentation, and pathomechanisms of human riboflavin transporter deficiency. J Inherit Metab Dis. 2019;42(4):598-607.
22. Udhayabanu T, Subramanian VS, Teafatiller T, Gowda VK, Raghavan VS, Varalakshmi P, et al. SLC52A2 [p.P141T] and SLC52A3 [p.N21S] causing Brown-Vialetto-Van Laere Syndrome in an Indian patient: First genetically proven case with mutations in two riboflavin transporters. Clin Chim Acta Int J Clin Chem. 2016;462:210-4.
23. Shi K, Shi Z, Yan H, Wang X, Yang Y, Xiong H, et al. A Chinese pedigree with Brown-Vialetto-Van Laere syndrome due to two novel mutations of *SLC52A2* gene: Clinical course and response to riboflavin. BMC Med Genet. 2019;20:76.
24. Gayathri S, Gowda VK, Udhayabanu T, O'Callaghan B, Efthymiou S, Varalakshmi P, et al. Brown–Vialetto–Van Laere and Fazio–Londe syndromes: SLC52A3 mutations with puzzling phenotypes and inheritance. Eur J Neurol. 2021;28(3):945-54.
25. Gorcenco S, Vaz FM, Tracewska-Siemiatkowska A, Tranebjærg L, Cremers FPM, Ygland E, et al. Oral therapy for riboflavin transporter deficiency —What is the regimen of choice? Parkinsonism Relat Disord. 2019;61:245-7.
26. Bamaga AK, Maamari RN, Culican SM, Shinawi M, Golumbek PT. Child Neurology: Brown-Vialetto-Van Laere syndrome. Neurology. 2018;91(20):938-41.

CHAPTER 9

Mitochondrial Disorders: A Neuromuscular Perspective

Madhu Nagappa

ABSTRACT

Mitochondrial myopathies are multisystemic disorders resulting from nuclear DNA (nDNA) and mitochondrial DNA (mtDNA) mutations, affecting oxidative phosphorylation (OXPHOS) function. Evaluation involves clinical assessment, metabolic screening, imaging, and pathological testing. These disorders are challenging to diagnose due to their dual genetic control, heteroplasmy, threshold effect, bottleneck effect, and unorthodox inheritance.

Keywords: Metabolic screening, OXPHOS, Threshold, nDNA, mtDNA, Mutations.

■ INTRODUCTION

Primary mitochondrial myopathies (PMMs) are defined as genetically determined disorders that lead to defective oxidative phosphorylation (OXPHOS) affecting predominantly, but not exclusively, skeletal muscle.[1] The mitochondria are under dual genetic control, i.e., encoded by nuclear DNA (nDNA) and mitochondrial DNA (mtDNA). Mutations in the nDNA or mtDNA can cause mitochondrial myopathies; some patients have multiple mutations.[2] Mutations in the nDNA are transmitted by Mendelian inheritance, which may be autosomal dominant, autosomal recessive, or X-linked. Mutations in the mtDNA are maternally inherited. Single mtDNA deletions occur sporadically. Heteroplasmy refers to the concomitant presence of wild-type (normal) and mutated mtDNA within the same cell. The number of copies of the mutated mtDNA should exceed a critical threshold within the cell to manifest the disease clinically. The "bottleneck" effect and mitotic segregation determine the inherited level and tissue distribution of the mutated mtDNA. Further, nuclear-mitochondrial intergenomic communication exists. Hence, mutations in the nDNA result in depletion and/or multiple deletions in the mtDNA and impair mitochondrial homeostasis.[3,4]

Myopathy is a common manifestation of mitochondrial disease because the skeletal muscle has a high energy demand. Exercise-induced symptoms are common in mitochondrial myopathies, and they reflect the lack of energy production due to mitochondrial dysfunction in the skeletal muscle, increased lactate production and depletion of phosphocreatine. Thus, patients have exercise intolerance, premature fatigue, exhaustion, tiredness, reduced energy levels, and dyspnea on exertion.[5] Muscle weakness occurs, but fatigue is often out of proportion to the degree of weakness. Recurrent rhabdomyolysis and myoglobinuria triggered by exercise are uncommon. When the onset is in infancy, the clinical manifestations include floppiness, developmental delay, and respiratory failure. Muscle weakness may be generalized or localized, taking the form of chronic progressive external ophthalmoplegia (CPEO).[6] The symptoms are insidiously progressive, with episodes of decompensation during periods of metabolic stress such as fever, due to which the apparently "relapsing" clinical course may be mistaken for an immune-mediated disorder. Spontaneous improvement has been uncommonly reported in mitochondrial myopathy due to *COXIII* mutations.[7] The range of age at onset is wide, and in general, an early age of onset is associated with a more severe phenotype. Clinical clues for an underlying mitochondrial pathology include the involvement of multiple organ systems that have a high energy demand, such as the heart, liver, and kidneys, besides the nervous system. These could range from rather benign symptoms, such as migrainous headaches, to life-threatening cardiomyopathies that carry a potential for sudden cardiac death.[8] Similarly, a family history of early-onset diabetes mellitus, CPEO, retinopathy, hearing loss, and cardiac involvement should alert the clinician of an underlying mitochondrial disorder.[9] This chapter highlights some mitochondrial syndromes with primary or predominant muscle involvement.

■ CHRONIC PROGRESSIVE EXTERNAL OPHTHALMOPLEGIA SYNDROMES

Mitochondrial myopathies classically affect the ocular muscles, leading to CPEO. This is seen in about two-thirds of the patients. Patients develop ptosis, the most prominent feature, due to weakness of the levator palpebrae superioris. It is bilateral and symmetrical. It may be mild to severe and complete, leading to significant obscuration of the visual field. Patients tend to have a compensatory frontalis muscle contraction and tilt the head backwards to overcome the ptosis. This is accompanied by ophthalmoplegia, wherein the eye movements are restricted symmetrically. This may progress to complete ophthalmoplegia, and the patients turn their heads to see the target, especially in the periphery of the visual field. This ophthalmoplegia rarely causes diplopia because of its symmetricity. Still, it has been noted that many patients complain of diplopia, especially in the initial stages when the restriction of eye movements is asymmetrical. Usually, ptosis occurs before or simultaneously with the ophthalmoplegia, and rarely, ophthalmoplegia occurs without the ptosis. These symptoms do not fluctuate, as happens in myasthenia gravis, which is the main differential diagnosis.[10]

A single deletion in the mtDNA often causes CPEO. Other ocular myopathies due to single mtDNA deletion include Pearson and Kearns–Sayre syndromes (KSS). The former is a severe disorder characterized by sideroblastic anemia, exocrine pancreatic insufficiency, lactic acidosis, renal and hepatic dysfunction, failure to thrive, and high mortality. Those who survive evolve into KSS. The "triad" of KSS comprises CPEO, onset before 20 years of age, and pigmentary retinopathy. Other features of KSS include short stature, ataxia, deafness, dementia, facial weakness, dysphagia, and weakness of the neck and limbs. Investigations show increased protein in cerebrospinal fluid and leukoencephalopathy on brain magnetic resonance imaging (MRI). Cardiac conduction defects may develop, which range from prolongation of PR interval to atrioventricular block and predispose to sudden cardiac death. Endocrine dysfunction manifests as diabetes, growth hormone insufficiency, adrenal sufficiency, hypoparathyroidism, and hypogonadotropic hypogonadism.[11,12]

Thus, CPEO may occur in isolation or as a part of a multisystem condition, where there is coexistence with extramuscular symptoms and signs. Thus, based on the phenotype, we can categorize patients with mitochondrial myopathy as follows:[13]

- CPEO, which is isolated, and there are no other neurological or systemic deficits.
- *CPEO-plus*: When CPEO is associated with other features of neuromuscular and multisystem involvement but excluding the central nervous system. These include dysphagia, impaired hearing, exercise intolerance, and weakness of other muscles.
- *Mitochondrial encephalomyopathy*: PEO + encephalomyopathy, with evidence of involvement of the CNS in the form of ataxia, cognitive impairment, seizures, pyramidal signs, tremor, impaired consciousness, dystonia, parkinsonism, etc.

Cross-sectional categorization into the above phenotypes may be difficult since some deficits may be subclinical and detectable only in investigations. So, the rigor and extent to which the investigations are done to look for a multiaxial or multisystem involvement also determine the phenotype. Besides, all the clinical features are not present at the onset or at the time of the first evaluation. Many clinical features evolve with time, and serial follow-up is necessary to define the phenotype fully. What is CPEO today may be reclassified as a CPEO-plus during follow-up.

■ MITOCHONDRIAL MYOPATHIES WITHOUT CPEO

Apart from CPEO, mitochondrial myopathy may manifest with the involvement of other muscles in the form of slowly progressive axial and proximal limb weakness, affecting predominantly the hip and shoulder girdles and neck flexor muscles, often with variable muscle wasting.[14] This nonspecific phenotype is often difficult to distinguish from other myopathies, especially when isolated. Muscle weakness may also cause dysphagia and dysarthria due to oropharyngeal weakness, as well as respiratory failure. Distal muscle weakness may be present but is rarely seen early in the disease. There are also uncommon reports where the phenotype resembled facioscapulohumeral muscular dystrophy (FSHD), but the inheritance pattern was maternal.

Mitochondrial Encephalomyopathy with Lactic Acidosis and Stroke-like Episodes

Mitochondrial encephalomyopathy with lactic acidosis and stroke-like episodes (MELAS) is considered to be one of the more prevalent mitochondrial disorders. The hallmark clinical feature is the presence of stroke-like episodes characterized by hemiparesis, hemianopia, and cortical blindness. These are called stroke-like episodes since there is no vascular occlusion, and the MRI changes during the episodes do not conform to any vascular territory. Besides, the MRI abnormalities resolve faster than in a typical stroke. Migrainous headaches, vomiting, and seizures may herald the onset of stroke-like episodes. In children, seizures are common, and they may be refractory to treatment. These patients eventually develop progressive cognitive decline.[15]

Other clinical features include short stature, optic atrophy, pigmentary retinopathy, impaired hearing, peripheral neuropathy, exercise intolerance, and proximal muscle weakness. Diabetes, gastrointestinal dysmotility, cardiac arrhythmias [Wolff–Parkinson–White (WPW) syndrome], and cardiomyopathy constitute the systemic manifestations. The onset is usually between 2 and 15 years of age and rarely in infancy or after adolescence. The initial development is normal or delayed. Failure to thrive, learning difficulty, and attention deficit hyperactivity may be present before the development of the stroke-like episodes. MELAS is caused by m.3243A>G in 80% while the rest have m.3271T>C mutation. Mutations in the nDNA causing MELAS are also reported.[16,17]

Myoclonic Epilepsy with Ragged Red Fibers

The canonical features of myoclonic epilepsy with ragged red fibers (MERRF), otherwise known as the Fukuhara syndrome, include myoclonus, epilepsy, ataxia, and ragged red fibers (RRFs) in muscle biopsy. This syndrome may manifest in childhood or adult life. Myoclonus is often the first symptom, and epilepsy may manifest as focal or generalized myoclonic, atonic, clonic, tonic-clonic seizures, and absence seizures. Other neurological features include exercise intolerance, ptosis, ophthalmoplegia, optic atrophy, pigmentary retinopathy, sensorineural hearing loss, myopathy, axonal neuropathy, pyramidal dysfunction, migraine, and dementia. General physical examination reveals short stature and lipomas commonly seen in the nuchal region. Other system involvement includes cardiac (dilated or hypertrophic cardiomyopathy, arrhythmias like WPW syndrome), and diabetes mellitus.[18]

The most common genetic mutation is m.8344A>G in the *MT-TK* gene, present in about 80% of the affected subjects. A similar phenotype is caused by other mutations such as m.8356T>C, m.8363G>A, m.3243A>G, m.3255G>A, and m.3291T>C.[12]

Mitochondrial Neurogastrointestinal Encephalomyopathy

This complex and extremely rare condition has a prevalence rate of less than one per million population. As the name suggests, mitochondrial neurogastrointestinal encephalomyopathy (MNGIE) manifests with gastrointestinal and neurological features. Gastrointestinal symptoms include severe dysmotility, vomiting, dysphagia, abdominal pain/cramps, intestinal pseudo-obstruction, borborygmi, bacterial overgrowth syndrome, diarrhea, and significant weight loss. The patients have frail and slender habitus. Neurological manifestations include ptosis, ophthalmoplegia, sensorineural hearing loss, seizures, impaired cognition, ataxia, and demyelinating neuropathy. Interestingly, these patients have leukoencephalopathy on brain MRI, which is clinically asymptomatic. Other clinical features include ocular (myopia, glaucoma, and pigmentary retinopathy), endocrine (exocrine pancreatic insufficiency and diabetes mellitus), cardiac (prolonged QT interval, supraventricular tachycardia, and cardiomyopathy) and recurrent infections. The onset is usually in the first or second decade. The course is progressive and is usually fatal by the fourth decade.[19]

Mutations in *TYMP* that encodes thymidine phosphorylase, which catalyzes the reversible phosphorylation of thymidine and deoxyuridine to thymine and uracil, respectively, lead to the accumulation of deoxyribonucleosides. This causes an imbalance in the deoxyribonucleotide pool, reduced ability of mtDNA for repair, and accumulation of multiple mutations within the mtDNA in the form of multiple deletions, depletion, and point mutations. Clinical manifestations occur when the threshold level of mutant mtDNA exceeds 80–90%.[20]

Coenzyme Q10 Deficiency

Mutations in genes involved in coenzyme Q10 (CoQ10) biosynthesis give rise to primary CoQ10 deficiency. This has a wide range of age at onset. Apart from isolated myopathy, the other phenotypes caused by primary CoQ10 deficiency include encephalomyopathy, cerebellar ataxia, infantile multisystemic disease, and nephropathy. Clinical manifestations include encephalopathy, optic atrophy, retinitis pigmentosa, sensorineural deafness, ataxia, seizures, stroke-like episodes, encephalopathy, rhabdomyolysis, cardiomyopathy, and nephropathy. Some patients may respond to CoQ10 supplementation if initiated early in the disease course.[21]

Leigh Syndrome

This manifests as a subacute encephalomyelopathy with onset usually in infancy or early childhood and rarely in adults. Clinical manifestations include delayed development, vomiting, dysphagia, failure to thrive, seizures, and neuroregression that may follow a period of metabolic stress. Examination may show hypotonia or spasticity, weakness of limbs, ataxia, chorea, dystonia and other movement disorders, peripheral neuropathy, and apneic spells. Ocular signs include ptosis, ophthalmoplegia, optic atrophy, nystagmus, and slow saccades. Cardiac, renal, hepatic, and gastrointestinal dysfunction may also be present. Adults have atypical presentations with cognitive decline, vertical gaze palsy, and psychiatric manifestations and may even be mistaken for acquired disorders such as multiple sclerosis. Brain MRI shows hyperintensities in the basal ganglia, thalami, brainstem, and cerebellum.[22]

Mitochondrial Peripheral Neuropathies

Mutations in genes involved in mitochondrial dynamics such as *MFN2*, *GDAP1*, *SLC25A46*, *OPA1*, and *DNM2* cause predominant neuropathy phenotype resembling Charcot–Marie–Tooth (CMT) disease, with distal predominant weakness and wasting and skeletal deformities. Additional features such as optic atrophy, sensorineural deafness, and pyramidal signs may also be present.

Mutations in *POLG1* cause the syndrome of sensory ataxic neuropathy, dysarthria, and ophthalmoplegia (SANDO).[23] The syndrome of neuropathy, ataxia, and retinitis pigmentosa (NARP) is characterized by developmental delay and ataxia, with sensory neuropathy, proximal neurogenic weakness, and retinitis pigmentosa during the second decade of life. NARP is caused by the m.8993T>C mutation. The same mutation also causes maternally inherited Leigh syndrome (MILS).[24] Leber's hereditary optic neuropathy (LHON) is characterized by sequential and painless impairment in vision, predominantly the central field, that develops over weeks to months. Males are particularly affected. The optic fundus shows optic disk hyperemia, dilatation, and tortuosity of peripapillary vessels, circum-papillary telangiectasia, nerve-fiber edema, and focal hemorrhages. Additional neurological features such as dystonia and peripheral neuropathy may also be present (LHON "plus"). The m.11778G>A, m.14484T>C, and m.3460G>A mutations account for most of the patients with LHON.[25]

■ LABORATORY EVALUATION

A panel of tests is used not only for diagnosing but also to define the phenotype as completely as possible. For example, biochemical tests detect hepatic/renal dysfunction, including renal tubular acidosis and Fanconi's syndrome, dyselectrolytemia, and endocrine abnormalities such as diabetes mellitus. Electrophysiological tests such as nerve conduction studies confirm and identify the pattern of neuropathy, while evoked potential studies assess the integrity of the visual, auditory, and somatosensory pathways. Audiometry is useful for detecting hearing loss. Cardiac evaluation by echocardiogram and electrocardiogram identifies cardiac conduction defects and structural changes such as cardiomyopathy. Several of these changes may be subclinical or asymptomatic and must be repeated periodically during follow-up to detect de novo abnormalities. Brain MRI shows the characteristic changes in Leigh's disease and shifting hyperintensities in MELAS, as well as asymptomatic leukoencephalopathy of MNGIE and KSS. MR spectroscopy is a noninvasive technique to measure the metabolites, which may show a lactate peak.[26]

■ BIOMARKERS OF MITOCHONDRIAL MYOPATHIES

There is no single biomarker for diagnosing mitochondrial disorder. Several molecules have been studied as potential biomarkers for diagnosing mitochondrial disorders. These include lactate, pyruvate, creatine, creatine kinase, amino acids, glutathione, and malondialdehyde. They reflect impaired electron transport chain and OXPHOS function. Since mitochondrial disorders are complex phenotypes affecting different parts of the neuraxis to varying extents and may have associated systemic manifestations with varying severity and clinical course/progression, it has not been possible to identify a single or perfect biomarker. These molecules can be altered in several nonmitochondrial disorders. For example, lactate and pyruvate may be elevated in the setting of infection, stroke, malignancy, inflammation, and seizures, as well as prolonged tourniquet application and struggling children. Pyruvate can also be increased in pyruvate dehydrogenase complex deficiency, pyruvate carboxylase deficiency, and biotinidase deficiency. Hence, the ratio of lactate-to-pyruvate may be more useful in distinguishing mitochondrial from other metabolic disorders. Creatine kinase is not increased in all mitochondrial disorders and is increased in muscular dystrophies and other nonmitochondrial disorders, and hence has very poor sensitivity and sensitivity for diagnosis of mitochondrial disorders. A number of amino acids have been studied since mitochondria have a role in their metabolism. Increased alanine, especially >450 µM, is considered to be highly specific for mitochondrial disorders. Arginine and citrulline are reduced in MELAS. However, none of the amino acids have consistent findings and are influenced by many environmental factors, including dietary intake.[27]

Recently, fibroblast growth factor 21 (FGF-21) and growth and differentiation factor 15 (GDF-15) have emerged as reliable biomarkers with high sensitivity and specificity for mitochondrial disorders.[28] These have important roles in glucose and lipid metabolism and immune regulation, respectively. They are increased in response to cellular stress. They are particularly increased in patients with muscle-manifesting mitochondrial disorders.[29] They can be used as a screening tool to triage patients to undergo further specialized workup such as muscle biopsy. Gelsolin, another marker of OXPHOS dysfunction, is reduced in the plasma and increased in the outer mitochondrial membrane in cell models. Reduced plasma gelsolin may be a useful biomarker, particularly when combined with GDF-15. Neurofilament light (Nfl), which is elevated in several neurodegenerative and inflammatory conditions, is also increased in mitochondrial disorders. However, it is not a good biomarker since it is increased in multisystem disorders as compared to myopathy phenotype. The role and utility of cell-free circulating mtDNA are being explored.[27]

■ MUSCLE BIOPSY

Muscle biopsy constitutes a crucial investigation in the workup of a patient with mitochondrial myopathy. Histological analysis may reveal specific findings of subsarcolemmal aggregation of abnormal mitochondria, which are seen as RRFs and ragged blue fibers (RBFs) in modified Gomori trichrome (MGT) and succinate dehydrogenase (SDH) stains, respectively. Muscle fibers deficient in cytochrome c oxidase (COX) can be identified by the combined COX-SDH histochemical stain, wherein the COX-deficient fibers appear blue in color due to the normal or high concentrations of SDH. In contrast, the normal fibers with COX and SDH appear brown.[30] Some of the patterns of histological changes that correlate with the phenotype and genetics include:

- *Segmental COX deficiency*: mtDNA mutation (due to heteroplasmy)
- *Global decrease in COX*: nDNA mutation
- *RRF, RBF, and COX deficiency*: mtDNA depletion disorders such as KSS and PEO, and tRNA mutations (e.g., MERRF)
- *Lipid droplets*: CoQ10 deficiency

These findings are neither specific nor sensitive since RRFs can be seen in other conditions, such as inflammatory and toxic myopathies, and normal aging. On the other hand, RRFs, RBFs, and COX-deficient fibers are not universally seen in all mitochondrial disorders; hence, their absence does not exclude the diagnosis. Nonspecific findings such as variation in fiber size, fiber atrophy, myofibrillar necrosis, regenerating fibers, fiber type grouping, and accumulation of lipid and glycogen can also be seen.[31] Ultrastructural studies reveal abnormal subsarcolemmal and intermyofibrillar proliferation of mitochondria, which are enlarged, elongated, or irregular in appearance with dystrophic cristae. Various morphological patterns such as paracrystalline inclusions, concentric cristae giving rise to onion-like mitochondria, linearized cristae with abnormal angular or geometric appearance, abnormal increase in the number of membrane-bound compartments within the mitochondria, nano-tunneling and hyperbranching of mitochondria as well as "donut"-shaped mitochondria due to self-fusion have been described.[32] Apart from histological and ultrastructural studies, the muscle tissue lends itself toward multiple diagnostic processes, including biochemical analysis of respiratory chain complex activity and molecular genetic studies.

■ GENETIC TESTING

The European Federation of Neurological Sciences (EFNS) provided the guidelines for the molecular diagnosis of mitochondrial disorders.[33] These guidelines emphasize stepwise and systematic genetic testing based on the phenotype. However, the phenotype-genotype correlation in mitochondrial disorders is rather complex—a single mutation causes several different clinical syndromes and different genetic alterations, leading to a common phenotype that cannot be distinguished at the bedside,[34] e.g., *POLG1* mutations most commonly cause the ataxia phenotype in adolescents and adults and CPEO in older subjects. But a range of clinical phenotypes is reported that include Alpers–Huttenlocher syndrome, childhood myocerebrohepatopathy spectrum, myoclonic epilepsy myopathy sensory ataxia (MEMSA), the ataxia neuropathy spectrum (ANS), etc. Besides, different members from a given family carrying a common mutation manifest differently, the so-called phenotypic heterogeneity, e.g., the MELAS-causing m.3243A>G mutation causes stroke-like episodes in one subject and isolated myopathy in another member of the same family. Thus, the phenotype is a poor predictor of the underlying molecular genetic defect in most cases.

However, sequencing the exome or the complete genome, including the mitochondrial genome, by high-throughput techniques, i.e., the next-generation sequencing (NGS), is effective and efficient in terms of yield, cost, and time. NGS, hence, is the preferred test for molecular genetic diagnosis.[35] However, it is important to test the relevant tissue, which is the one that expresses the disease, i.e., the muscle. The skeletal muscle is a postmitotic terminally differentiated tissue with limited regenerative capacity. It has a fairly stable ratio of wild-type to mutant mtDNA throughout life. So, the percentage of mutant mtDNA is higher in muscle than in the blood or skin fibroblasts because of altered heteroplasmy, given the higher tissue regeneration rate of blood cells and fibroblasts. So, mtDNA point mutations, deletions, and depletion are most reliably detected in the muscle.[36] Determining the size of deletion and heteroplasmy provides some important information regarding the disease's severity and progression, at least in some instances. This is also useful for the functional characterization of the variants of "uncertain" significance detected by NGS.[37]

■ TREATMENT PERSPECTIVES

There is no single or common pharmacotherapy for mitochondrial disorders because they have varied phenotypic manifestations that evolve with time. Hence, the treatment has to be tailored to the individual patient and modified periodically depending on the clinical status. A multidisciplinary team comprising a neurologist and a geneticist together with a physician/pediatrician, cardiologist, pulmonologist, gastroenterologist, endocrinologist, ophthalmologist, otorhinolaryngologist, and physical rehabilitation experts is necessary. Appropriate genetic counseling regarding the nature of the disease and prognosis needs to be provided together with adequate psychosocial support. Broadly, the treatment can be classified as symptomatic and mitochondrial-specific. The former includes eyelid crutches (for ptosis), hearing aids/cochlear implants (for sensorineural hearing loss), cardiac pacemakers (for conduction blocks), anticonvulsants (for seizures) and antispastic agents (for spasticity), etc. Exercise therapy, including aerobic, endurance, and resistance training, has been shown to overcome physical deconditioning, increase mitochondrial biogenesis and oxidative capacity, and thereby improve fatigue and quality of life; however, a patient should be warned not to exercise to the point of exhaustion. A number of vitamins and supplements that are collectively referred to as the mitochondrial "cocktail" are administered to improve mitochondrial function and overcome the biochemical defect in the electron transport chain. This "cocktail" includes levocarnitine, riboflavin (B2), vitamins B1, B2, B3, B5, E and C, β-carotene, alpha-lipoic acid, and selenium.[38]

Specific therapies such as supplementation with CoQ may improve the symptoms of CoQ deficiency when administered early and hence are recommended to be given even on an empirical basis in patients with a compatible phenotype. Additionally, arginine, nicotinamide, and succinate may reduce the stroke-like episodes and encephalopathy in MELAS. Therapeutic options in MNGIE include dialysis to remove the excess thymidine nucleosides, enzyme replacement, and platelet infusion. The ketogenic diet not only improves mitochondrial biogenesis but also causes a shift in heteroplasmy with an increase in wild-type mtDNA. Other agents that have been tried to improve mitochondrial biogenesis and function include bezafibrate, acipimox, omaveloxolone, vatiquinone, elamipretide, and idebenone. Among these, idebenone is licensed for use in LHON. Importantly, agents that worsen mitochondrial function, such as sodium valproate, propofol, etc., should be avoided. Further, gene therapies that target the underlying genetic defect and assisted reproductive techniques that prevent the transmission of mutant mtDNA, such as spindle transfer and nuclear transfer, are also being developed.[39]

CONCLUSION

Mitochondrial myopathies comprise a spectrum of phenotypes that range from pure myopathy to multisystemic disorders, with a wide range of age at onset, severity, and progression. They arise from impaired OXPHOS function due to mutations in nDNA and mtDNA. The current practice for evaluating a patient with mitochondrial myopathy involves a multipronged approach, including clinical assessment, metabolic screening, imaging, and pathological, functional, and biochemical testing to get as comprehensive a phenotype as possible. Dual genetic control, heteroplasmy, threshold effect, bottleneck effect, and unorthodox inheritance are peculiar characteristics of these disorders, because of which these disorders are often challenging to diagnose and prognosticate.

REFERENCES

1. Mancuso M, McFarland R, Klopstock T, Hirano M; consortium on Trial Readiness in Mitochondrial Myopathies. International Workshop: Outcome measures and clinical trial readiness in primary mitochondrial myopathies in children and adults. Consensus recommendations. 16-18 November 2016, Rome, Italy. Neuromuscul Disord. 2017;27(12):1126-37.
2. DiMauro S, Gurgel-Giannetti J. The expanding phenotype of mitochondrial myopathy. Curr Opin Neurol. 2005;18(5):538-42.
3. Ahmed ST, Craven L, Russell OM, Turnbull DM, Vincent AE. Diagnosis and treatment of mitochondrial myopathies. Neurotherapeutics. 2018;15(4):943-53.
4. Rusecka J, Kaliszewska M, Bartnik E, Tońska K. Nuclear genes involved in mitochondrial diseases caused by instability of mitochondrial DNA. J Appl Genet. 2018;59(1):43-57.
5. Olimpio C, Tiet MY, Horvath R. Primary mitochondrial myopathies in childhood. Neuromuscul Disord. 2021;31(10):978-87.
6. de Barcelos IP, Emmanuele V, Hirano M. Advances in primary mitochondrial myopathies. Curr Opin Neurol. 2019;32(5):715-21.
7. Horváth R, Lochmüller H, Hoeltzenbein M, Müller-Höcker J, Schoser BG, Pongratz D, et al. Spontaneous recovery of a childhood onset mitochondrial myopathy caused by a stop mutation in the mitochondrial cytochrome c oxidase III gene. J Med Genet. 2004;41(6):e75.
8. Nardin RA, Johns DR. Mitochondrial dysfunction and neuromuscular disease. Muscle Nerve. 2001;24(2):170-91.
9. Witters P, Saada A, Honzik T, Tesarova M, Kleinle S, Horvath R, et al. Revisiting mitochondrial diagnostic criteria in the new era of genomics. Genet Med. 2018;20(4):444-51.
10. McClelland C, Manousakis G, Lee MS. Progressive external ophthalmoplegia. Curr Neurol Neurosci Rep. 2016;16(6):53.
11. Björkman K, Vissing J, Østergaard E, Bindoff LA, de Coo IFM, Engvall M, et al. Phenotypic spectrum and clinical course of single large-scale mitochondrial DNA deletion disease in the paediatric population: A multicentre study. J Med Genet. 2023;60(1):65-73.
12. Mancuso M, Orsucci D, Angelini C, Bertini E, Carelli V, Comi GP, et al. Redefining phenotypes associated with mitochondrial DNA single deletion. J Neurol. 2015;262(5):1301-9.
13. Orsucci D, Angelini C, Bertini E, Carelli V, Comi GP, Federico A, et al. Revisiting mitochondrial ocular myopathies: a study from the Italian Network. J Neurol. 2017;264(8):1777-84.
14. Lin Y, Wang J, Ren H, Ma X, Wang W, Zhao Y, et al. Mitochondrial myopathy without extraocular muscle involvement: a unique clinicopathologic profile. J Neurol. 2024;271(2):864-76.
15. Lorenzoni PJ, Werneck LC, Kay CS, Silvado CE, Scola RH. When should MELAS (Mitochondrial myopathy, Encephalopathy, Lactic Acidosis, and Stroke-like episodes) be the diagnosis? Arq Neuropsiquiatr. 2015;73(11):959-67.
16. Chakrabarty S, Govindaraj P, Sankaran BP, Nagappa M, Kabekkodu SP, Jayaram P, et al. Contribution of nuclear and mitochondrial gene mutations in mitochondrial encephalopathy,

lactic acidosis, and stroke-like episodes (MELAS) syndrome. J Neurol. 2021;268(6):2192-207.
17. Sproule DM, Kaufmann P. Mitochondrial encephalopathy, lactic acidosis, and strokelike episodes: basic concepts, clinical phenotype, and therapeutic management of MELAS syndrome. Ann N Y Acad Sci. 2008;1142:133-58.
18. Finsterer J, Zarrouk-Mahjoub S, Shoffner JM. MERRF Classification: Implications for Diagnosis and Clinical Trials. Pediatr Neurol. 2018;80:8-23.
19. Hirano M, Carelli V, De Giorgio R, Pironi L, Accarino A, Cenacchi G, et al. Mitochondrial neurogastrointestinal encephalomyopathy (MNGIE): Position paper on diagnosis, prognosis, and treatment by the MNGIE International Network. J Inherit Metab Dis. 2021;44(2):376-87.
20. Hirano M, Lagier-Tourenne C, Valentino ML, Martí R, Nishigaki Y. Thymidine phosphorylase mutations cause instability of mitochondrial DNA. Gene. 2005;354:152-6.
21. Emmanuele V, López LC, Berardo A, Naini A, Tadesse S, Wen B, et al. Heterogeneity of coenzyme Q10 deficiency: Patient study and literature review. Arch Neurol. 2012;69(8):978-83.
22. Baertling F, Rodenburg RJ, Schaper J, Smeitink JA, Koopman WJ, Mayatepek E, et al. A guide to diagnosis and treatment of Leigh syndrome. J Neurol Neurosurg Psychiatry. 2014;85(3):257-65.
23. Sharma G, Pfeffer G, Shutt TE. Genetic neuropathy due to impairments in mitochondrial dynamics. Biology (Basel). 2021;10(4):268.
24. Pareyson D, Piscosquito G, Moroni I, Salsano E, Zeviani M. Peripheral neuropathy in mitochondrial disorders. Lancet Neurol. 2013;12(10):1011-24.
25. Carelli V, La Morgia C, Yu-Wai-Man P. Mitochondrial optic neuropathies. Handb Clin Neurol. 2023;194:23-42.
26. Milone M, Wong LJ. Diagnosis of mitochondrial myopathies. Mol Genet Metab. 2013;110(1-2):35-41.
27. Shayota BJ. Biomarkers of mitochondrial disorders. Neurotherapeutics. 2024;21(1):e00325.
28. Suomalainen A, Elo JM, Pietiläinen KH, Hakonen AH, Sevastianova K, Korpela M, et al. FGF-21 as a biomarker for muscle-manifesting mitochondrial respiratory chain deficiencies: a diagnostic study. Lancet Neurol. 2011;10(9):806-18.
29. Suomalainen A. Blood biomarkers of mitochondrial disease-One for all or all for one? Handb Clin Neurol. 2023;194:251-7.
30. Phadke R. Myopathology of Adult and Paediatric Mitochondrial Diseases. J Clin Med. 2017;6(7):64.
31. Lu JQ, Mubaraki A, Yan C, Provias J, Tarnopolsky MA. Neurogenic muscle biopsy findings are common in mitochondrial myopathy. J Neuropathol Exp Neurol. 2019;78(6):508-14.
32. Vincent AE, Ng YS, White K, Davey T, Mannella C, Falkous G, et al. The spectrum of mitochondrial ultrastructural defects in mitochondrial myopathy. Sci Rep. 2016;6:30610.
33. Finsterer J, Harbo HF, Baets J, Van Broeckhoven C, Di Donato S, Fontaine B, et al; European Federation of Neurological Sciences. EFNS guidelines on the molecular diagnosis of mitochondrial disorders. Eur J Neurol. 2009;16(12):1255-64.
34. Arena IG, Pugliese A, Volta S, Toscano A, Musumeci O. Molecular genetics overview of primary mitochondrial myopathies. J Clin Med. 2022;11(3):632.
35. Stenton SL, Prokisch H. Genetics of mitochondrial diseases: Identifying mutations to help diagnosis. EBioMedicine. 2020;56:102784.
36. Mavraki E, Labrum R, Sergeant K, Alston CL, Woodward C, Smith C, et al. Genetic testing for mitochondrial disease: the United Kingdom best practice guidelines. Eur J Hum Genet. 2023;31(2):148-63.
37. Mahmud S, Biswas S, Afrose S, Mita MA, Hasan MR, Shimu MSS, et al. Use of Next-Generation Sequencing for Identifying Mitochondrial Disorders. Curr Issues Mol Biol. 2022;44(3):1127-48.
38. Hassani A, Horvath R, Chinnery PF. Mitochondrial myopathies: Developments in treatment. Curr Opin Neurol. 2010;23(5):459-65.
39. Tinker RJ, Lim AZ, Stefanetti RJ, McFarland R. Current and Emerging Clinical Treatment in Mitochondrial Disease. Mol Diagn Ther. 2021;25(2):181-206.

Therapeutic Advances in Nodoparanodopathies

Satish Khadilkar, Varsha Patil, Jharna Mahajan

ABSTRACT

In clinical practice, patients with acute to subacute onset, aggressive neuropathy, respiratory involvement, or acute inflammatory demyelinating polyneuropathy (AIDP) or chronic inflammatory demyelinating polyneuropathy (CIDP), with atypical features such as tremors and severe sensory ataxia, should be tested for nodal and paranodal antibodies. Treatment should include corticosteroids, intravenous immunoglobulin (IVIg), and plasma exchange (PLEX) as the initial lines of therapy. Some cases are severe and refractory, in such patients, rituximab can be beneficial. Newer monoclonal antibodies are also being considered in this group of diseases.

Keywords: Nodoparanodopathies, AIDP, CIDP, Neurofascin, Contactin, Ganglioside antibodies, IVIg, PLEX, Corticosteroids, Rituximab.

■ INTRODUCTION

The node of Ranvier and the paranodal structures have received attention for their molecular structure and role in the pathophysiology of immune neuropathies.[1] As shown in **Figure 1**, the nodal, paranodal, and juxtaparanodal areas have been studied in detail and various antigens have been localized. **Figure 1** shows a simplified representation of the molecular organization at the nodal region. The nodal Na+ channels (Nav) are anchored to spectrin of the axonal cytoskeleton via ankyrin G and to gliomedin of the Schwann cell microvilli via neurofascin-186 (NF186). At the paranode, axonal contactin-associated protein (CASPR) and contactin are tightly connected to neurofascin 155 (NF155) of paranodal myelin loops. This complex forms septate-like junctions, which separate the nodal Na+ channel clusters from the juxta paranodal K+ channels (Kv). Immune-mediated attacks on these antigens lead to various changes in the nodal and paranodal organization and the interaction of myelin and axon, leading to clinical and electrophysiological abnormalities. With this information, the pathophysiological mechanisms have become clearer. The distinction between demyelinating and axonal processes has merged with the advent of this clarity of the targets. The following paragraph gives the perspective of the evolution of nodo-paranodopathies over the last decade, with timelines.

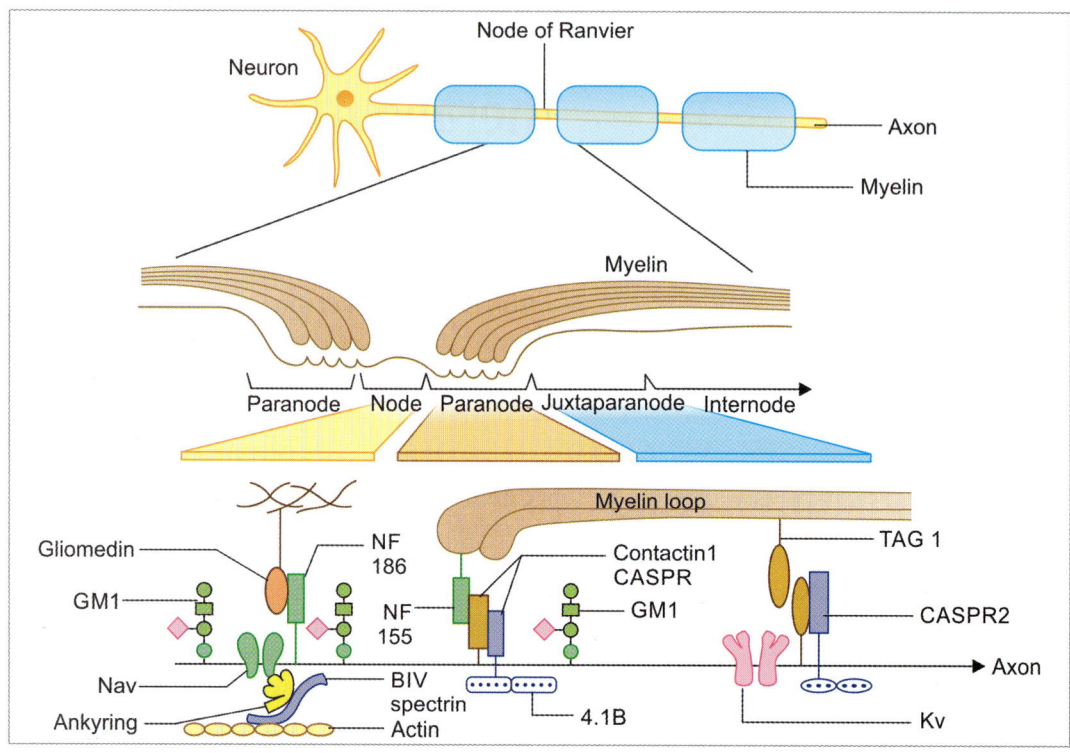

FIG. 1: Organization of nodal and paranodal antigens.

In 2009, Pillai and colleagues studied the rapid conduction in nerves in rat experiments and described a myelin-dependent organization of axons into distinct molecular domains.[2] Their study of nodal and paranodal domains led to the discovery of glial isoforms of NF155. In 2012, Devaux and colleagues demonstrated the presence of antibodies such as NF186, gliomedin, and contactin in the sera of patients suffering from Guillain–Barré syndrome (GBS) and chronic inflammatory demyelinating polyneuropathy (CIDP).[3] In 2012, Yuki reviewed his journey with antiganglioside antibodies in GBS.[4] In this review, he discussed the rationale of therapies in various subtypes of GBS. Further in 2013, Uncini (in a landmark paper) discussed the details of antigens responsible for autoimmune nodoparanodopathies and elucidated "the node" as the bridge between the electrophysiological classification of demyelinating and axonal neuropathies.[5] The initial observations in GBS were followed quickly by studies on antineurofascin antibodies in CIDP by Querol and colleagues.[6] They identified a subgroup with tremors and poor response to intravenous immunoglobulins (IVIg). Their study included four patients who had anti-NF155 antibodies, which are more frequent than others in most studies. Around this time, a proportion of patients with multifocal motor neuropathy (MMN) were shown to have anti-NF186 or contactin antibodies in their sera and demonstrated activation of the complement by these antibodies.[7] But this observation was challenged by another group that did not find the antibodies in their cohort.[8] Ogata and colleagues characterized various aspects of a cohort of anti-NF155-associated neuropathies in 2015 and commented upon the distal dominant nature and nerve thickening.[9] Interestingly, Devaux and colleagues studied Japanese patients with CIDP having anti-NF155 antibodies to highlight the typical features such as tremors, sensory ataxia, and documented central nervous system demyelination with poor response to IVIg.[10] Delmont's investigation focused on the clinical features of anti-NF186 and anti-NF140 positive neuropathies and compared them with those having anti-NF155 positivity.[11] A variety of antibodies other than neurofascin such as contactin 1 (CNTN1), ganglioside antibodies, and CASPR1 have been associated with autoimmune nodoparanodopathies.

Clinically, nodoparanodopathies can be suspected in acute or subacute, predominantly distal motor neuropathies with rapid progression, severe disabilities, and in chronic neuropathies with severe sensory ataxia, tremors, and early atrophy. Associated systemic features such as membranous nephropathy can be a clue.

Electrophysiological features such as reduced motor conduction velocities, marked prolongation of distal motor latencies, marked prolongation of F wave latencies, early axonal loss, and decreased compound motor action potentials and conduction block without temporal dispersion can be suggestive of a nodoparanodopathy. Kouton et al. in the year 2020, compared the electrophysiological features of CIDP with antibodies against NF and contactin with CIDP without antibodies. They concluded that patients with positive antibodies had more prolonged distal latencies, F waves, and markedly reduced conduction velocities.[12]

The therapeutic perspectives of neurofascin and contactin-related neuropathies started appearing in 2016, and some information on conditions such as MMN was available even earlier. Garg and colleagues gave information on the therapy response in 55 patients of CIDP who tested positive for anti-NF155 immunoglobulin G4 (IgG4) antibody.[13] In 2022, Aguilar et al. studied significant long-term follow-up of 48 months of treatment in 45 patients with anti-NF155 antibody-related autoimmune paranodopathy.[14] Their observations suggested a good response to first-line therapies (IVIg and steroids), but a better response was noted in patients treated with rituximab (RTX) (class IV evidence). In a review paper 10 years after his first review, Uncini discussed various evolved clinical and therapeutic aspects of different nodoparanodopathies.[15] Delmont and colleagues studied a large cohort of CIDP patients with positive anti-NF antibodies and compared them with CIDPs with negative antibodies.[16] By now, some information on the therapy aspects of these neuropathies has accumulated and is discussed below.

■ THERAPY OF NODOPARANODOPATHIES

General Comments

Most patients with autoimmune nodoparanodopathies are initially treated with steroids with some benefits. The response is often partial and not well sustained. IVIg and plasma exchange (PLEX) have been used to bind or filter the circulating antibodies and reduce the load, respectively. All first-line therapies such as IVIg, steroids, and PLEX have proven to be successful, except in patients with anti-NF155 antibody-related neuropathies.[6] IgG4 antibodies are produced by CD20 positive plasma cells, hence B-cell depletion strategies stand to reason. In keeping with this, patients with autoimmune nodoparanodopathies are noted to respond to medications such as RTX, even after poor response to initial IVIg or steroid therapy.[17-19] This led to a thought process that RTX could be started early in the therapy paradigm, but has not been tested adequately, yet.[14] RTX is known to show effects by 3 months and the benefits can go on for 12–24 months. After induction with RTX, maintenance can also be done with RTX, decisions based on the improvements in the scoring systems such as Inflammatory Rasch-built Overall Disability Scale (I-RODS), Inflammatory Neuropathy Cause and Treatment (INCAT), and Expanded Disability Status Scale (EDSS). While antibody levels do not generally correlate with the disease activity and course, in each case, tracking over time shows the antibody levels to reduce.[14] Relapses have not been fully studied but a significant proportion of patients are believed to relapse and recur, adding to the ultimate disabilities. Cyclophosphamide, mycophenolate, and azathioprine have also been used with variable success rates.[20] Beyond RTX, newer molecules such as eculizumab and methods such as immunoadsorption are being tested. The summary of therapeutic advances in autoimmune nodopathy over the period of last decade is described in **Table 1**. A broad protocol for therapy has been proposed earlier.[1]

Neurofascin Neuropathies

Anti-NF155-associated autoimmune paranodopathy has been the most studied of the neuropathies, in terms of therapeutics. The initial observations by Querol *et al.* in four cases of IgG4 predominant anti-NF155 positive CIDP seem pertinent. They reported poor response to IVIg, but partial response to steroids in one patient, and good response to PLEX in two of them.[6] This same group later described three patients (two with anti-NF155 and one with anti-CNTN1 antibodies) with good response to RTX. Later, Devaux et al. described 38 IgG4 NF155 antibody-positive patients with CIDP. In their cohort, five of 25 patients (20%) responded to IVIg and 15 out of 29 (51.7%) responded to steroids.[10] Nidhi Garg et al. described three anti-NF155-positive patients with good responses to PLEX.[13] In a study by Davies and colleagues, it was shown that repeated PLEX may be required to induce sustained suppression of antibody levels and thus clinical improvement.[33] Thus, it is seen from the above studies that the highest response rates for IgG NF155-associated paranodopathy are seen with PLEX (78%) followed by RTX (75%), steroids (56%), and IVIg (32%).[34] Recently, Aguilar and colleagues published their data on a large cohort of anti-NF155 positive patients to show low response rates to IVIg and corticosteroids, but 70.5% of their patients responded to RTX.[14] A single case report of telitacicept (a dual inhibitor of B lymphocyte stimulator and A proliferation-inducing ligand) in NF155 antibody-positive patient has recently been published, in cases refractory to RTX.[29]

Patients with IgG CNTN1 antibodies are refractory to treatment with IVIg but have good responses to steroids, RTX, and PLEX. A recent case report has documented the efficacy of low-dose RTX therapy.[31] Recently, two patients having anti-CNTN1 antibodies have been successfully treated with low-dose RTX therapy. Both patients had sensory ataxia, tremors, and nephropathy. Both patients had received corticosteroids and RTX. The improvement began after 2 weeks and after a 6-month review, they were ambulant.[35] Another patient having cerebellar dysarthria in addition to severe demyelinating neuropathy has been shown to have benefits after RTX therapy.[36] Response to immunoadsorption has been recently documented in a patient having anti-CaSPR1 antibody positivity.[37]

There are only a few papers on the therapy of NF186.[27] A single patient having NF186, and 140 antibodies has been described in detail.[38] This patient initially responded partially to IVIg but worsened again and did not respond to the second course of IVIg, PLEX, and corticosteroids. He improved spontaneously

TABLE 1: Summary of therapeutic advances in autoimmune nodopathy.

Authors	Year	Number of patients	Antibodies	Therapy
Querol[6]	2014	2	Anti-NF155	Class IV evidence that autoantibodies to NF155 should be identified as a CIDP subtype characterized by severe neuropathy and poor response to IVIg
Ogata[9]	2015	13	Anti-NF155 IgG4	IVIg 4/13 (30.8%), IV pulse CST 3/8(37.5%), oral CST 5/8 (62.5%), and PE–4/6 (66.7%)
Querol[17]	2015	9	Anti-NF155 and anticontactin	Four received RTX–(two each of anticontactin and anti-NF-positive patients)—three-fourths improved with RTX significantly
Devaux[10]	2016	51	38 with positive anti-NF155, 13 with positive anticontactin IgG4	Poor response to IVIg compared to antibody-negative CIDP (20% vs. 60%). Anti-NF155 group had a poorer response to IVIg (20%) compared to anticontactin group (40%)
Nidhi Garg[13]	2016	3	Anti-NF155 IgG4	Two patients responded to steroids and one patient improved after receiving multiple immunosuppressants including RTX
Kuwahara[21]	2018	4	Anti-NF155 IgG4	Patients with long duration of illness responded poorly to all treatments. Response to usual immunotherapies like IVIg was poor with decent response with CST and PE
Cortese[22]	2020	13	Seven (anti-NF155), three (anticontactin), three (anti-CASPR1)	Patients with positive paranodal antibodies showed 8% improvement with IVIg and 67% in the seronegative CIDP group
Delmont[16]	2020	27	Anti-NF155, anticontactin, anti-CASPR1 antibodies	IVIg was ineffective in most seropositive patients. Rituximab resulted in dramatic improvements in disability and decreased antibody titers in 13 seropositive patients (8 with anti-Nfasc155 and 5 with anti-CNTN1 antibodies)
Chong Xie[23]	2021	16	Anti-NF186 IgG antibodies—nine had CNS features	13 patients received immunomodulating treatments, and patients with the chronic onset and the progressive course showed poor responses to the therapies

Continued

Continued

Authors	Year	Number of patients	Antibodies	Therapy
Sahar Shelly[24]	2021	32	Anti-NF155 (IgG4 and IgM)	NF155—IgG4-positive cases responded favorably to immunotherapy compared to MAG-IgM-seropositive cases with distal acquired demyelinating symmetric neuropathy and had better long-term clinical outcomes compared to contactin-1 IgG
Aguilar[14]	2022	40	Anti-NF 155 IgG4	IVIg response rates 13%, CST 27.8%, PE 38.8%, and RTX 77.3%. Autoantibody titers and sNfL are useful to monitor disease status in these patients
Meng Dong[25]	2022	11	Five patients had IgG against NF155, three against CASPR1, two against NF186, and one against CNTN1	CST was effective in 42.9%, IVIg in 14.3%, and RTX in 75.0% of patients. They also documented, the damage on nerves is more severe in anti-NF155-positive patients than that in anti-CASPR1-positive patients during electrophysiological diagnosis
Luise Appeltshauser[26]	2023	18	11 patients of pan-NF antibodies, seven of anti-NF155 only	PE response rates in the Pan NF group 45.5% IVIg 20%, CST 14.3%, and RTX 80%. This subset of patients may benefit from early antibody-depleting therapy
Bingyou Liu[27]	2023	33	13 with anti-NF186, 20 with anti-NF155	IVIg response rates in 186 group 55.6%, CST 80%, and RTX 100%
Yunfei Bai[28]	2023	1 case report	Refractory anti-NF155	In this study, anti-RTX antibodies (ARAs) presented in a patient with anti-NF155 nodopathy undergoing rituximab treatment showed an unfavorable impact on rituximab efficacy
Yijun Ren[29]	2023	1 case report	Anti-NF155 ab	Telitacicept, a dual inhibitor of B lymphocyte stimulator (BLyS) and A proliferation-inducing ligand (APRIL) administered 160 mg, subcutaneous injection, demonstrated a significant response in INCAT and IRODS in patients who were refractory to all other immunomodulatory therapies

Continued

Continued

Authors	Year	Number of patients	Antibodies	Therapy
Bingyou Liu[18]	2023	19	16 anti-NF155, 3 anti-contactin	Participants received IV RTX treatment of 100 mg the first day and 500 mg the next day and given every 6 months. In patients who received more than one RTX infusion, the improvement of INCAT score and I-RODS at the last assessment was higher than that after the first infusion
Hyun Ji Lyoua[30]	2024	6	Anti-NF155	5/6 showed partial response to CST and IVIg. 3/6 patients treated with RTX showed a significant response
Ivan Kmezic[31]	2024	1 case report	Anti-NF155	A clinical and serological good response to low-dose RTX (500 mg) given twice with a 6-month interval
20. Efficacy and safety of rituximab in refractory CIDP with or without IgG4 autoantibodies (RECIPE)[32]			Ongoing RCT phase 2 ongoing	

(CASPR1: contactin-associated protein-1; CIDP: chronic inflammatory demyelinating polyneuropathy; CNS: central nervous system; CNTN1: contactin 1; CST: contraction stress test; IVIg: intravenous immunoglobulin; NF155: neurofascin 155; PE: preeclampsia; RCT: randomized controlled trial; RTX: rituximab; sNfL: serum neurofilament light chain) after a few months but attained significant ambulation.

In personal data (unpublished) from a study of 22 patients having NF186 antibodies, approximately one-third responded partially to the first immunosuppressant medication (corticosteroids, IVIg, or PLEX). The choice of the second immunosuppressant was variable, and among the resistant group, 50% responded to RTX therapy.

Few patients with pan NF antibody positivity have been reported on their therapy features. Some of these respond to IVIg, but not to corticosteroids. Relapses and deteriorations are common and may not respond to second courses of IVIg, PLEX, and steroids. RTX has been known to help some of these patients.[26]

Ganglioside Antibodies

Patients having GBS-like presentation and testing positive for ganglioside antibodies have been treated with IVIg or PLEX with variable results. Two trials of eculizumab are available on this group of patients. The first study had only eight randomized patients and hence was inconclusive.[15,39] In the second trial, the primary outcome measure was 50% of patients regaining the ability to walk by 4 weeks. This was not achieved but 74% fulfilled the secondary outcome measure, the ability to run after 24 weeks. Further studies are required to establish the doses and the safety of eculizumab in this group of patients.[40]

The lack of response to corticosteroids is well-recognized in MMN. Steroids may worsen the disease, and the explanation may be in the increasing sodium-potassium pump activity in the axons. The primary treatment is IVIg at periodic intervals.[41] Cyclophosphamide has also been used but the side effect profile can be limiting. Some studies have used cyclophosphamide to increase the gap between IVIg courses. RTX and eculizumab have not been effective in small trials.[39]

In a recent review of a large cohort, Broers and colleagues have stressed the importance of identifying autoimmune neuropathies in a cohort of CIDP patients, as they are less responsive to conventional therapies and require more intense and longer therapies.[42]

■ NEWER THERAPIES

Recently, RTX has been used in combination with bortezomib in a patient of anti-pan NF antibodies with severe and refractory inflammatory neuropathy.[43] Scheibe et al. studied the response of treatment-refractory antibody-mediated neurological diseases with daratumumab. In this, they report a patient with CIDP with neurofascin antibody with nemaline myopathy.[44] Both agents cause clinically relevant depletion of autoreactive long-lived plasma cells. Both the patients showed a significant clinical improvement with a reduction in titers of antibodies. Other B-cell-depleting therapies such as ofatumumab and ocrelizumab, Bruton kinase inhibitors such as tolebrutinib and zanubrutinib, and anti-FcRn agents are potential candidates for therapy in immune nodopathies.[26] Recently, the complement system has been shown to be affected in these conditions and complement inhibitors may be useful. As mentioned earlier, eculizumab is one such agent studied in two trials.

■ CONCLUSION

Thus, in clinical practice, it is recommended to test for nodal and paranodal antibodies if the patient has acute to subacute onset, aggressive, distal, and motor predominant neuropathy and associated cranial neuropathy, and respiratory involvement or is initially diagnosed as acute inflammatory demyelinating polyneuropathy (AIDP) or

CIDP, particularly with atypical features such as sensory ataxia and tremors. Patients should be started on first-line therapies such as corticosteroids with or without IVIg depending on severity. If a patient is refractory to IVIg/steroids, then treatment should be rapidly escalated to other methods such as PLEX. If a patient does not respond to first-line therapies during the first 8 weeks of illness or the clinical phenotype is aggressive at the onset with evidence of early axon loss, then RTX should be considered.

REFERENCES

1. Khadilkar S, Kamat S, Patel R. Nodo-paranodopathies: Concepts, clinical implications, and management. Ann Indian Acad Neurol. 2022;25(6):1001-8.
2. Pillai AM, Thaxton C, Pribisko AL, Cheng G, Dupree JL, Bhat MA. Spatiotemporal ablation of myelinating glia-specific neurofascin (NfascNF155) in mice reveals gradual loss of paranodal axoglial junctions and concomitant disorganization of axonal domains. J Neurosci Res. 2009;87(8):1773-93.
3. Devaux JJ, Odaka M, Yuki N. Nodal proteins are target antigens in Guillain-Barré syndrome. J Peripher Nerv Syst. 2012;17(1):62-71.
4. Yuki N. Guillain-Barré syndrome and anti-ganglioside antibodies: A clinician-scientist's journey. Proc Jpn Acad Ser B Phys Biol Sci. 2012;88(7):299-326.
5. Uncini A, Susuki K, Yuki N. Nodo-paranodopathy: Beyond the demyelinating and axonal classification in anti-ganglioside antibody-mediated neuropathies. Clin Neurophysiol. 2013;124:1928-34.
6. Querol L, Nogales-Gadea G, Rojas-Garcia R, Diaz-Manera J, Pardo J, Ortega-Moreno A, et al. Neurofascin IgG4 antibodies in CIDP associated with disabling tremors and poor response to IVIg. Neurology. 2014;82(10):879-86.
7. Notturno F, Di Febo T, Yuki N, Fernandez Rodriguez BM, Corti D, Nobile-Orazio E, et al. Autoantibodies to neurofascin-186 and gliomedin in multifocal motor neuropathy. J Neuroimmunol. 2014;276(1–2):207-12.
8. Doppler K, Appeltshauser L, Krämer HH, Ng JKM, Meinl E, Villmann C, et al. Contactin-1 and neurofascin-155/-186 are not targets of auto-antibodies in Multifocal motor neuropathy. PLoS One. 2015;10(7):e0134274.
9. Ogata H, Yamasaki R, Hiwatashi A, Oka N, Kawamura N, Matsuse D, et al. Characterization of IgG4 anti-neurofascin 155 antibody-positive polyneuropathy. Ann Clin Transl Neurol. 2015;2(10):960-71.
10. Devaux JJ, Miura Y, Fukami Y, Inoue T, Manso C, Belghazi M, et al. Neurofascin-155 IgG4 in chronic inflammatory demyelinating polyneuropathy. Neurology. 2016;86(9):800-7.
11. Delmont E, Manso C, Querol L, Cortese A, Berardinelli A, Lozza A, et al. Autoantibodies to nodal isoforms of neurofascin in chronic inflammatory demyelinating polyneuropathy. Brain. 2017;140(7):1851-8.
12. Kouton L, Boucraut J, Devaux J, Rajabally YA, Adams D, Antoine JC, et al. Electrophysiological features of chronic inflammatory demyelinating polyradiculoneuropathy associated with IgG4 antibodies targeting neurofascin 155 or contactin 1 glycoproteins. Clin Neurophysiol. 2020;131(4):921-7.
13. Garg N, Park SB, Yiannikas C, Vucic S, Howells J, Noto YI, et al. Neurofascin-155 IGG4 neuropathy: Pathophysiological insights, spectrum of clinical severity and response to treatment. Muscle Nerve. 2018;57(5):848-51.
14. Martín-Aguilar L, Lleixà C, Pascual-Goñi E, Caballero-Ávila M, Martínez-Martínez L, Díaz-Manera J, et al. Clinical and laboratory features in anti-NF155 autoimmune nodopathy. Neurol Neuroimmunol Neuroinflamm. 2022;9(1):e1098.
15. Uncini A. Autoimmune nodo-paranodopathies 10 years later: Clinical features, pathophysiology and treatment. J Peripher Nerv Syst. 2023:28 Suppl 3:S23-S35.
16. Delmont E, Brodovitch A, Kouton L, Allou T, Beltran S, Brisset M, et al. Antibodies against the node of Ranvier: a real-life evaluation of incidence, clinical features and response to treatment based on a prospective analysis of 1500 sera. J Neurol. 2020;267(12):3664-72.
17. Querol L, Rojas-García R, Diaz-Manera J, Barcena J, Pardo J, Ortega-Moreno A, et al. Rituximab in treatment-resistant CIDP with antibodies against

paranodal proteins. Neurol Neuroimmunol Neuroinflamm. 2015;2(5):e149.
18. Liu B, Hu J, Sun C, Qiao K, Xi J, Zheng Y, et al. Effectiveness and safety of rituximab in autoimmune nodopathy: a single-center cohort study. J Neurol. 2023;270(9):4288-95.
19. Hu J, Sun C, Lu J, Zhao C, Lin J. Efficacy of rituximab treatment in chronic inflammatory demyelinating polyradiculoneuropathy: a systematic review and meta-analysis. J Neurol. 2022;269(3):1250-1263.
20. Gupta P, Mirman I, Shahar S, Dubey D. Growing spectrum of autoimmune nodopathies. Curr Neurol Neurosci Rep. 2023;23(5):201-12.
21. Kuwahara M, Suzuki H, Oka N, Ogata H, Yanagimoto S, Sadakane S, et al. Electron microscopic abnormality and therapeutic efficacy in chronic inflammatory demyelinating polyneuropathy with anti-neurofascin155 immunoglobulin G4 antibody. Muscle Nerve. 2018;57(3):498-502.
22. Cortese A, Lombardi R, Briani C, Callegari I, Benedetti L, Manganelli F, et al. Antibodies to neurofascin, contactin-1, and contactin-associated protein 1 in CIDP: Clinical relevance of IgG isotype. Neurol Neuroimmunol Neuroinflamm. 2020;7(1):E639.
23. Xie C, Wang Z, Zhao N, Zhu D, Zhou X, Ding J, et al. From PNS to CNS: characteristics of anti-neurofascin 186 neuropathy in 16 cases. Neurol Sci. 2021;42(11):4673-81.
24. Shelly S, Shouman K, Paul P, Engelstad J, Amrami KK, Spinner RJ, et al. Expanding the spectrum of chronic immune sensory polyradiculopathy. Neurol. 2021;96(16):e2078-89.
25. Dong M, Tai H, Yang S, Gao X, Pan H, Zhang Z. Characterization of the patients with antibodies against nodal-paranodal junction proteins in chronic inflammatory demyelinating polyneuropathy. Clin Neurol Neurosurg. 2022;223:107521.
26. Appeltshauser L, Junghof H, Messinger J, Linke J, Haarmann A, Ayzenberg I, et al. Anti-pan-neurofascin antibodies induce subclass-related complement activation and nodo-paranodal damage. Brain. 2023;146(5):1932-49.
27. Liu B, Zhou L, Sun C, Wang L, Zheng Y, Hu B, et al. Clinical profile of autoimmune nodopathy with anti-neurofascin 186 antibody. Ann Clin Transl Neurol. 2023;10(6):944-52.
28. Bai Y, Li W, Yan C, Hou Y, Wang Q. Anti-rituximab antibodies in patients with refractory autoimmune nodopathy with anti-neurofascin-155 antibody. Front Immunol. 2023;14:1121705.
29. Ren Y, Chen S, Yang H. Case Report: Telitacicept in treating a patient with NF155+ autoimmune nodopathy: A successful attempt to manage recurrent elevated sero-anti-NF155 antibodies. Front Immunol. 2023;14:1279808.
30. Lyou HJ, Chung YH, Kim MJ, Kim M, Jeon MY, Kim SW, et al. Clinical features of autoimmune nodopathy with anti-neurofascin-155 antibodies in South Koreans. J Clin Neurol. 2024;20(2):186.
31. Kmezic I, Press R, Glenewinkel H, Doppler K, Appeltshauser L. Low-dose rituximab treatment in a patient with anti-neurofascin-155 IgG4 autoimmune nodopathy. J Neuroimmunol. 2024;389:578326.
32. Shimizu S, Iijima M, Fukami Y, Tamura N, Nakatochi M, Ando M, et al. Efficacy and Safety of Rituximab in Refractory CIDP With or Without IgG4 Autoantibodies (RECIPE): Protocol for a Double-Blind, Randomized, Placebo-Controlled Clinical Trial. JMIR Res Protoc. 2020;9(4):e17117.
33. Davies AJ, Fehmi J, Senel M, Tumani H, Dorst J, Rinaldi S. Immunoadsorption and Plasma Exchange in Seropositive and Seronegative Immune-Mediated Neuropathies. J Clin Med. 2020;9(7):2025.
34. Vizcarra JA, Harrison TB, Garcia-Santibanez R. Update on nodopathies of the peripheral nerve. Curr Treat Options Neurol. 2021;23(8):25.
35. Hou Y, Zhang C, Yu X, Wang W, Zhang D, Bai Y, et al. Effect of low-dose rituximab treatment on autoimmune nodopathy with anti-contactin 1 antibody. Front Immunol. 2022;13:939062.
36. Chen J, Liu L, Zhu H, Han J, Li R, Gong X, et al. Autoimmune nodopathy with anti-contactin 1 antibody characterized by cerebellar dysarthria: a case report and literature review. Front Immunol. 2024;15:1308068.
37. Liu L, Chen J, Zhang Y, Wu J, Hu J, Lin Z. Case report: Immunoadsorption therapy for anti-caspr1 antibody-associated nodopathy. Front Immunol. 2022;13:986018.
38. Vallat JM, Mathis S, Magy L, Bounolleau P, Skarzynski M, Heitzmann A, et al. Subacute nodopathy with conduction blocks and anti-neurofascin 140/186 antibodies: An ultrastructural study. Brain. 2018;141(7):e56.
39. Misawa S, Kuwabara S, Sato Y, Yamaguchi N, Nagashima T, Katayama K, et al. Safety and efficacy of eculizumab in Guillain-Barré syndrome: a multicentre, double-blind, randomised phase 2 trial. Lancet Neurol. 2018;17(6):519-29.

40. Davidson AI, Halstead SK, Goodfellow JA, Chavada G, Mallik A, Overell J, et al. Inhibition of complement in Guillain-Barré syndrome: the ICA-GBS study. J Peripheral Nerv Syst. 2017;22(1):4-12.
41. Keddie S, Eftimov F, van den Berg LH, Brassington R, de Haan RJ, van Schaik IN. Immunoglobulin for multifocal motor neuropathy. Cochrane Database Syst Rev. 2022;1(1):CD004429.
42. Broers MC, Wieske L, Erdag E, Gürlek C, Bunschoten C, van Doorn PA, et al. Clinical relevance of distinguishing autoimmune nodopathies from CIDP: Longitudinal assessment in a large cohort. J Neurol Neurosurg Psychiatry. 2024;95(1):52-60.
43. Fels M, Fisse AL, Schwake C, Motte J, Athanasopoulos D, Grüter T, et al. Report of a fulminant anti- pan-neurofascin-associated neuropathy responsive to rituximab and bortezomib. J Peripheral Nerv Syst. 2021;26(4):475-80.
44. Scheibe F, Ostendorf L, Prüss H, Radbruch H, Aschman T, Hoffmann S, et al. Daratumumab for treatment-refractory antibody-mediated diseases in neurology. Eur J Neurol. 2022;29(6):1847-54.

CHAPTER 11

Chronic Inflammatory Demyelinating Polyradiculoneuropathy and its "Variants": Current Treatment Recommendations

Rakesh K Singh, Anuradha Mahto

ABSTRACT

The traditional therapies for typical chronic inflammatory demyelinating polyradiculoneuropathy (CIDP) are available since many years. It has not only proven effective in reducing the disabilities, but also helped characterize CIDP-mimics recently, which did not respond very well. Recent guidelines have stressed on using the objective scales for response documentation. The most used therapies, intravenous immunoglobulin (IVIg) and steroids, however, pose lot of practical difficulties. IVIg effectiveness is proven by randomized trials, but the high cost and need for prolonged usage appears impractical for regular use in our patients. Steroids benefits, backed by vast clinical experience, can cause side effects in the long run. The definition of various CIDP variants is still being elucidated. Their treatment meanwhile remains same as of typical CIDP.

In this chapter, we looked at various nuances of the two mainline therapies (IVIg and steroids) along with other immunosuppressives and attempted to find the cost-effective, yet evidence-based therapy, for our patients.

Keywords: Chronic inflammatory demyelinating polyneuropathy, Treatment, Intravenous Immunoglobulins, Monitoring.

INTRODUCTION

"Typical" chronic inflammatory demyelinating polyradiculoneuropathy (CIDP) is chronic, progressive (beyond 8 weeks), relapsing, sensory-motor, and weakness of limbs, both proximal and distal. The "variants" are phenotypically different but share with "typical" CIDP a common pathophysiology of macrophage mediated segmental demyelination and response to immunotherapy. Recent European Academy of Neurology/Peripheral Nerve Society guidelines have attempted to make the diagnosis more specific, but misdiagnosis is common, especially of "variants" CIDP. The treatment involves intravenous immunoglobulin (IVIg), plasma exchange (PLEX), and corticosteroids, with other immunosuppressives, as "sparing" agents. Addition of subcutaneous immunoglobulin (SCIg) is a boon to patients, but cost concerns remain. Choosing the most cost-effective treatment continues to pose a challenge. This chapter will cover various aspects of "typical" and "variant" CIDP treatment.

First-line therapies for CIDP include IVIg, steroids, and PLEX, for both induction and maintenance.[1] The goals of treatment are disability reduction and achieving long-term remission, without therapy. Counseling should be done about the prolonged course of treatment with fluctuations in weakness, risk of side effects, and need for a regular follow-up.

■ INTRAVENOUS IMMUNOGLOBULINS IN CHRONIC INFLAMMATORY DEMYELINATING POLYRADICULONEUROPATHY

Standard Guideline

Intravenous immunoglobulin is considered the main first-line treatment in CIDP. It got the Food and Drug Administration (FDA) approval in 2008, after the Intravenous CIDP Efficacy (ICE) trial.[2] Since then, multiple studies have confirmed both short- and long-term effectiveness of IVIG.[3,4] The standard dose advocated for induction (initial push, in a treatment naïve patient) is loading of 2 g/kg over 2–5 days, followed by maintenance of 1 g/kg every 3 weeks. More than half will improve (54% as per ICE trial)[2] significantly, as measured by objective disability scales, over the next 24 weeks. The benefits begin about 6–8 weeks into therapy[4] and are often sustained over prolonged periods, with continued injections. Once in remission or has stable deficits, without further worsening, the dose of IVIg is gradually tapered (20–25% reduction for subsequent doses), to total stoppage, unless relapse occurs. For 15%, one or two infusions are enough to enter remission,[5] but in general, 30% will achieve remission, over 12–15 months, which can persist for about 5 years, without any further treatment ("true" remission).[6]

Real-life Intravenous Immunoglobulin Usage

The real-life usage of IVIg in CIDP is different from standard advice. Attempts are being made to individualize the therapy, using different regimes, while maintaining effectiveness. While the loading dose of 2 g/kg remains standard and most effective in rapidly inducing the initial response (lower doses failing to do so), the maintenance doses may range from 0.4 to 2 g/kg every 2–6 weeks. It appears that lower, less frequent doses, used for shorter duration, may be noninferior to the standard regime.[7] Similarly, some patients may need more frequent infusions to control disease.[8,9] The wide range of effective maintenance doses for disease control is partly explained by the fact that the pharmacodynamics (and kinetics) of IVIg differs among patients. Also, it appears that the minimum threshold level of serum immunoglobulin G (IgG) needed for improvement, below which patient relapses, differs among patients.[10]

Concept of "Dosing Weight"

Given the fact that IVIg therapy is exorbitantly costly and is in limited supply, attempts to reduce the dosage have been made by using the "dosing weight (DW)", rather than the usual recorded weight, for calculating the IVIg dose. DW is equal to "ideal" body weight + 0.4 × (recorded weight – ideal body weight), where ideal body weight can be easily calculated as per height and weight of an individual. DW, often lesser, is considered clinically equivalent to the recorded weight, in CIDP treatment.[11,12] Use of DW would mean less IVIg dose requirement and so less cost burden and better safety.

Drawbacks of Intravenous Immunoglobulin Therapy

Despite high costs, IVIg remains the most sought-after therapy, not only as the initial choice (induction), in a treatment naïve patient, especially for rapid improvement of severe disability, but also for long-term "maintenance", due to better safety profile. However, it has few drawbacks which are as follows:
- *Not everybody responds*: Despite being highly recommended as the first-line therapy with an impressive number needed to treat (NNT) of three (need to give three IVIg courses for 1 improvement), if 10 patients are treated, only three will improve, two will improve spontaneously and approximately 4 will not respond, needing additional treatments. This certainly questions the cost effectiveness of IVIg therapy.[5]
- *Less chance of "true" remission*: With IVIg therapy, despite a robust short-term improvement, achieving "true" remission (meaning, a stable and improved deficits, without therapy) is difficult, in the long run. This results in prolonged and continuous IVIg therapy, with huge cost implications.[2,13]
- *"Wearing off" or treatment-related fluctuations*:[13] The serum levels of IgG fluctuate a lot with IVIg therapy. With peak levels soon after the infusion, it falls to very low toward the end of the month (half-life of IVIg is 3–4 weeks), just before the next dose. This "wearing off" may lead to clinical worsening, often needing increasing the infusion frequency to more than once a month or shifting to SCIg **(Fig. 1)**.

Mechanism of Action

Intravenous immunoglobulin, derived from normal healthy volunteers, comprises of unfractionated polyclonal IgG. Immunomodulatory actions include neutralization and inhibition of autoantibodies, abolition of activated complement, and alteration of FcR expression. Its limited supply advocates judicious use.[14]

Adverse Effects of Intravenous Immunoglobulin Therapy

The IVIg therapy is usually safe, even in the long term. Minor infusion-related reactions such as headaches, fever, chills, and flushing are common. Rarely, serious side effects

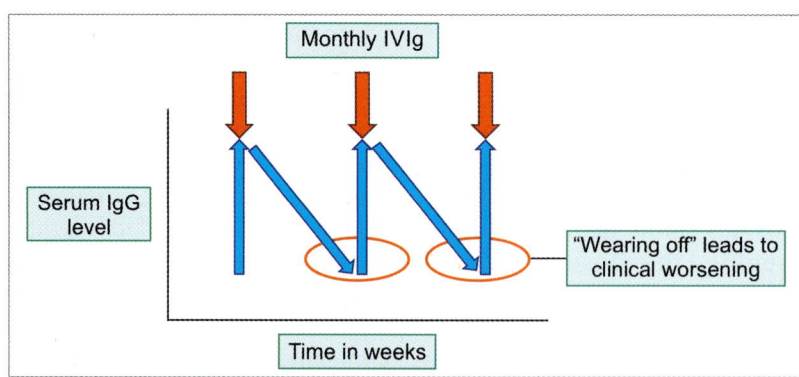

FIG. 1: "Wearing off" phase shown as red ovals, toward the end of the month, just before the next infusion. Inverted red arrows show the monthly IVIg infusion. Blue arrows show the rising and falling levels, toward the end of the month.
(IgG: immunoglobulin G; IVIg: intravenous immunoglobulin)

such as aseptic meningitis, renal failure, thromboembolism, and hemolysis can develop.[15] Caution should be exercised in patients with previous history of stroke or thrombosis.

Monitoring Treatment Response

In a suspected "clinical" CIDP (as per the clinical criteria of "typical" CIDP), documenting a "clinically meaningful improvement" or "an objective response" to a CIDP therapy, nearly confirms the diagnosis. It is considered a crucial supportive criterion for CIDP diagnosis.[1] Even without supportive electrophysiology, a "clinical" CIDP diagnosis can be upgraded to a "possible" CIDP, merely by showing an objective treatment response, in association with one or more other supportive criteria.[1] Relying on merely "subjectively" feeling better can lead to misdiagnosis of CIDP.[16]

When to assess the treatment response is also critical. CIDP therapies, including IVIg, may take a few months (usually <3 months or two to three IVIg infusions) to show the meaningful response, but should act by 6 months, if effective.[2,3] Too soon an evaluation would render an effective therapy erroneously labeled "ineffective". Failure to respond should prompt reconsidering the diagnosis but does not rule out CIDP.

Most of the studies use disability scales such as Inflammatory Neuropathy Cause and Treatment (INCAT) and Inflammatory Rasch-built Overall Disability Scale (I-RODS) **(Table 1)**, as primary outcome measure. INCAT is the oldest scale, developed in 2001, very easy to use in clinical settings, but like I-RODS, it is patient reported scale, so prone to flaws. Impairment scales such as Grip Dynamometer and Medical Research Council (MRC) sum score are clinician assessed scores. A minimal clinical important difference (MCID) is recorded and used as a cut-off to define improvement.[17]

■ SUBCUTANEOUS IMMUNOGLOBULINS IN CHRONIC INFLAMMATORY DEMYELINATING POLYRADICULONEUROPATHY

Subcutaneous immunoglobulin is the latest entry in CIDP therapeutics. Although it is being used for various immunodeficiency diseases since many years, FDA approval, as maintenance therapy in adults, came only in 2018, after the PATH study.[18] Patients who are already stabilized on IVIg can be given the option of shifting to weekly 0.2–0.4 g/kg SCIg (or the total monthly IVIg dose divided into weekly SCIg). Patients continue to remain

TABLE 1: Disability and impairment scales used in assessing improvement in CIDP.[17]

Scale	MCID	Remarks
INCAT	↓ > or =1 point	• UL and LL disabilities are scored on a 0–5 scale • Easy to use, but patient reported scale
I-RODS	↑ 4 points (raw score)	24-item questionnaires, scaled on 0–2 (0 being impossible to do). May not reflect all disabilities
Grip dynamometer	↑ 10% change	Useful for detecting "wearing off" phase. Average of three values used. Impractical for severe grip weak case
MRC SS	↑ 2–4 points	Total 60 (six paired muscle groups, three each in upper and lower limb). Poor interrater correlation

(CIDP: chronic inflammatory demyelinating polyradiculoneuropathy; INCAT: Inflammatory Neuropathy Cause and Treatment; I-RODS: Inflammatory Rasch-built Overall Disability Scale; LL: lower limb; MCID: minimal clinical important difference; MRC SS: Medical Research Council sum score; UL: upper limb)

in remission, more often with the higher dose (0.4 g/kg weekly) of SCIg. Later, the weekly dose can be reduced by 20–25% and slowly tapered off, unless relapse occurs. The decision to shift to SCIg should be an informed decision, based on either patient's preference or doctor's advice in case of difficult venous access or side effects or significant wearing off with IVIg.[19]

Although SCIg is tried as an initial treatment, with noninferior results, it is not approved for induction therapy, where IVIg is preferred.[20] Due to slow absorption from the subcutaneous site, it cannot help achieving the "rapid" and "higher" peak levels of serum IgG (about 30 g/dL), needed for the induction (or the initial "push"). However, for long-term maintenance therapy, clinical efficacy of SCIg is comparable to IVIg,[19] with the following advantages:

- Patient enjoys independent home therapy, without the need of venous access.
- Safety from infusion-related side effects of IVIg, such as headaches, nausea, and flu-like reactions. These reactions occur due to the rapid peak levels of serum IgG, after IVIg infusion. Risk of major side effects with IVIg such as thromboembolism, renal failure, aseptic meningitis, and hemolysis are rare with SCIg, but can still occur.
- SCIg is slowly absorbed from the subcutaneous site, thus maintains a "steady state" level of serum IgG throughout, thus avoiding the fluctuations and the "wearing off" worsening in weakness, seen often with IVIg therapy **(Fig. 2)**.

Overall, quality of life is better with SCIg. However, IVIg may be continued for those who are unable to self-administer due weakness or lack the self-drive. Some may still feel safe in hospital settings.

■ CORTICOSTEROIDS IN CHRONIC INFLAMMATORY DEMYELINATING POLYRADICULONEUROPATHY

Steroids are the least expensive and most widely used among the CIDP therapies. It was way back in 1958, when it was first shown effective,[21] but since then large retrospective series, observational studies, and clinical experience have confirmed its effectiveness. Despite lack of randomized controlled trials,[22] steroids continue to be the cornerstone of CIDP treatment, for both induction and maintenance.

Mechanism of action involves binding to the glucocorticoid receptor in the cytoplasm

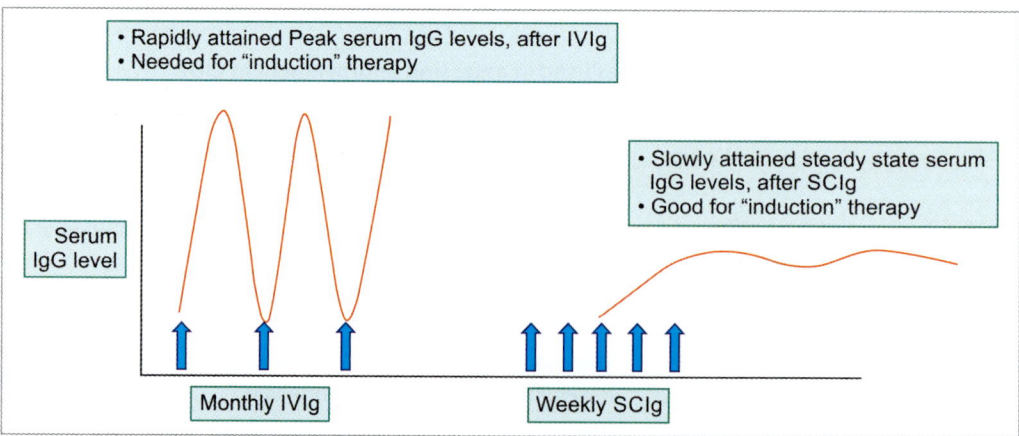

FIG. 2: Difference in serum immunoglobulin G (IgG) levels after intravenous immunoglobulin (IVIg) and subcutaneous immunoglobulin (SCIg) therapy.[19]

and altering the gene transcription inside nucleus, thus inhibiting the release of inflammatory mediators.

Three regimens are commonly used which are as follows:[1]
1. Oral daily prednisolone, 1–1.5 mg/kg, usually 60 mg (or 48 mg methylprednisolone) gradually tapered over 4–6 months. Higher initial doses like 120 mg daily have not shown any added benefit.
2. Pulsed oral dexamethasone, 40 mg daily for 4 days every month for 6 months.
3. Pulsed intravenous (IV) methylprednisolone, 500 mg daily for 4 days every month for 6 months.

Initial disability reduction is noted in about 60% patients (comparable to IVIg), similar with all three regimens. However, the "pulsed" regimens may induce more frequent and prolonged remission, compared to the daily steroids.[23] Also, the side effects are more in daily therapy, due to higher cumulative dose of steroids used. Daily calcium 600–800 mg with vitamin D supplementation is advised.

How do corticosteroids compare with intravenous immunoglobulin?
Intravenous immunoglobulin is preferred over steroids in the following situations:
- *In severe weakness*: In treatment naïve patient, guidelines do not favor either IVIg or steroids (or PLEX), as both induce similar improvement in disability in 60–70% cases.[24,25] But IVIg is preferred if weakness is severe and fast worsening, as it is rapidly effective. In case of no response to IVIg, steroids or PLEX can be used.[1]
- *For motor CIDP variant*: IVIg is the most recommended. Steroids-induced worsening of the motor variant CIDP is however debatable.
- In patients where steroids-induced side effect risks are considered high, especially development of osteoporosis and diabetes, IVIg is favored.

Are steroids a better long-term immunosuppressive?
It is in the ability to bring about more frequent long-term remission that steroids score over IVIg.[26] Long-term follow-up of initial treatment responders (approximately 50–60%) to immunotherapy, either IVIg or steroids, reveals that about 40% remain on treatment (treatment-dependent group) even after 1–2 years, while another 40% have gone into complete remission (treatment-withdrawal group). It is important to note that almost 79% in the "dependent" group were on IVIg responsive and 42% in the "withdrawal" group were on steroids **(Fig. 3)**. This implies that chances of remission are lesser with IVIg use and patients need to continue the therapy to prevent relapse.[26]

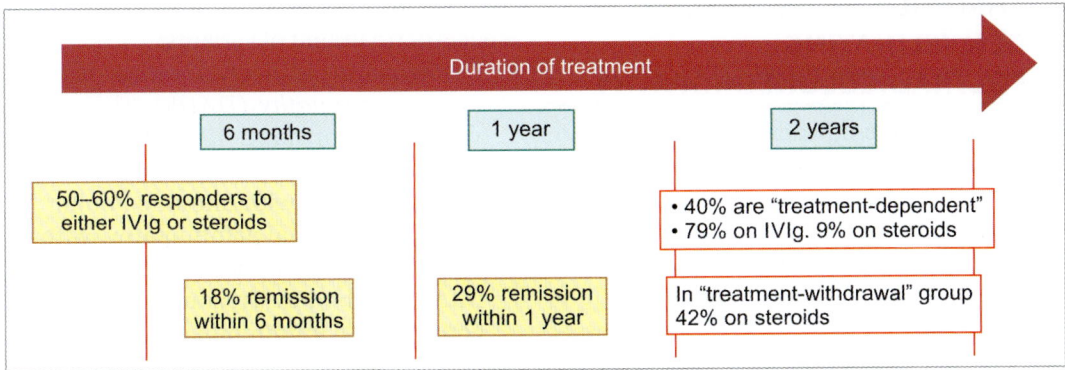

FIG. 3: Chances of remission with intravenous immunoglobulin (IVIg) compared to steroids.

Similar dependency on IVIg was noted in ICE trial,[2] where 45% relapsed when IVIg was withdrawn and converted to placebo (in 24 weeks extension phase). In a prospective randomized controlled trial,[12] 38% worsened when IVIg was withdrawn. Overall long-term remission rates with IVIg are around 26–40%, compared to impressive 61% with steroids.[27] Time to relapse after withdrawal of IVIg versus "pulsed" IV methylprednisolone, after improvement was found to be median 4.5 months and 14 months, respectively.[12] In the PREDICT study,[23] 40% were still in remission, 6 months after the steroid withdrawal. Thus, it appears that steroids are better long-term immunosuppressive, compared to IVIg. Steroid responsiveness is a predictor of long-term remission.

Combined Use of Steroids and Intravenous Immunoglobulin

Combining the rapid effectiveness of IVIg with better long-term remitting ability of steroids, a pilot study (OPTIC protocol) was done, in which both IVIg and IV methylprednisolone (1 g) were given as "combined" induction treatment, followed by 3 weekly infusions (of both) as maintenance, for 18 weeks. The results showed an impressive 60% remission rate, at the end of one year.

■ PLASMA EXCHANGE IN CHRONIC INFLAMMATORY DEMYELINATING POLYRADICULONEUROPATHY

Plasma exchange efficacy is comparable to IVIg and steroids for short-term benefits.[1] Usually, five cycles are done over 2 weeks, followed by twice weekly.[29] Long-term use is limited due to technical problems. PLEX is usually resorted to when the main first-line therapies fail.

■ OTHER IMMUNOSUPPRESSIVES

Azathioprine, mycophenolate, and cyclosporine can be used as immunoglobulin and steroid-sparing agents. Methotrexate may be useful.[1]

Rituximab is reserved for refractory cases only. Hematopoietic stem cell transplantation can be used as a last resort.[1]

■ SHORT- AND LONG-TERM PROGNOSIS

Overall, all three therapies (IVIg, steroids, or PLEX) are similar in efficacy, for short-term benefits.[1] The choice depends on the clinical factors, cost burden, and risk of side effects. Over the next 5 years, 26% will achieve total remission (with normal electrophysiology) and 61% will get "partial" remission (ambulatory) with (26%) or without (34%) treatment. 39% will remain chronically dependent on therapy. 13% will be severely disabled.[30]

■ TREATMENT OF CHRONIC INFLAMMATORY DEMYELINATING POLYRADICULONEUROPATHY "VARIANTS"

Understanding and treatment of CIDP variants are still evolving.[31] They are frequently misdiagnosed. Following are some aspects of treatment of variants:
- *Distal acquired demyelinating sensorimotor neuropathy (DADS)*: This distal variant, comprising 2–15% of CIDP, shares common phenotype of distal, predominantly sensory, with immunoglobulin M (IgM) monoclonal gammopathy, with or without myelin-associated glycoprotein (MAG) antibodies. Treatment response to conventional immunotherapy is excellent

(70–80% response rate).[32] It is important to rule out secondary causes of distal presentation, such as anti-MAG neuropathy and nodo-paranodopathies, due to therapy implications. Milder and nondisabling phenotypes are known to occur, which can be treated conservatively.

- *Multifocal acquired demyelinating sensory and motor neuropathy (MADSAM)*: MADSAM, the most common variant, usually shows excellent response to routine therapies (response rate of 56% with IVIg and 50% with prednisolone).[33] However, overall response is inferior, compared to typical CIDP.[30] Interestingly, different muscle groups may respond differently.
- *"Pure" sensory*: Controlled trials are lacking, but most respond to conventional immunotherapy.[34] Almost 70% of sensory variant will evolve into typical CIDP.[35]
- *"Pure" motor*: Pure motor CIDP closely mimics multifocal motor neuropathy (MMN) in having conduction blocks sans sensory abnormalities. Steroid resistance in motor CIDP is contentious. The reports of unresponsiveness or worsening with steroids,[36] may have inadvertently included cases of MMN, which is typically steroid resistant and can even worsen. Later studies did not substantiate steroid failure,[37] and in fact showed significant improvement.[31] The current, however, recommend IVIg as an ideal choice of treatment for pure motor variant, as distinction from MMN is clinically difficult.[1]
- *"Focal" CIDP*: Focal CIDP is a minimally understood variant with limited cases. But they respond regularly to treatment, like typical CIDP.[38] Long-term therapy is needed, as relapses are high.

Table 2 summarizes the "variants" treatment.

CASE VIGNETTE

A 74-year-old male, diabetic, came with 4 days of left foot drop, in October 2021. MRI showed enhancing cauda equina roots. Nerve conduction velocity (NCV) was inconclusive. 1 week later, left hand became weak with paresthesia, followed by right upper limb weakness. NCV now showed asymmetrical

TABLE 2: Summary of treatment and special considerations.

CIDP variants	Treatment and prognosis	Snippets
DADS	• Conventional immunotherapy • Prognosis is like CIDP	Regular hematological evaluation
MADSAM	• Conventional immunotherapy • Other agents—rituximab, cyclophosphamide, and azathioprine in refractory cases	Overall remissions and outcome inferior to CIDP
Pure sensory	Conventional immunotherapy and treatment response like CIDP	Most will convert to typical CIDP
Pure motor	IVIg is the first recommendation	Worsening with steroids debatable. Response better, if sensory affection present
Focal CIDP	Conventional immunotherapy, prognosis, and treatment response like CIDP	Relapse rate high, if therapy stopped

(CIDP: chronic inflammatory demyelinating polyradiculoneuropathy; DADS: distal acquired demyelinating sensorimotor neuropathy; IVIg: intravenous immunoglobulin; MADSAM: multifocal acquired demyelinating sensory and motor neuropathy)

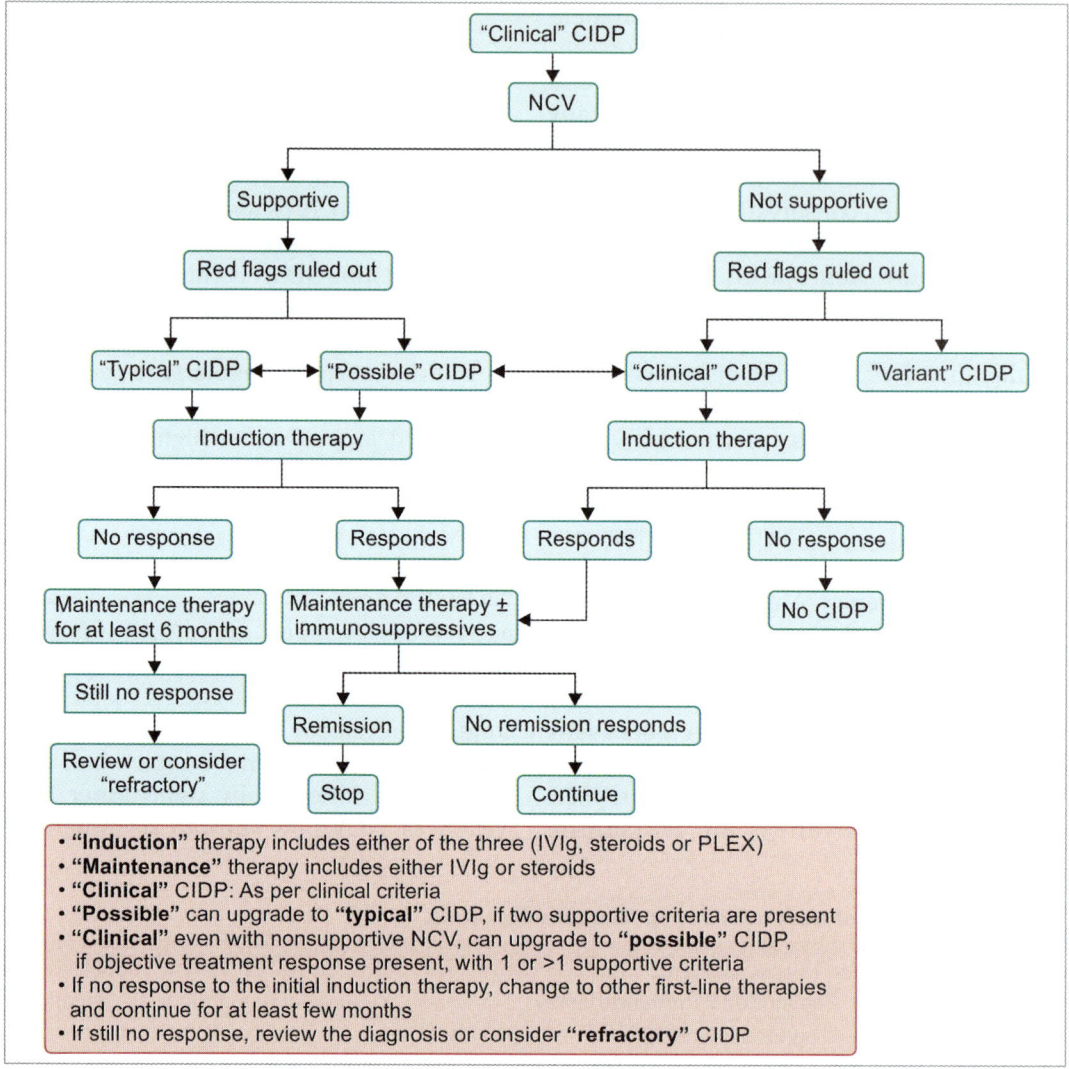

FLOWCHART 1: Chronic inflammatory demyelinating polyradiculoneuropathy (CIDP) therapy
(IVIg: intravenous immunoglobulin; NCV: nerve conduction velocity; PLEX: plasma exchange)

sensory-motor conduction blocks. Atypical CIDP of MADSAM type was suspected. Vasculitis panel, whole body positron emission tomography (PET), and lumbar puncture were all normal. He responded to IVIg, followed by steroids. Presently, he is in remission on low doses of steroids and mycophenolate.

Flowchart 1 depicts the bed-side approach to CIDP therapy.

CONCLUSION

It is quite evident that there is no difference between the therapies (IVIg or steroids or PLEX) in their ability to reduce the short-term disability. Either of them can be chosen as an initial treatment, depending upon the cost, comorbidities, and availability. Long-term remission appears clearly more likely with steroids usage, compared to IVIg. This fact, added to its low cost, easy availability, and ease of use, steroids can be considered as a cost-effective first-line option for our patients, with close monitoring of the potential side effects. IVIg (or PLEX) can be used as a "rescue" therapy for severe relapses. The availability of subcutaneous Ig for maintenance therapy, though costly, will surely improve the quality of life. There remain, however, many unmet needs in CIDP therapy, like management of "refractory" cases, which pose difficulties. As we continue to understand the disease better, novel treatment options will emerge to fill these gaps.

REFERENCES

1. Van den Bergh PYK, van Doorn PA, Hadden RDM, Avau B, Vankrunkelsven P, Allen JA, et al. European Academy of Neurology/Peripheral Nerve Society guideline on diagnosis and treatment of chronic inflammatory demyelinating polyradiculoneuropathy: report of a joint task force—second revision. J Peripher Nerv Syst. 2021;26(3):242-68.

2. Hughes RA, Donofrio P, Bril V, Dalakas MC, Deng C, Hanna K, et al. Intravenous immune globulin (10% caprylate chromatography purified) for the treatment of chronic inflammatory demyelinating polyradiculoneuropathy (ICE study): a randomised placebo-controlled trial. Lancet Neurol. 2008;7:136-44.

3. Léger JM, de Bleecker JL, Sommer C, Robberecht W, Saarela M, Kamienowski J, et al. Efficacy and safety of Privigen(*) in patients with chronic inflammatory demyelinating polyneuropathy: results of a prospective, single-arm, open label phase III study (the PRIMA study). J Peripher Nerv Syst. 2013;18:130-40.

4. Nobile-Orazio E, Pujol S, Kasiborski F, Ouaja R, Corte GD, Bonek R, et al. An international multicenter efficacy and safety study of IqYmune in initial and maintenance treatment of patients with chronic inflammatory demyelinating polyradiculoneuropathy: PRISM study. J Peripher Nerv Syst. 2020;25:356-65.

5. Eftimov F, Winer JB, Vermeulen M, de Haan R, van Schaik IN. Intravenous immunoglobulin for chronic inflammatory demyelinating polyradiculoneuropathy. Cochrane Database Syst Rev. 2013;(12):CD001797.

6. Gorson KC, van Schaik IN, Merkies ISJ, Lewis RA, Barohn RJ, Koski CL, et al. Chronic inflammatory demyelinating polyneuropathy disease activity status: recommendations for clinical research standards and use in clinical practice. J Peripher Nerv Syst. 2010;15(4):326-33.

7. Rajabally YA, Afzal S. Clinical and economic comparison of an individualised immunoglobulin protocol vs. standard dosing for chronic inflammatory demyelinating polyneuropathy. J Neurol. 2019;266(2):461-7.

8. Lunn MP, Ellis L, Hadden RD, Rajabally YA, Winer JB, Reilly MM. A proposed dosing algorithm for the individualized dosing of human immunoglobulin in chronic inflammatory neuropathies. J Peripher Nerv Syst. 2016;21:33-7.

9. Debs R, Reach P, Cret C, Demeret S, Saheb S, Maisonobe T, et al. A new treatment regimen with high-dose and fractioned immunoglobulin in a special subgroup of severe and dependent CIDP patients. Int J Neurosci. 2017;127:864-72.

10. Kuitwaard K, van Doorn PA, Vermeulen M, van den Berg LH, Brusse E, van der Kooi AJ, et al. Serum IgG levels in IV immunoglobulin treated chronic inflammatory demyelinating polyneuropathy. J Neurol Neurosurg Psychiatry. 2013;84:859-61.

11. Rajabally YA, Seow H, Wilson P. Dose of intravenous immunoglobulins in chronic inflammatory demyelinating polyneuropathy. J Peripher Nerv Syst. 2006;11:325-9.

12. Nobile-Orazio E, Cocito D, Jann S, Uncini A, Beghi E, Messina P, et al. Intravenous immunoglobulin versus intravenous methylprednisolone for chronic inflammatory demyelinating polyradiculoneuropathy: a randomised controlled trial. Lancet Neurol. 2012;11:493-502.

13. Allen JA, Pasnoor M, Dimachkie MM, Ajroud-Driss S, Brannagan TH, Cook AA, et al. Quantifying Treatment-Related Fluctuations in CIDP: Results of the GRIPPER Study. Neurology. 2021;96(14):e1876-86.

14. Arnson Y, Shoenfeld Y, Amital H. Intravenous immunoglobulin therapy for autoimmune diseases. Autoimmunity. 2009;42:553-60.

15. Orbach H, Katz U, Sherer Y, Shoenfeld Y. Intravenous immunoglobulin: Adverse effects and

safe administration. Clin Rev Allergy Immunol. 2005;29:173-84.
16. Allen JA. The Misdiagnosis of CIDP: A Review. Neurol Ther. 2020;9(1):43-54.
17. Allen JA, Eftimov F, Querol L. Outcome measures and biomarkers in chronic inflammatory demyelinating polyradiculoneuropathy: from research to clinical practice. Expert Rev Neurother. 2021;21(7):805-16.
18. van Schaik IN, Bril V, van Geloven N, Hartung HP, Lewis RA, Sobue G, et al. Subcutaneous immunoglobulin for maintenance treatment in chronic inflammatory demyelinating polyneuropathy (PATH): a randomised, double-blind, placebo controlled, phase 3 trial. Lancet Neurol. 2018;17(1):35-46.
19. Goyal NA, Karam C, Sheikh KA, Dimachkie MM. Subcutaneous immunoglobulin treatment for chronic inflammatory demyelinating polyneuropathy. Muscle Nerve. 2021;64(3):243-54.
20. Markvardsen LH, Sindrup SH, Christiansen I, Olsen NK, Jakobsen J, Andersen H; Danish CIDP and MMN Study Group. Subcutaneous immunoglobulin as first-line therapy in treatment-naive patients with chronic inflammatory demyelinating polyneuropathy: randomized controlled trial study. Eur J Neurol. 2017;24(2):412-8.
21. Austin JH. Recurrent polyneuropathies and their corticosteroid treatment; with five-year observations of a placebo-controlled case treated with corticotrophin, cortisone and prednisone. Brain. 1958;81(2):157-92.
22. Dyck PJ, O'Brien PC, Oviatt KF, Dinapoli RP, Daube JR, Bartleson JD, et al. Prednisone improves chronic inflammatory polyradiculoneuropathy more than no treatment. Ann Neurol. 1982;11(2):136-41.
23. Eftimov F, Vermeulen M, van Doorn PA, Brusse E, van Schaik IN; PREDICT. Long-term remission of CIDP after pulsed dexamethasone or short-term prednisolone treatment. Neurology. 2012;78:1079-84.
24. Viala K, Maisonobe T, Stojkovic T, Koutlidis R, Ayrignac X, Musset L, et al. A current view of the diagnosis, clinical variants, response to treatment and prognosis of chronic inflammatory demyelinating polyradiculoneuropathy. J Periph Nerv Syst. 2010;15:50-6.
25. Kuitwaard K, Hahn AF, Vermeulen M, Venance SL, van Doorn PA. Intravenous immunoglobulin response in treatment-naïve chronic inflammatory demyelinating polyradiculoneuropathy. J Neurol Neurosurg Psychiatry. 2015;86:1331-6.
26. Rabin M, Mutlu G, Stojkovic T, Maisonobe T, Lenglet T, Fournier E, et al. Chronic inflammatory demyelinating polyradiculoneuropathy: search for factors associated with treatment dependence or successful withdrawal. J Neurol Neurosurg Psychiatry. 2014;85:899-904.
27. van Lieverloo GGA, Peric S, Doneddu PE, Gallia F, Nikolic A, Wieske L, et al. Corticosteroids in chronic inflammatory demyelinating polyneuropathy: A retrospective, multicentre study, comparing efficacy and safety of daily prednisolone, pulsed dexamethasone, and pulsed intravenous methylprednisolone. J Neurol. 2018;265(9):2052-9.
28. Adrichem ME, Bus SR, Wieske L, Mohammed H, Verhamme C, Hadden R, et al. Combined intravenous immunoglobulin and methylprednisolone as induction treatment in chronic inflammatory demyelinating polyneuropathy (OPTIC protocol): a prospective pilot study. Eur J Neurol. 2020;27(3):506-13.
29. Mehndiratta MM, Hughes RA, Pritchard J. Plasma exchange for chronic inflammatory demyelinating polyradiculoneuropathy. Cochrane Database Syst Rev. 2015;2015(8):CD003906.
30. Kuwabara S, Misawa S, Mori M, Tamura N, Kubota M, Hattori T. Long- term prognosis of chronic inflammatory demyelinating polyneuropathy: a five year follow up of 38 cases. J Neurol Neurosurg Psychiatry. 2006;77:66-70.
31. Doneddu PE, Cocito D, Manganelli F, Fazio R, Briani C, Filosto M, et al; Italian CIDP Database study group. Atypical CIDP: diagnostic criteria, progression and treatment response. Data from the Italian CIDP Database. J Neurol Neurosurg Psychiatry. 2019;90(2):125-32.
32. Katz JS, Saperstein DS, Gronseth G, Amato AA, Barohn RJ. Distal acquired demyelinating symmetric neuropathy. Neurology. 2000;54(3):615-20.
33. Saperstein DS, Amato AA, Wolfe GI, Katz JS, Nations SP, Jackson CE, et al. Multifocal acquired demyelinating sensory and motor neuropathy: the Lewis-Sumner syndrome. Muscle Nerve. 1999;22:560-6.
34. Oh SJ, Joy JL, Kuruoglu R. "Chronic sensory demyelinating neuropathy": chronic inflammatory demyelinating polyneuropathy presenting as a pure sensory neuropathy. J Neurol Neurosurg Psychiatry. 1992;55:677-80.
35. van Dijk GW, Notermans NC, Franssen H, Wokke JH. Development of weakness in patients with chronic inflammatory demyelinating polyneuropathy and only sensory symptoms

at presentation: a long-term follow-up study. J Neurol. 1999;246(12):1134-9.
36. Donaghy M, Mills KR, Boniface SJ, Simmons J, Wright I, Gregson N, et al. Pure motor demyelinating neuropathy: deterioration after steroid treatment and improvement with intravenous immunoglobulin. J Neurol Neurosurg Psychiatry. 1994;57(7):778-83.
37. Kimura A, Sakurai T, Koumura A, Yamada M, Hayashi Y, Tanaka Y, et al. Motor-dominant chronic inflammatory demyelinating polyneuropathy. J Neurol. 2010;257:621-9.
38. Ayrignac X, Bienvenu SR, Morales R, Renard D, Labauge P. Focal CIDP presenting as chronic progressive monomelic sensory neuropathy. Muscle Nerve. 2013;47:143-4.

CHAPTER 12

Neuromuscular Imaging: MRI and Ultrasound

Lokesh Bathala, Y Muralidhar Reddy

ABSTRACT

Ultrasonography (USG) and magnetic resonance imaging (MRI) assessment of neuromuscular diseases add value to the traditional clinical and electrodiagnostic evaluation by providing important structural information about the nerves and muscles. Recent advancements in USG and MRI have made this assessment accurate and precise. Although USG is cost-effective, safe, convenient, repeatable, dynamic, and point-of-care, and offers excellent spatial resolution, the latter provides a distinct benefit in assessing structures at greater depths. This chapter reviews the application of both imaging techniques in different neuromuscular conditions.

Keywords: Ultrasonography, Magnetic resonance imaging, Neuromuscular disorders, Electrodiagnostics, Point-of-care imaging.

■ INTRODUCTION

Neuromuscular disorders (NMDs) are traditionally evaluated by clinical examination, electrodiagnostic, and pathological studies. However, the noninvasive structural evaluation of muscle and nerve, facilitated by ultrasonography (USG) and magnetic resonance imaging (MRI), is increasingly being used to complement these methods in the comprehensive evaluation of neuropathies, myopathies, and motor neuron diseases.[1,2] This chapter aims to provide the latest updates in the screening, diagnosis, and monitoring of NMDs by imaging.

■ BASIC PRINCIPLES OF NEUROMUSCULAR IMAGING

Ultrasonography

The USG transducer crystal uses the piezoelectric effect to create images of the bodily tissues. The differences in acoustic impedance at tissue boundaries determine the brightness of the image. Tissues such as bone appear white (hyperechoic), and fluids appear dark (hypoechoic). Linear arrayed transducers with an adjustable frequency range of 18–6 MHz are commonly used for neuromuscular imaging. Doppler imaging identifies direction-dependent blood flow. Power Doppler is direction-independent and is useful in detecting blood flow in nerves and muscles.[3] On axial view, nerves appear rounded structures with hypoechoic fascicles surrounded by hyperechoic perineurium and epineurium. This gives the appearance of a "honeycomb". On the longitudinal view, nerves appear as multiple hypoechoic streaks enclosed by hyperechoic epineurium **(Figs. 1A and B)**. Nerves inherently are less anisotropic than tendons, so they do not change echogenicity significantly with transducer tilt. Blood vessels are identified by their pulsatility, collapsibility, and presence of flow on color Doppler. Normal muscle on the USG appears anechoic (muscle fascicles) with hyperechoic speckles (intervening connective tissue). This gives a characteristic appearance of a "starry sky" **(Figs. 2A and B)**. The overall echogenicity of a muscle depends on factors such as age, gender, and body mass index.[3]

Magnetic Resonance Imaging

3T MRI is favored for nerve imaging because it has a higher signal-to-noise ratio, which improves temporal, spatial, and contrast resolution. The frequently used sequences are constructive interference in steady state (CISS) three-dimensional (3D) for

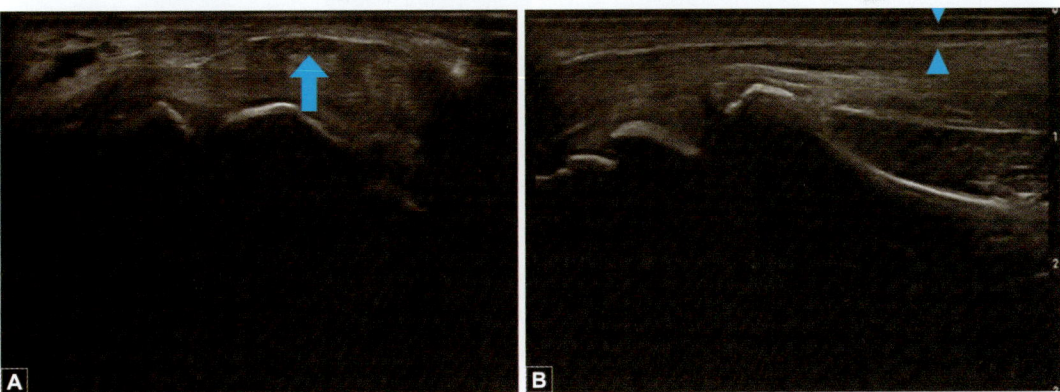

FIGS. 1A AND B: Ultrasound images showing the normal appearance of the median nerve at the wrist in axial (A) and longitudinal views (B).

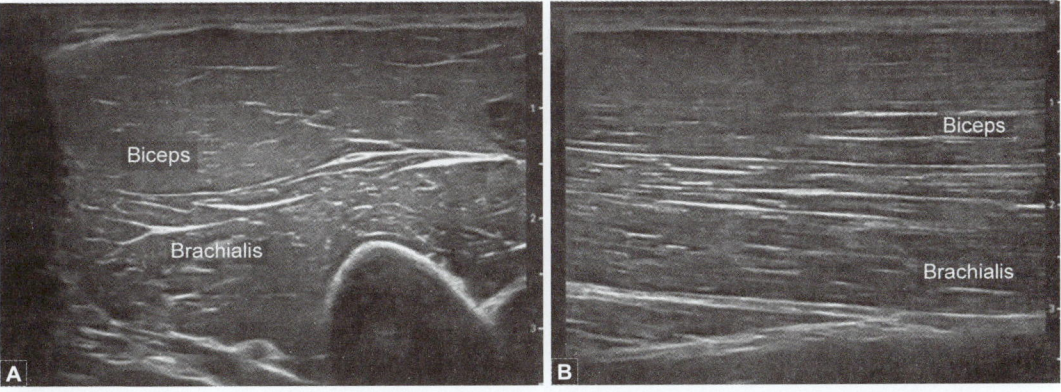

FIGS. 2A AND B: Ultrasound images showing normal biceps/brachialis muscle in axial (A) and longitudinal (B) views.

preganglionic segments, T2-weighted (T2W) sequences with fat suppression or short tau inversion recovery (STIR) for postganglionic segments, and T1-gadolinium sequences for any areas of nerve enhancement.[4] An optimal MRI protocol for muscle imaging typically consists of T1W and T2W sequences with fat suppression or STIR. Axial sections of the regions of interest are the mainstay of diagnosis; coronal sections may be acquired better to demonstrate any proximal-distal gradient in the involvement of muscles. Normal peripheral nerves are isointense to muscle, exhibit a fascicular pattern, and are often surrounded by a thin rim of adipose tissue **(Figs. 3A and B)**.[4] Normal skeletal muscle has an isointense signal on MRI, and it is used as a reference tissue to determine the signal properties of other tissues and organs. On T1, normal muscle looks hypointense **(Figs. 4A and B)**. T1W sequences assess the anatomy, muscle

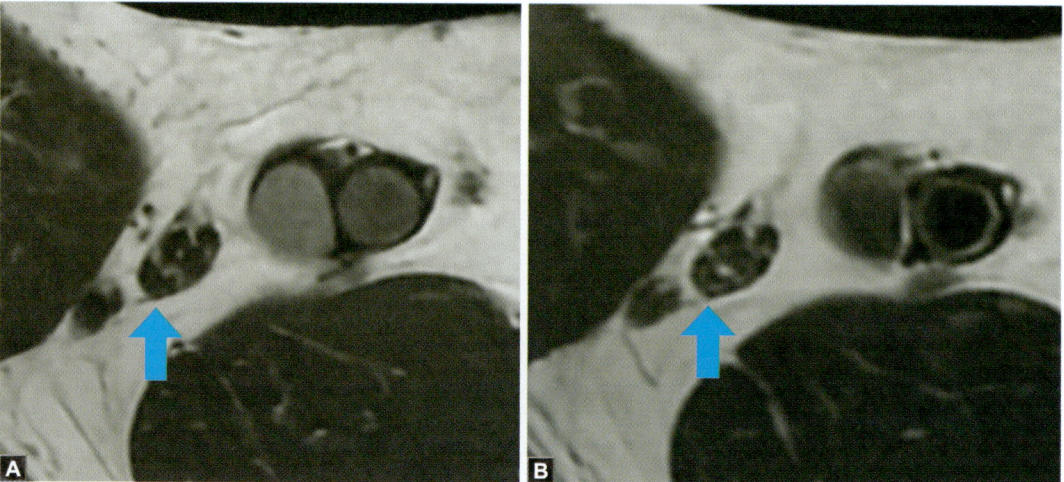

FIGS. 3A AND B: Normal appearance of the sciatic nerve (with two divisions) in the lower thigh on axial T2 (A) and T1 (B).

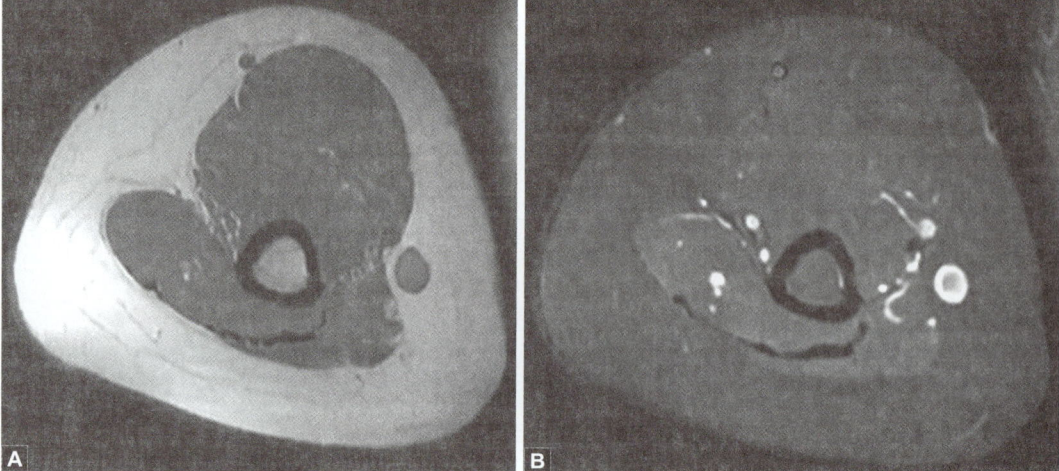

FIGS. 4A AND B: Normal appearance of arm muscles on axial T1 (A); and short tau inversion recovery (STIR) (B).

volume, and degree of fatty infiltration, and STIR or T2W sequences assess edema and ongoing inflammation.[2]

PARAMETERS OF INTEREST IN NERVE AND MUSCLE IMAGING

Nerve Imaging

The most important measure in USG is the cross-sectional area (CSA) of the nerve. It is measured within the hyperechoic rim with the transducer placed orthogonal to the nerve. Fascicular architecture and fascicle size are other parameters that indicate the amount of nerve damage. Intraneural vascularity, assessed through color or power Doppler, is another notable feature, especially in infectious neuritis.[3] The evaluation of structures around the nerve is an integral part of the evaluation of focal neuropathies. The most important measure in MRI is the nerve thickness along the peripheral nerve. Other parameters that point to an abnormal nerve are asymmetry and nonuniformity of nerve thickening, T2/STIR hyperintense signal, and contrast enhancement.

Muscle Imaging

On USG, muscle echogenicity is the most important parameter. Various methods are used to assess muscle echogenicity. The first technique is simply eyeballing the muscle on the USG. The second is the semiquantitative muscle grading per the four-point Heckmatt scale.[5] These two techniques have a sensitivity of around 70%. The third is a quantitative method based on the z-score of the gray-scale images of muscle. Apart from echogenicity, other notable parameters include muscle thickness and CSA. On MRI, the three important parameters are: (1) muscle bulk, (2) degree of fatty infiltration, and (3) T2/STIR hyperintensity. Noting preferentially involved and spared muscles can help to understand the disease pattern. The amount of fatty infiltration in each muscle is graded using a six-point Mercuri scale.[2]

FOCAL PERIPHERAL NEUROPATHIES

Entrapment Neuropathies

Peripheral nerves can get compressed at fibromuscular and fibro-osseous tunnels along the course, resulting in entrapment. This results in myelin disruption and microvascular damage. Imaging helps to identify the site and cause of compression. Although MRI is useful in assessing focal nerve regions, USG has a high-spatial resolution and provides dynamic details. The increase in nerve CSA and loss of fascicular architecture are the common USG features of entrapment. We discussed the most commonly encountered entrapment neuropathies in clinical practice here.

Carpal Tunnel Syndrome

Over the past decade, many studies have stressed the diagnostic value of USG in carpal tunnel syndrome (CTS).[6] The median nerve CSA with a cut-off of >11 mm^2 at the carpal tunnel showed high sensitivity and specificity in diagnosing idiopathic CTS **(Fig. 5)**.[7] However, this cut-off value

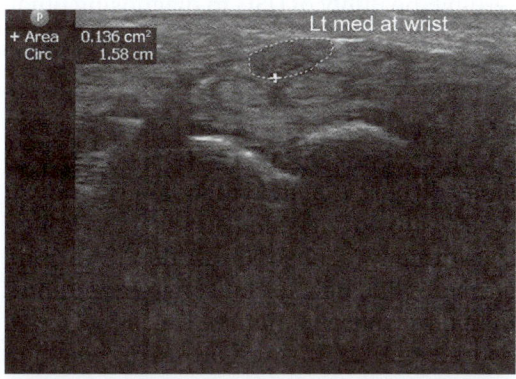

FIG. 5: Ultrasound axial image showing enlarged median nerve at the wrist in carpal tunnel syndrome (CTS).

does not apply to the Asian population, children, patients with bifid nerve **(Fig. 6)**, polyneuropathy, and those who underwent surgery.[8,9] Nerve enlargement correlates with the electrophysiological severity of CTS. The reliability of USG in diagnosing CTS is similar to electromyography (EMG).[10] Other well-studied USG parameters include the swelling ratio (CSA at the inlet/CSA at the outlet) and the flattening ratio (transverse diameter/anteroposterior diameter) of the median nerve at the wrist. Studies showed decreased sonoelasticity and increased intraneural vascularity in severe CTS. USG is helpful in postoperative cases with renewed or persistent symptoms. It can identify scar tissue, hematoma, and the transverse carpal ligament. It is also beneficial in detecting structural abnormalities in secondary CTS, such as bifid median nerve, persistent median artery, tenosynovitis, accessory muscle, and mass lesions. MRI has good sensitivity and specificity (over 85%) for diagnosing idiopathic CTS at a median nerve CSA cut-off >15 mm^2 at the carpal tunnel. A cut-off >19 mm^2 indicates severe CTS. MRI can also detect tumors, arthritis, and normal anatomical variants.

Ulnar Neuropathy

Extensive research has been published concerning the utility of USG in diagnosing ulnar nerve entrapment at the cubital tunnel, also known as ulnar neuropathy at the elbow (UNE).[11] The most reliable measure of UNE is the nerve enlargement at the tunnel, with a CSA >10 mm^2 **(Fig. 7)**.[12] In addition to nerve CSA, nerve diameter and the swelling ratio (CSA at the cubital tunnel/CSA above the medial epicondyle or mid-forearm) are also used.[13] They have comparable sensitivity and specificity to nerve CSA at the cubital tunnel. USG can also identify ganglion cysts, neuromas, and schwannomas. USG is of immense value in diagnosing ulnar nerve snapping during flexion movement at the elbow. Increased intraneural vascularity and fascicular effacement indicate severe UNE. USG can localize the disease in patients with nonlocalizable findings on electrodiagnostic studies. MRI in UNE may show nerve thickening, T2 hyperintensity, and denervation changes in innervated muscles.

The USG can be used to diagnose ulnar nerve entrapment at the wrist. However, systematic studies and disease-specific cut-off values are lacking. A focal increase in the nerve size at the wrist suggests entrapment. MRI is only indicated in patients with persistent symptoms following surgery or with a clinical suspicion of the tumor.

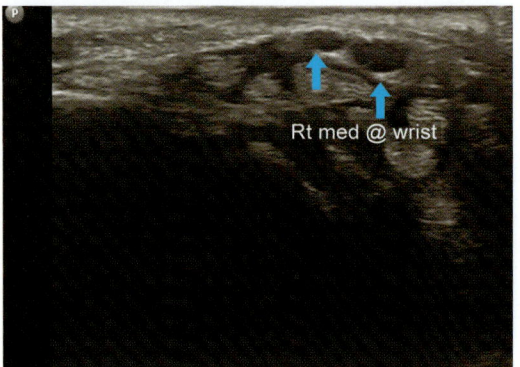

FIG. 6: Ultrasound axial image of Bifid median nerve (arrows) at the wrist.

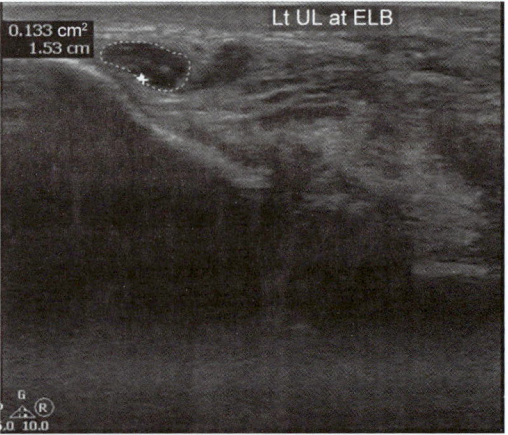

FIG. 7: Ultrasound axial image showing discrete enlargement of the ulnar nerve at the elbow.

Radial Neuropathy

The USG can diagnose radial neuropathy due to compression at the spiral groove and posterior interosseous nerve (PIN) entrapment at the arcade of Frohse.[14] CSA of the normal radial nerve ranges from 5 to 11 mm^2 at the spiral groove and 2–3 mm^2 for PIN and superficial radial nerve **(Figs. 8A and B)**. Normative data on radial nerve CSA in Indian subjects is lacking. An inter-side difference of >2 mm^2 or a focal size change is also considered significant. USG is more accurate than EMG and can aid in localization and finding the etiology. MRI helps to confirm the USG findings and provides additional details about the surrounding soft tissue. Muscle denervation edema or atrophy of muscles innervated by PIN distribution is the most common MRI finding in PIN entrapment. Compressive anatomical entities are often difficult to visualize with MRI.

Peroneal Neuropathy and Tarsal Tunnel Syndrome

The increased CSA of the common peroneal nerve at the fibular head and above on USG suggests entrapment of the nerve at the neck of the fibula.[15] USG can identify intraneural ganglion and schwannomas. Like other pressure palsies, nerve enlargement, high T2W signal intensity, and loss of fascicular architecture are the MR findings of peroneal entrapment. MRI can also help to identify mass lesions.

Tarsal tunnel syndrome has long been controversial due to the lack of a good diagnostic test. However, several studies have shown USG to be more sensitive and specific than often technically challenging EMG. USG-measured nerve CSA of the posterior tibial nerve at the tarsal tunnel seems reliable. An interside difference in CSA of >2 mm^2 is an important criterion.[16]

Traumatic Neuropathies

Both USG and MRI are highly effective for imaging peripheral nerve injuries. On USG, traumatized nerves appear enlarged and hypoechoic with an effaced fascicular pattern. Traumatic neuroma typically appears as a fusiform-shaped structure with varying echogenicity **(Fig. 9)**. The traumatized nerves appear enlarged on MRI with hyperintense or heterogenous signal intensity on T2W

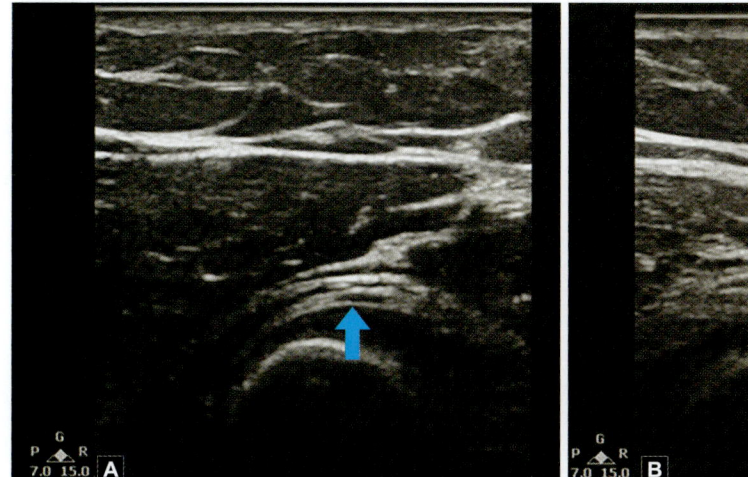
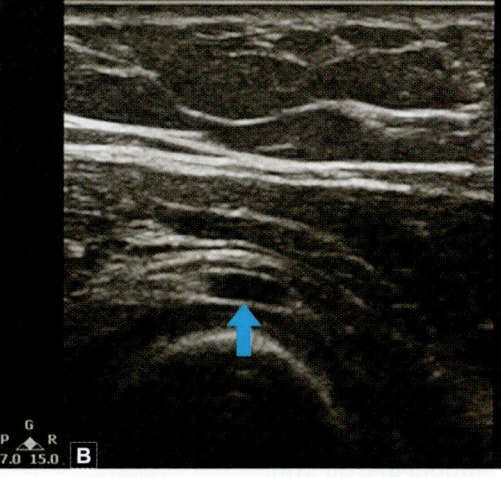

FIGS. 8A AND B: Ultrasound axial image showing normal (A), and enlarged posterior interosseous nerve (B) (arrows).

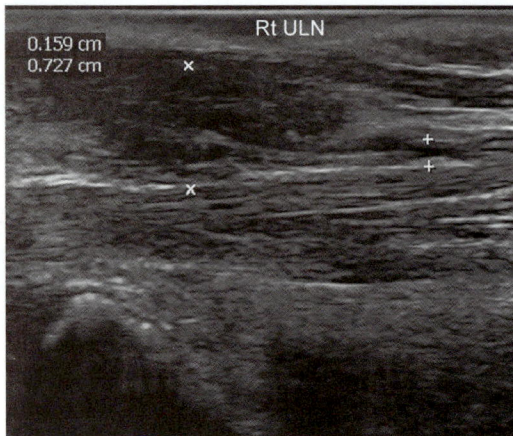

FIG. 9: Ultrasound longitudinal image showing right ulnar nerve in the distal forearm with neuroma in continuity in a patient due to glass cut injury.

sequences. Neuroma appears fusiform, with a heterogenous signal on T2, and does not show contrast enhancement. Denervated muscles either show a bright T2 signal or atrophy and fatty infiltration, depending on the disease duration. In the early phase of trauma, imaging has replaced EMG. USG is widely available and can be easily performed at the bedside; MRI provides better visualization of deeper nerves and plexuses. Both can accurately locate and identify the nature of the injury and can give beneficial information to the surgeon. It is essential to assess nerve size, continuity, and surrounding tissues for abnormalities, including foreign bodies and hematoma, and screen proximal and distal nerve segments. Differentiating between neuropraxia and axonotmesis can be challenging if edema disrupts the internal fascicular structure. Furthermore, an overlying hematoma can complicate the USG assessment of nerve integrity. USG can be handy when susceptibility artifacts due to metal plates and screws obscure the injured nerve in MRI. Other bony and soft-tissue abnormalities are better visualized and reproducible on MRI.[10]

Nerve Tumors

Here, we discussed the commonly encountered peripheral nerve tumors in clinical practice. The location, size, and shape of the tumor, MRI signal changes and enhancement pattern, and vascularity on USG are important diagnostic clues.[17]

Pseudotumors

Traumatic neuromas appear as globular lesions with heterogeneous echogenicity. *Morton's neuromas* appear as sharply demarcated, homogeneous, hypoechoic, and fusiform lesions in continuity with the digital plantar nerve. MRI and USG are comparable in sensitivity and specificity. *The intraneural ganglion* appears as a sharply demarcated cyst with preserved fascicular architecture and no vascularity. It is closely related to the intra-articular branch. MRI can depict the intraneural ganglia.

Benign Tumors

Neural lipomatosis appears as a fusiform nerve thickening, enlarged fascicles surrounded by fat without any vascularity. *Schwannoma* appears as a void hypoechogenic mass with smooth contour, sharp boundaries, and displacement of fascicular structures **(Figs. 10A to E)**. MRI features include split-fat and fascicular signs. *Neurofibromas* appear as a fusiform mass, homogeneous, or inhomogeneous, with lobulated boundaries and a target sign. Small nodular lesions are well capsulated. Cysts are also found in some neurofibromas. MRI shows similar shape aspects, with inhomogeneous signals on T1 and a target sign on T2.

Malignant Tumors

Malignant peripheral nerve sheath tumors appear as large fusiform masses, heterogeneous echogenicity, irregular cystic necrotic degeneration, calcifications, internal bleeding,

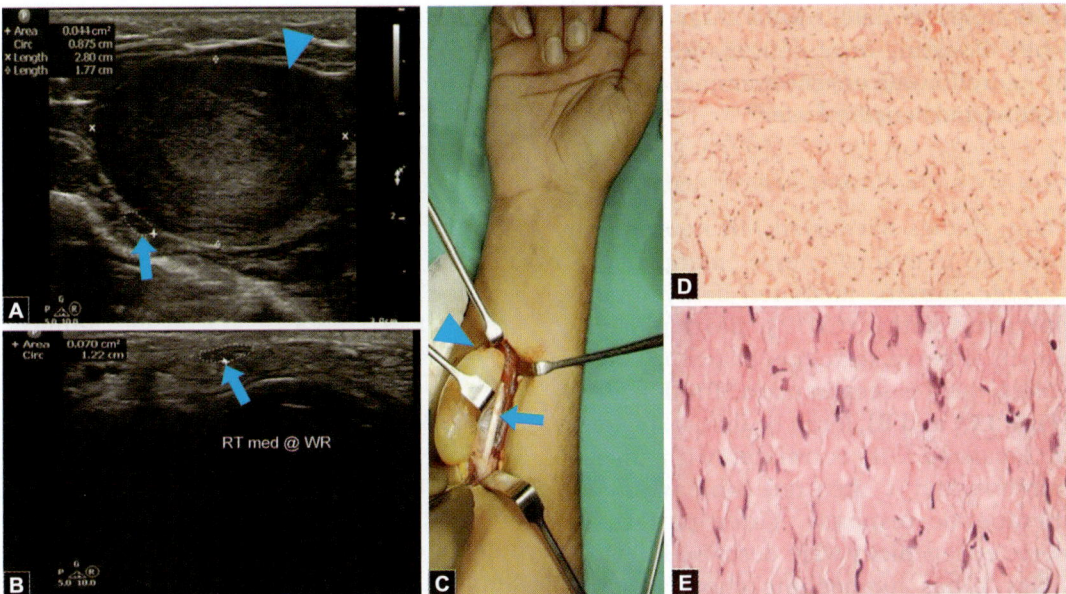

FIGS. 10 A TO E: Ultrasound axial images of neurofibroma (arrow head) compressing median nerve at 7'O clock position (arrow) (A); The normal appearance of the median nerve at the wrist (B); Pero-operative photograph showing neurofibroma arising from median nerve (C); Histopathological pictures showing elongated cells over a collagenous background in low and high-power view (D and E).

heterotopic tissue, and hypervascularization. USG characteristics of *neurolymphomatosis and carcinoma metastasis* in peripheral nerves are not specific. The sensitivity of nerve USG for tumor infiltration detection is unknown. MRI can aid in diagnosis.

■ POLYNEUROPATHIES

Inherited Neuropathies

Charcot–Marie–Tooth (CMT), hereditary neuropathy with pressure palsies (HNPP), and neurofibromatosis (NF) are the most extensively studied hereditary neuropathies. USG is potentially an effective screening method for genetic demyelinating CMT mutations, especially CMT1A. Peripheral nerves and plexuses frequently exhibit nerve expansion across their whole length.[18] USG, therefore, can serve as an excellent tool for screening children suspected to have CMT1A or relatives of genetically confirmed patients.

Patients with CMT1B show nerve enlargement, but the degree of enlargement is not as significant as that of CMT1A.[19] USG can help determine the efficacy of immunomodulatory treatment in CMT-overlapping neuropathies. In addition to nerve enlargement, CMT1 may show fascicular enlargement and hypoechogenicity. Multiple MRI studies on demyelinating CMT variants have identified similar patterns of nerve thickening. In cases with axonal CMT, there is a limited increase in the size of nerves, but certain groups of nerve fibers may undergo enlargement. HNPP is distinguished by a unique pattern of nerve enlargement at sites of nerve compression.[19] USG helps detect nerve enlargements, schwannomas, and neurofibromas in individuals with NF1 and NF2. Although USG helps to monitor nerves in NF, it is crucial to acknowledge that MRI is preferable since it enables evaluation of both the central and peripheral nervous systems. However,

USG helps to detect individuals with NF while assessing focal neuropathies caused by neurofibroma or schwannoma, offering a distinct and beneficial use.[20]

Immune-mediated Neuropathies

Many studies have used MR neurography and USG to evaluate nerve enlargement in chronic immune-mediated demyelinating polyneuropathy (CIDP), particularly in proximal nerve segments and roots. Nerve enlargement is seen in up to 90% of patients **(Figs. 11A and B)**. It can be diffuse, regional, or localized.[21] It correlates with disease duration and is often reversible with good therapeutic response. Three patterns of nerve echogenicity were described in CIDP. Class 1 has hypoechoic characteristics, class 2 has a mixed pattern with hypoechoic and hyperechoic fascicles, and class 3 has minimal or no nerve enlargement. Patients with class 3 patterns respond poorly to therapy, and those with class 1 architecture respond well. The pattern of nerve enlargement in paranodopathies is similar to that of CIDP. However, the literature on this is very limited.[22] Patients with Lewis–Sumner syndrome (LSS) have a similar pattern to CIDP but with a greater degree of asymmetry in distribution and sometimes involving distal nerve segments. Nerve enlargement may regress with successful therapy.[23] Multifocal motor neuropathy (MMN) must be differentiated from amyotrophic lateral sclerosis (ALS) and pure motor CIDP. In MMN, nerve enlargement is usually isolated and involves few fascicles, contrary to LSS and CIDP. Identifying multifocal nerve enlargement also helps to distinguish it from ALS.[24] Most patients with Guillain–Barré syndrome (GBS) show cervical nerve root and vagus nerve enlargement. The latter correlates with autonomic dysfunction. Nerve root enlargement decreases within 3 months after successful treatment.[25] The nerve enlargement pattern resembles CIDP in immunoglobulin M (IgM) paraproteinemia and antimyelin-associated glycoprotein (MAG).[26] MRI is of immense value in chronic immune sensory polyradiculoneuropathies and related diseases, which show thickened and enhancing nerve roots.[27]

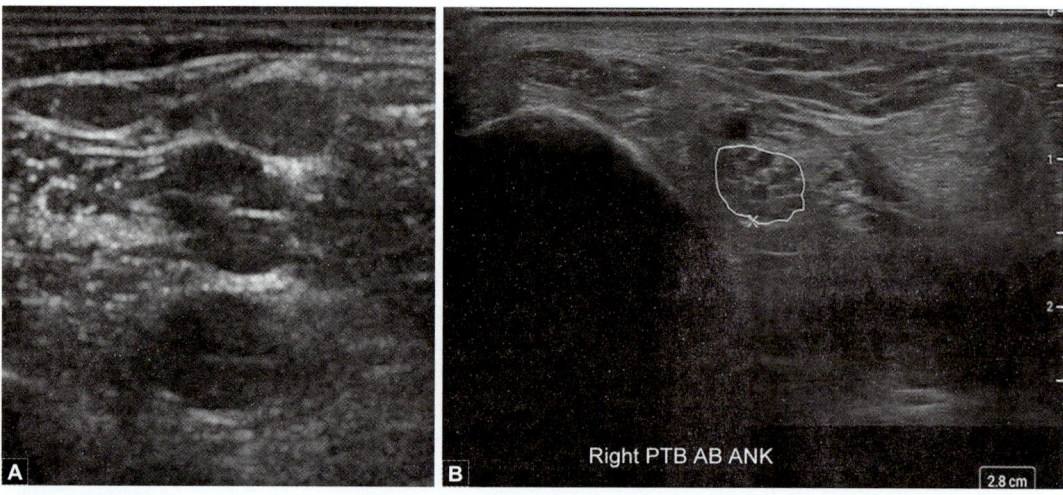

FIGS. 11A AND B: Axial ultrasound images showing enlarged brachial plexus trunks (A) and posterior tibial nerve with fascicular enlargement (B) in a patient of chronic immune-mediated demyelinating polyneuropathy (CIDP).

Leprosy

The USG is superior to clinical examination alone in identifying abnormal nerves in leprosy.[28] It can help to identify clinically silent neuropathy. Leprosy usually causes fusiform nerve enlargements, a few centimeters proximal to fibro-osseous canals, such as the ulnar sulcus and carpal tunnel **(Fig. 12)**.[29,30] Nerve thickening is more prevalent in patients with paucibacillary leprosy, lepra reactions, and longer disease duration. USG also reveals isolated anechoic regions suggestive of abscesses. In addition to nerve enlargement, one may see hypoechoic fascicles, disruption of fascicular architecture, thickened epineurium, and abnormally increased intraneural and perineural vascularity. Increased vascularity correlates with disease activity **(Fig. 13)**.[31] MRI is very helpful to detect plexus involvement **(Figs. 14A and B)**.

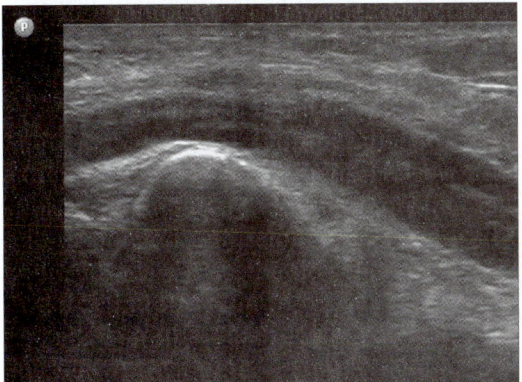

FIG. 12: Longitudinal ultrasound image showing enlarged posterior tibial nerve at the ankle in leprosy.

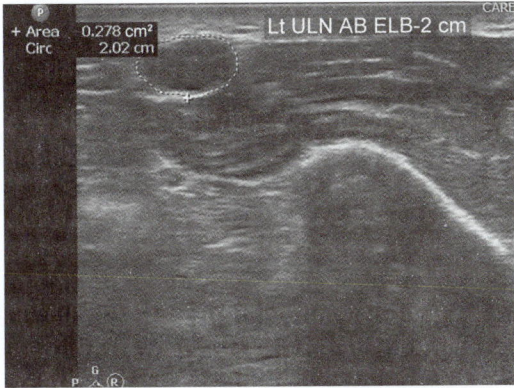

FIG. 13: An axial ultrasound image showing an enlarged ulnar nerve in the arm above the medial epicondyle with completely effaced fascicular architecture in a patient with Hansen's disease.

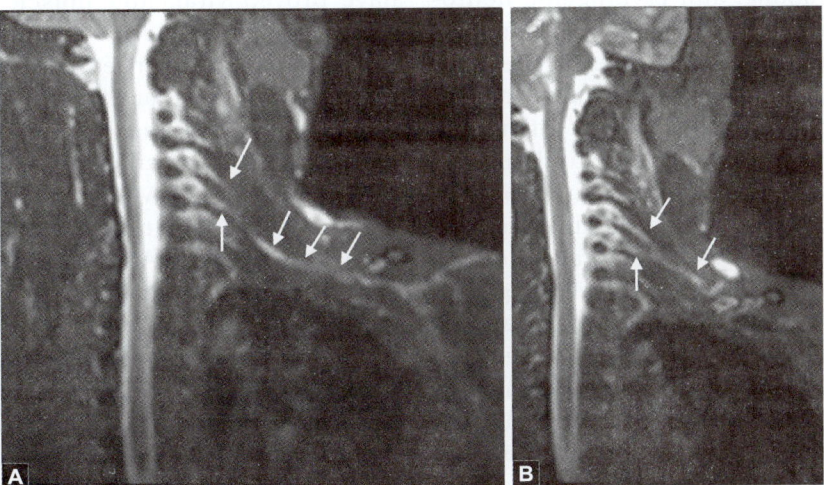

FIGS. 14A AND B: Oblique reconstruction of 3D short tau inversion recovery (STIR) showing the formation and course of left upper trunk and roots (A); upper trunk shows prominent thickening and hyperintensity approaching the signal intensity of vascular structures (B) in a patient with Hansen's disease.

Diabetic Neuropathies

Diabetic neuropathies (DNs) constitute a significant subset of peripheral neuropathies, yet USG literature is scarce. Some authors report no nerve enlargement in DN, apart from entrapment sites. Some authors report an increase in nerve size, depending on the severity and glycated hemoglobin. However, nerve enlargement in DN never exceeds the upper limit of the normal range.[32] Significant nerve enlargements beyond the usual entrapment locations in a patient with diabetes may indicate non-DN.

Vasculitis Neuropathies

Multifocal thickening of peripheral nerves can also be seen in vasculitis-associated neuropathy (systemic and nonsystemic). The plexus often appears to be spared, and parts of the enlarged nerves may also show intraneural vascularity. In suspected vasculitis-associated neuropathy, including the sural nerve in the USG examination may be useful in locating the site for biopsy.[33]

Miscellaneous

Toxic, metabolic, and cryptogenic neuropathies are mostly axonal and do not show nerve enlargement or changes in the USG. Studies in chemotherapy-induced neuropathies are inconsistent. Patients with taxane treatment showed smaller sural nerves, while oxaliplatin-treated patients showed a slight increase. Neurodegenerative diseases showed small nerves, and storage diseases often showed nerve enlargement **(Fig. 15)**. Studies showed nerve enlargement in proximal segments and plexus, suggesting USG is an important tool for early treatment of transthyretin amyloidosis. Finally, multifocal thickenings of nerves and/or plexuses can also occur in neuralgic amyotrophy, diabetic amyotrophy, sarcoidosis, and neurolymphomatosis. However, literature on all these disorders is limited to case reports.

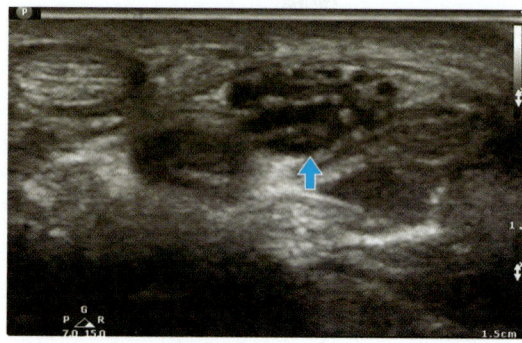

FIG. 15: Ultrasound axial image showing enlarged median nerve (arrow) at the wrist in a child with mucopolysaccharidosis.

■ AMYOTROPHIC LATERAL SCLEROSIS

Amyotrophic lateral sclerosis is diagnosed using the revised El Escorial and Awaji-Shima criteria. Clinical examination and electrodiagnostic testing are insensitive to early diagnosis and tracking the longitudinal progression of ALS. USG offers considerable promise as a point-of-care tool for nerve and muscle imaging, potentially revolutionizing ALS diagnosis and monitoring.[34]

When diagnosing ALS, fasciculations have proven vital, and muscle USG has emerged as the superior method for their detection, surpassing needle EMG. Research has demonstrated that USG offers a broader field of view than needle EMG, leading to more accurate detection rates. Combined muscle USG and EMG have significantly increased the diagnostic sensitivity for probable or definite ALS.[35] Muscle USG can also assess both muscle quantity and quality in ALS. Muscle quantity is measured by Echo intensity (EI). Muscle quantity is measured by muscle thickness and CSA. The potential of USG-measured muscle quantity and quality measures to enhance ALS diagnosis and track disease progression is encouraging. Greater baseline EI values were shown to predict shorter survival. USG-measured muscle thickness, EI, and fasciculations

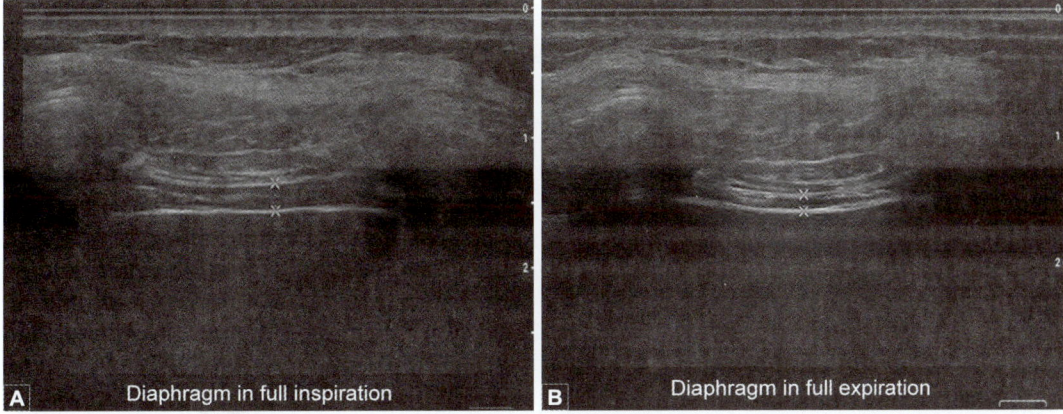

FIGS. 16A AND B: Diaphragmatic ultrasound showing diaphragm thickness in maximal inspiration (A) and expiration (B) in a patient with ALS.

might also predict ALS survival. Respiratory and diaphragmatic muscle weakness is a major cause of ALS mortality. Diaphragmatic USG can identify respiratory insufficiency. Studies have shown a correlation between USG-measured diaphragmatic thickness and thickening ratio with the vital capacity and partial pressure of carbon dioxide. However, not all studies have been encouraging **(Figs. 16A and B)**.

■ MYOPATHIES

Muscle Ultrasound

Muscle ultrasound is a widely used screening tool for NMDs, particularly in children. It has a good positive predictive value in detecting the presence of an NMD.[36] It can detect changes in echogenicity across the ages in various NMDs, such as Duchenne muscular dystrophy, congenital myopathies, Pompe disease, facioscapulohumeral dystrophy (FSHD), inflammatory myopathies, spinal muscular atrophy, and ALS.

Muscle fibers are replaced by fat and fibrosis in muscular dystrophies. These changes are reflected on USG as homogenously increased echogenicity with loss of architectural features, giving a "rubbed paper" or "ground-glass" appearance **(Fig. 17)**.

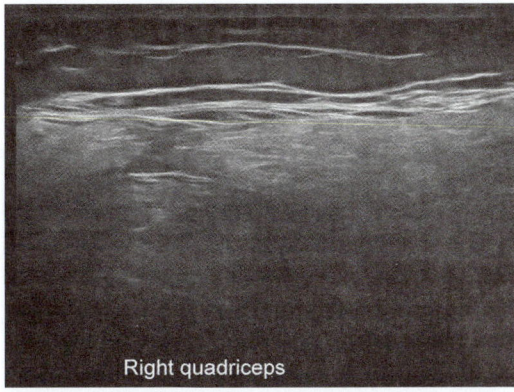

FIG. 17: Ultrasound image showing the patchy hyperechogenicity in a patient with dermatomyositis.

These changes may be found in specific regions of muscle that expand with disease progression or the entire muscle. Atrophy is a variable feature in muscle dystrophies. Inflammatory myopathies show features of edema and focal hypoechogenic areas in the initial phases, giving a "see-through" appearance **(Fig. 18)**. With progression, entire muscle could be involved. USG findings can identify occult muscle involvement. USG is useful in locating the site for performing biopsy in inflammatory myopathies. Studies have shown that muscle echogenicity can be reversible with successful treatment in dermatomyositis, and USG findings can also be used to assess clinical disease activity.[37]

Inclusion body myositis (IBM) involves the selective involvement of quadriceps, gastrocnemius, and flexor digitorum profundus, which can be readily appreciated in the USG.[38] Muscle ultrasound is used for diagnosing and monitoring connective tissue diseases such as deep morphea, myositis, and systemic lupus erythematosus. Neurogenic disorders have a variable appearance in the USG, depending on the severity of axonal loss and the extent of reinnervation. Patients with denervation and incomplete reinnervation characteristically show a "moth-eaten" pattern.

Textural analysis, machine learning, contrast-enhanced USG, and elastography techniques are promising for evaluating muscle quality in myositis. The USG is a valuable tool for studying muscle diseases, allowing targeted tissue acquisition and noninvasive assessment of muscle skeletal architecture. However, challenges such as operator dependence, subjectivity, and inadequate knowledge hinder its widespread use.

Muscle Magnetic Resonance Imaging

Muscle MRI has limitations in distinguishing between types of inflammatory myopathy. T2/STIR hyperintensity is the notable finding.[2] Dermatomyositis may show calcinosis in the subcutaneous tissue in addition to muscle involvement. Necrotizing autoimmune myopathy affects predominantly proximal and axial muscles with prominent edema. In contrast, IBM shows fatty infiltration of muscles, especially the flexor digitorum profundus, quadriceps, and gastrocnemius **(Figs. 19A and B)**.[2] Some patients with sarcoidosis show nodular muscle involvement.

Dystrophinopathies typically affect the glutei and adductor magnus muscles, but the sartorius and gracilis muscles are spared. In more advanced stages, it might show involvement of the quadriceps and biceps femoris muscles. The gastrocnemius and peroneus longus muscles are mostly affected in the leg, whereas the tibialis anterior

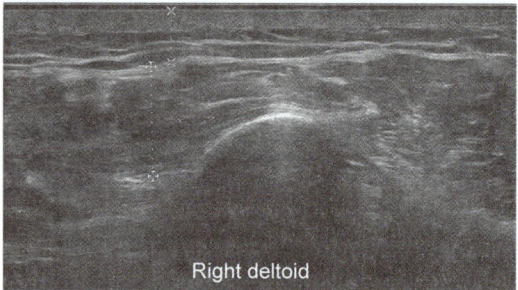

FIG. 18: Ultrasound image showing "ground glass appearance" of vastus lateralis in a patient with dysferlinopathy.

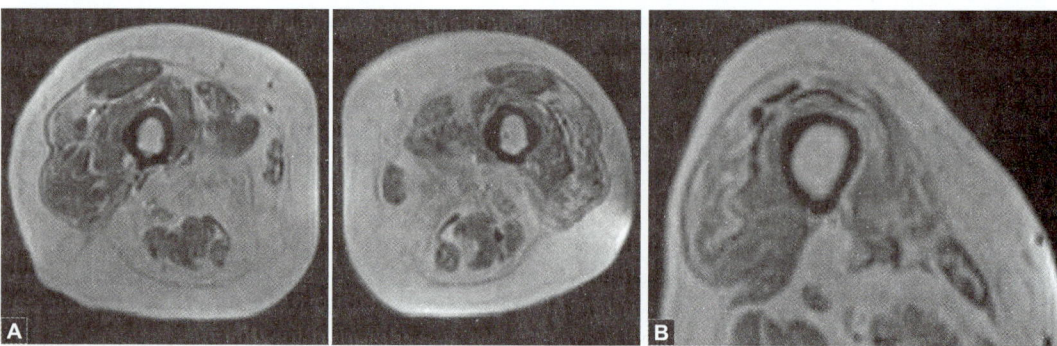

FIGS. 19A AND B: Magnetic resonance imaging (MRI) thigh shows severe fatty infiltration of the bilateral posterior and anterior compartment.

muscle remains unaffected. Myotonic dystrophy type I is characterized by the selective involvement of the flexor digitorum profundus in the upper limb and the gastrocnemius and soleus in the lower limb. The tibialis anterior is affected to a lesser extent, whereas the tibialis posterior remains unaffected. The quadriceps femoris muscles are involved, particularly the regions closer to the femur. FSHD mostly affects the pectoralis, periscapular, and leg muscles. MRI reveals the involvement of semimembranosus in the thigh and the medial gastrocnemius and tibialis anterior muscles in the leg. The deltoid, supraspinatus, infraspinatus, and subscapularis muscles are usually unaffected.[39]

While MRI cannot discriminate between different kinds of limb–girdle muscular dystrophy (LGMD), it can be highly useful in differentiating LGMD from other myopathies. They mostly affect proximal upper and lower limb muscles. Hamstrings, adductors, and glutei are primarily affected in most LGMDs, including those related to mutations in calpainopathy, dysferlinopathy, anoctaminopathy, and fukutin-related protein (FKRP) myopathy. Calf muscles are most affected in the leg, except for FKRP-related muscular dystrophy, where the involvement is diffuse. Sarcoglycanopathies have a distinct pattern, with leg muscles being unaffected. They show a distal-to-proximal gradient with the distal part of the vastus lateralis spared. The quadriceps, adductor magnus, and glutei are the initial and most severely affected muscles.[40]

Diverse genes, such as *SELENON*, *collagen VI*, and *RYR1*, cause congenital myopathies and muscular dystrophies, each associated with distinct MRI findings. SELENON-related myopathies affect the semimembranosus, sartorius, and sternocleidomastoid. Preferential involvement of the periphery of the muscles (vastus, gastrocnemius, and soleus) gives a characteristic appearance of "tigroid or rolled cake" in collagen VI-related myopathies. In contrast, protein-O-glucosyltransferase 1-related myopathy shows the involvement of the central part of the muscles and sparing of the periphery. RYR1 mutations result in varied clinical phenotypes, but muscle involvement on MRI looks similar. Myofibrillar myopathies are related to Z-disk-associated protein aggregation. Despite clinical and pathological similarities, they exhibit different imaging patterns. Desminopathies mainly affect the peroneal muscles, while myotilinopathies involve the posterior compartment.[40]

■ CONCLUSION

Both MRI and USG are highly effective for imaging peripheral nerves and muscles. Neuromuscular imaging is sometimes diagnostic but more often reveals patterns that help to narrow down the differential and aid in assessing the disease progression and treatment response. While USG is easy to perform, convenient, cost-effective and offers high spatial resolution, MRI is superior in evaluating deeper and proximal nerves and surrounding soft tissues.

REFERENCES

1. Goedee HS, van der Pol WL, Hendrikse J, van den Berg LH. Nerve ultrasound and magnetic resonance imaging in the diagnosis of neuropathy. Curr Opin Neurol. 2018;31(5):526-33.
2. Nicolau S, Naddaf E. Muscle MRI for Neuromuscular Disorders. Pract Neurol. 2020:27-32.
3. van Alfen N, Mah JK. Neuromuscular ultrasound: A new tool in your toolbox. Can J Neurol Sci. 2018;45(5):504-15.
4. Jung JY, Lin Y, Carrino JA. An updated review of magnetic resonance neurography for plexus imaging. Korean J Radiol. 2023;24(11):1114-30.

5. Heckmatt JZ, Leeman S, Dubowitz V. Ultrasound imaging in the diagnosis of muscle disease. J Pediatr. 1982;101(5):656-60.
6. Yoshii Y, Zhao C, Amadio PC. Recent advances in ultrasound diagnosis of carpal Tunnel syndrome. Diagnostics (Basel). 2020;10(8):596.
7. Cartwright MS, Hobson-Webb LD, Boon AJ, Alter KE, Hunt CH, Flores VH, et al. Evidence-based guideline: Neuromuscular ultrasound for the diagnosis of carpal tunnel syndrome. Muscle Nerve. 2012;46(2):287-93.
8. Burg EW, Bathala L, Visser LH. Difference in normal values of median nerve cross-sectional area between Dutch and Indian subjects. Muscle Nerve. 2014;50(1):129-32.
9. Yerasu MR, Ali M, Rao R, Murthy JMK. Bifid median nerve: A notable anomaly in carpal tunnel syndrome. BMJ Case Rep. 2022;15(5):e249220.
10. Padua L, Di Pasquale A, Liotta G, Granata G, Pazzaglia C, Erra C, Briani C, et al. Ultrasound as a useful tool in the diagnosis and management of traumatic nerve lesions. Clin Neurophysiol. 2013;124(6):1237-43.
11. Beekman R, Visser LH, Verhagen WI. Ultrasonography in ulnar neuropathy at the elbow: A critical review. Muscle Nerve. 2011;43(5):627-35.
12. Reddy YM, Murthy JMK, Suresh L, Jaiswal SK, Pidaparthi L, Kiran ESS. Diagnosis and Severity Evaluation of Ulnar Neuropathy at the Elbow by Ultrasonography: A Case-Control Study. J Med Ultrasound. 2021;30(3):189-95.
13. Bäumer P, Dombert T, Staub F, Kaestel T, Bartsch AJ, Heiland S, et al. Ulnar neuropathy at the elbow: MR neurography--nerve T2 signal increase and caliber. Radiology. 2011;260(1):199-206.
14. Song S, Yoo Y, Won SJ, Park HJ, Rhee WI. Investigation of the diagnostic value of ultrasonography for radial neuropathy located at the spiral groove. Ann Rehabil Med. 2018;42(4):601-8.
15. Visser LH, Hens V, Soethout M, De Deugd-Maria V, Pijnenburg J, Brekelmans GJ. Diagnostic value of high-resolution sonography in common fibular neuropathy at the fibular head. Muscle Nerve. 2013;48(2):171-8.
16. Fantino O. Role of ultrasound in posteromedial tarsal tunnel syndrome: 81 cases. J Ultrasound. 2014;17(2):99-112.
17. Abreu E, Aubert S, Wavreille G, Gheno R, Canella C, Cotten A, et al., Peripheral tumor and tumor-like neurogenic lesions. Eur J Radiol. 2013;82(1):38-50.
18. Goedee, SH, Brekelmans GJ, van den Berg LH, Visser LH. Distinctive patterns of sonographic nerve enlargement in Charcot-Marie-Tooth type 1A and hereditary neuropathy with pressure palsies. Clin Neurophysiol. 2015;126(7):1413-20.
19. Noto Y, Shiga K, Tsuji Y, Mizuta I, Higuchi Y, Hashiguchi A, et al. Nerve ultrasound depicts peripheral nerve enlargement in patients with genetically distinct Charcot-Marie-Tooth disease. J Neurol Neurosurg Psychiatry. 2015;86:378-84.
20. Telleman JA, Stellingwerff MD, Brekelmans GJ, Visser LHi. Nerve ultrasound shows subclinical peripheral nerve involvement in neurofibromatosis type 2. Muscle Nerve. 2018;57(2):312-6.
21. Fisse AL, Pitarokoili K, Motte J, Gamber D, Kerasnoudis A, Gold R, et al. Nerve echogenicity and intranerve CSA variability in high-resolution nerve ultrasound (HRUS) in chronic inflammatory demyelinating polyneuropathy (CIDP). J. Neurol. 2019;266:468-75.
22. Athanasopoulos D, Motte J, Fisse AL, Grueter T, Trampe N, Sturm D, et al. Longitudinal study on nerve ultrasound and corneal confocal microscopy in NF155 paranodopathy. Ann Clin Transl Neurol. 2020; 7(6):1061-8.
23. Neubauer C, Gruber H, Bauerle J, Egger K. Ultrasonography of multifocal acquired demyelinating sensory and motor neuropathy (MADSAM). Clin Neuroradiol. 2015;25:423-5.
24. Loewenbruck KF, Liesenberg J, Dittrich M, Schafer J, Patzner B, Trausch B, et al. Nerve ultrasound in the differentiation of multifocal motor neuropathy (MMN) and amyotrophic lateral sclerosis with predominant lower motor neuron disease (ALS/LMND). J Neurol. 2016;263:35-44.
25. Razali SNO, Arumugam T, Yuki N, Rozalli FI, Goh KJ, Shahrizaila N. Serial peripheral nerve ultrasound in Guillain–Barré syndrome. Clin Neurophysiol. 2016;127:1652-6.
26. Athanasopoulou IM, Rasenack M, Grimm C, Axer H, Sinnreich M, Décard BF, et al et al. Ultrasound of the nerves-An appropriate addition to nerve conduction studies to differentiate paraproteinemic neuropathies. J Neurol Sci. 2016;362:188-95.
27. Shelly S, Shouman K, Paul P, Engelstad J, Amrami KK, Spinner RJ, et al. Expanding the Spectrum of Chronic Immune Sensory Polyradiculopathy: CISP-Plus. Neurology. 2021;96(16):e2078-89.
28. Jain S, Visser LH, Yerasu MR, Raju R, Meena AK, Lokesh B, et al. Use of high resolution ultrasonography as an additional tool in the diagnosis of primary neuritic leprosy: A case report. Lepr Rev. 2013;84(2):161-5.

29. Bathala L, N Krishnam V, Kumar HK, Neladimmanahally V, Nagaraju U, Kumar HM, et al. Extensive sonographic ulnar nerve enlargement above the medial epicondyle is a characteristic sign in Hansen's neuropathy. PLoS Negl Trop Dis. 2017;11(7):e0005766.
30. Reddy YM, Murthy JMK, Pidaparthi L, Jaiswal SK, Kiran ESS, Penneru A, et al. Sonographic characteristics of median nerve neuropathy in Hansen's disease: a case-control study. Leprosy Rev. 2021;92(3):207-17.
31. Y MR, Pidaparthi L, Tourani V, Penneru A, Murthy J. High-resolution ultrasound features of greater auricular nerve in leprosy. Postgrad Med J. 2020;96(1137):443.
32. Kang S, Kim SH, Yang SN, Yoon JS. Sonographic features of peripheral nerves at multiple sites in patients with diabetic polyneuropathy. J Diabetes Complicat. 2016;30:518-23.
33. Goedee HS, van der Pol WL, van Asseldonk JH, Vrancken A, Notermans, NC, Visser LH, et al. Nerve sonography to detect peripheral nerve involvement in vasculitis syndromes. Neurol Clin Pract. 2016;6:293-303.
34. Hobson-Webb LD, Simmons Z. Ultrasound in the diagnosis and monitoring of amyotrophic lateral sclerosis: A review. Muscle Nerve. 2019;60(2):114-23.
35. Misawa S, Noto Y, Shibuya K, Isose S, Sekiguchi Y, Nasu S, et al. Ultrasonographic detection of fasciculations markedly increases diagnostic sensitivity of ALS. Neurology. 2011;77:1532-7.
36. Pillen S, Arts IMP, Zwarts MJ. Muscle ultrasound in neuromuscular disorders. Muscle Nerve. 2008;37:679-93.
37. Habers GEA, Van Brussel M, Bhansing KJ, Hoppenreijs EP, Janssen AJWM, Van Royen-Kerkhof A, et al. Quantitative muscle ultrasonography in the follow-up of juvenile dermatomyositis. Muscle Nerve. 2015;52:540-6.
38. Noto Y, Shiga K, Tsuji Y, Kondo M, Tokuda T, Mizuno T, et al. Contrasting echogenicity in flexor digitorum profundus-flexor carpi ulnaris: a diagnostic ultrasound pattern in sporadic inclusion body myositis. Muscle Nerve. 2014;49(5):745-8.
39. Leung DG. Magnetic resonance imaging patterns of muscle involvement in genetic muscle diseases: A systematic review. J Neurol. 2017;264(7):1320-33.
40. Tasca G, Monforte M, DiazManera J, Brisca G, Semplicini C, D'Amico A, et al. MRI in sarcoglycanopathies: a large international cohort study. J Neurol Neurosurg Psychiatry. 2018;89(1):72-77.

CHAPTER 13

Hirayama Disease/Monomelic Amyotrophy: Recent Advances and Surgical Management

Atchayaram Nalini, Dipti Baskar, Nupur Pruthi, Dhananjay Bhat, Seena Vengalil

ABSTRACT

Hirayama disease (HD) or monomelic amyotrophy affects young males and is a cervical flexion-induced myelopathy (CFIM) characterized by progressive unilateral or more commonly bilateral asymmetrical/symmetrical weakness and atrophy of distal forearm and hand muscles. Magnetic resonance imaging demonstrates classical forward displacement of posterior dura in the lower cervicothoracic cord on neck flexion resulting in ischemic-atrophy of the anterior horn cells and other tracts in the region. Currently surgical intervention is the choice of treatment for patients diagnosed in the early progressive phase of the illness. The damage and disability can be stalled or reversed by cervical decompressive surgeries.

Keywords: Hirayama disease, Cervical flexion-induced myelopathy, Monomelic amyotrophy, Bimelic amyotrophy, Proximal bimelic amyotrophy.

INTRODUCTION

Hirayama disease (HD) is a cervical flexion-induced myelopathy (CFIM) and predominantly affects young Asian males and is characterized by progressive unilateral or more commonly bilateral asymmetrical weakness and atrophy of distal forearm and hand muscles without clinical sensory disturbance or lower limb involvement.[1,2] Since its initial description by Dr Keizo Hirayama and colleagues in 1959, it is described by various namessuch as juvenile nonprogressive monomelic amyotrophy (JNPMA), juvenile asymmetric segmental spinal muscular atrophy (JASSMA), juvenile muscular atrophy of the distal upper extremity (JMADUE), benign juvenile brachial spinal muscular atrophy (SMA), oblique atrophy, benign focal amyotrophy, and monomelic amyotrophy. The disease has a progressive course with possible spontaneous arrest after several years but resulting in significant disability in the majority. Therefore, early recognition and intervention is imperative to prevent progression and functional impairment. With the advent of magnetic resonance imaging (MRI) in 1980s, it is shown that HD patients demonstrate characteristic forward displacement of posterior dura in the lower cervicothoracic cord on neck flexion resulting in ischemicatrophy of the anterior horn cells (AHCs) in the region. Currently surgical intervention is the choice of treatment for patients diagnosed in the early phase of the illness. This damage can be stalled or reversed by cervical decompressive surgeries.

EPIDEMIOLOGY

The majority of cases of HD are from Asia with only a few reports from other countries such as Europe, Australia, and North America.[3-5] The disease has striking male predominance with male to female ratios of 8.3:1 and 20:1 in Japan; 11:1 and 31.6:1 in China; and in India ratio ranges from 9:1 to only males.[6-9] In the nationwide epidemiological survey in Japan done by Tashiro and colleagues, the male preponderance was speculated to be due to rapid height gain as compared to females at puberty.[6] The onset of symptoms is mainly in the late second or early third decade ranging from 15 to 20 years in various cohorts.[6,8] The age of onset peaks around pubertal growth spurt which is attributed to disproportionate growth of vertebral column and spinal canal contents, especially the dural sac. Though initially HD was considered a sporadic disease, there are reports of familial clustering with two candidate genes identified, *KIAA1377* [also known as centrosomal protein 126 (CEP 126)] and chromosome 5 open reading frame 42 (*C5orf42*) and suggested as susceptibility genes to develop HD.[10] The basis for familial occurrence and genetic factors that affect growth and development of vertebral column and contents are yet to be elucidated.

Etiopathogenesis

The central pathogenesis of dynamic cord compression has been postulated and hypothesized by various theories such as dural sac theory, nerve root theory, dural structural abnormality, abnormal venous engorgement, immunological theory, and incongruous strength of cervical spine muscle with weak superficial extensors than flexors contributing to spine instability. However, venous stasis-ischemia hypothesis is the most plausible explanation for the occurrence of HD and can lead to venous congestive myelopathy due to venous stasis and ischemia.[11]

CLINICAL FEATURES

The typical HD, also known as brachial monomelic amyotrophy (BMMA) has the following clinical features **(Figs. 1A to I)**:
- Insidious onset with progression initially for 3–5 years followed by arrest. The motor disability is variable from mild to severe.
- Unilateral or asymmetrical bilateral wasting and weakness of the distal upper limbs (ULs), with predominant wasting of the ulnar aspect of the hand resulting in characteristic "reverse split hand syndrome" in contrast to "split hand" noted in amyotrophic lateral sclerosis (ALS) with thenar wasting. This is hypothesized due to hypothenar AHC susceptibility in HD compared to thenar AHC susceptibility to apoptosis in ALS. There is also characteristic sparing of brachioradialis muscle in the forearm resulting in "oblique atrophy".
- Coarse irregular tremors called minipolymyoclonus of the affected hands.
- Cold paresis, noted in 97% of HD patients. Previous study on axonal excitability on cold exposure has shown increased refractoriness of sodium channels on immature sprouting neurons.[12]
- Absence of objective sensory disturbance.

VARIANTS OF HIRAYAMA DISEASE

In addition to the typical clinical features of HD described earlier, there are various atypical features which have to be borne in mind during diagnosis.

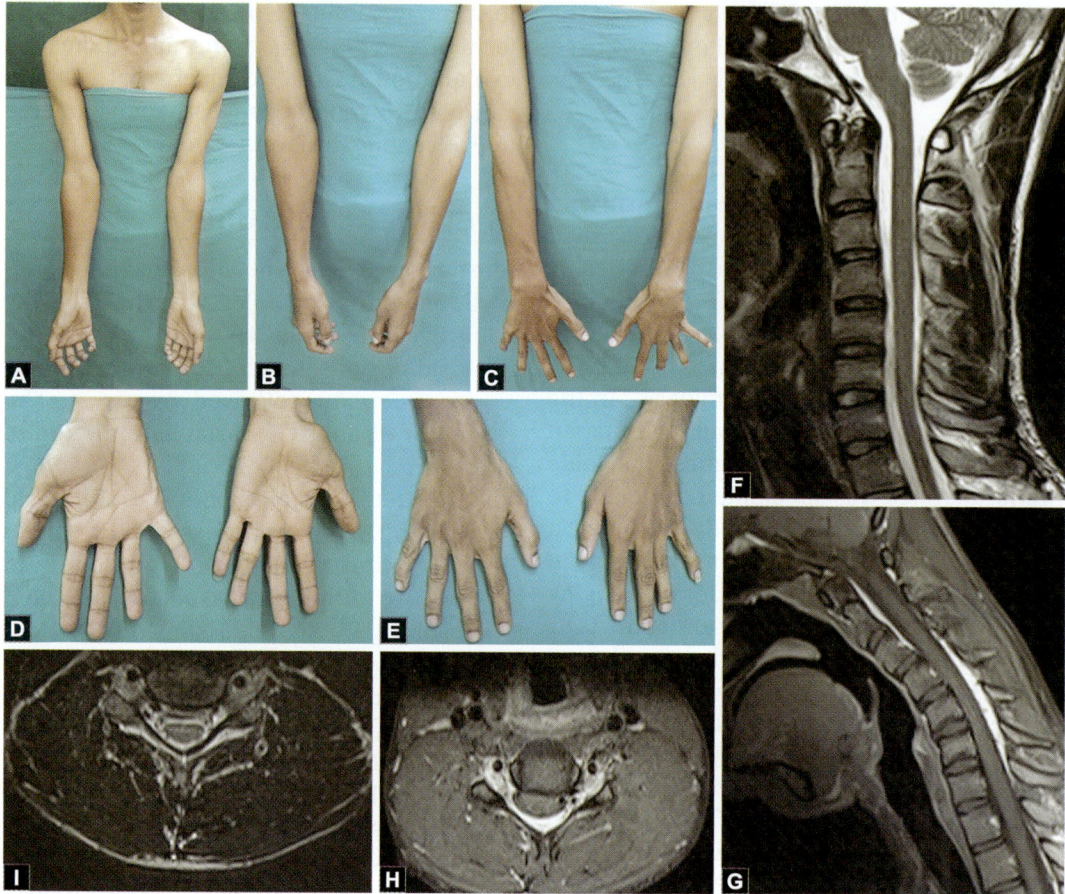

FIGS. 1A TO I: Clinical and MRI images of typical brachial monomelic amyotrophy (BMMA). (A to C) Oblique atrophy of forearm with sparing of brachioradialis; (D and E) Hypothenar wasting noted in right hand (reverse split hand); (F) T2-weighted (T2W) showing loss of cervical lordosis. (G) T1 postcontrast shows posterior crescentic enhancement; (H) T1-weighted (T1W); and (I) T2W—flattening and asymmetric cord atrophy.

Distal Bimelic Amyotrophy (Figs. 2A to H)

Classical HD/BMMA is primarily unilateral even though with later involvement of the contralateral UL, it grossly remains asymmetrical. In distal bimelic amyotrophy (DBMA), there is symmetrical bilateral severe distal UL involvement with affection of C7-T1 AHCs. However, DBMA carries all other typical features of HD/BMMA such as onset in early 20s, arrest after initial progression for 2–3 years, significant disability, and dynamic cervical MRI features.[13]

Crural Monomelic Amyotrophy (Figs. 3A to D)

Similar to classical brachial variant, crural phenotype causes muscle atrophy and

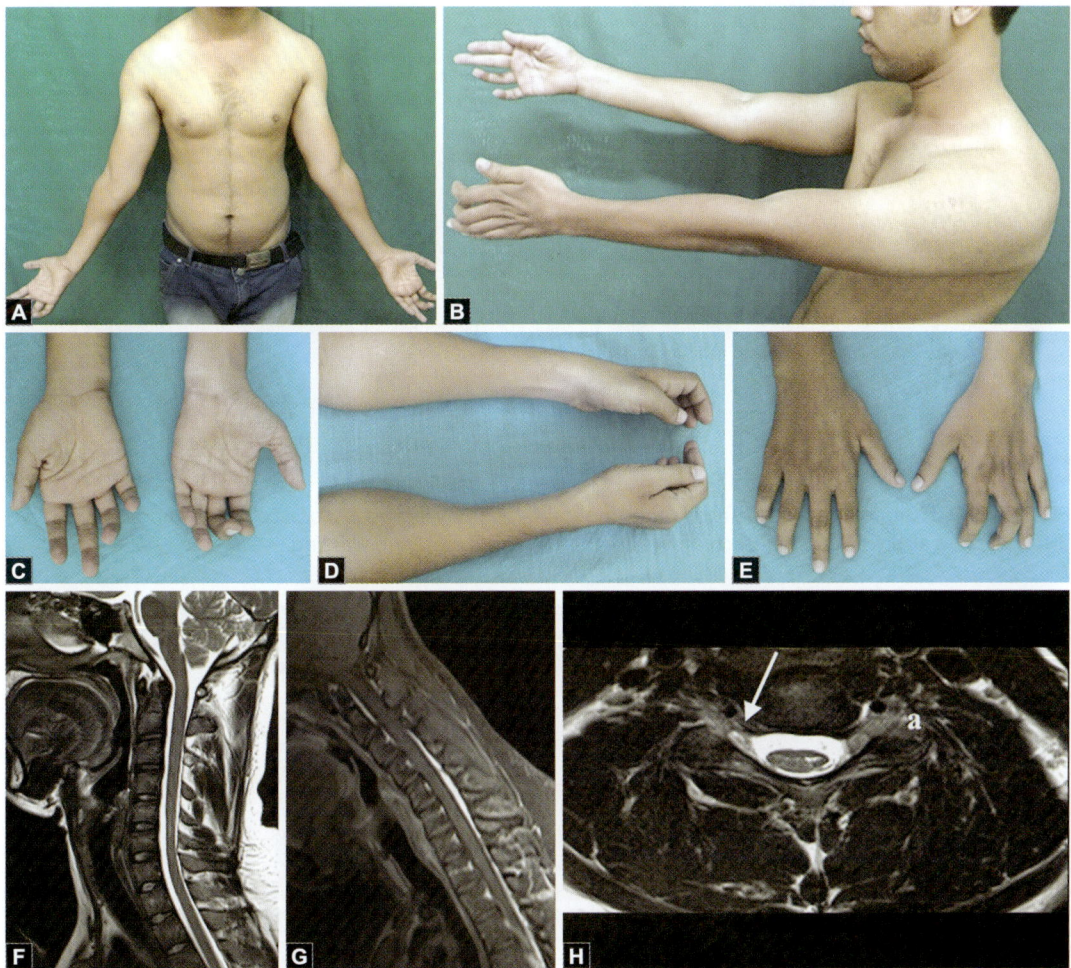

FIGS. 2A TO H: Clinical and MRI images of distal bimelic amyotrophy (DBMA). (A to E) Symmetrical forearm atrophy with brachioradialis sparing and hypothenar wasting. (F) T2-weighted (T2W)—cord atrophy from C6 to T1; (G) T1-weighted (T1W) postcontrast—posterior crescentic enhancement; and (H) (T2W)—cord flattening with anterior horn enhancement.

weakness involving unilateral or asymmetrical bilateral lower limbs[8] although MRI features are not detectable.

Upper Motor Neuron Involvement

Severe cord involvement in HD can result in hyperreflexia and inverted tendon reflexes, especially of lower limbs. Previous studies have reported pyramidal involvement in HD ranging from 2.4 to 18%.[6,14,15]

Proximal Variant (Figs. 4A to J)

Proximal bimelic amyotrophy (PBMA) and proximo-distal bimelic amyotrophy (PDBMA) are uncommon variants with wasting and weakness of shoulder girdle muscles.[7] They can be unilateral or bilaterally asymmetrical and have severe motor disability similar to DBMA. Compared to BMMA and DBMA, proximal variants have higher cervical level compression at C4–C5 levels.[13,16]

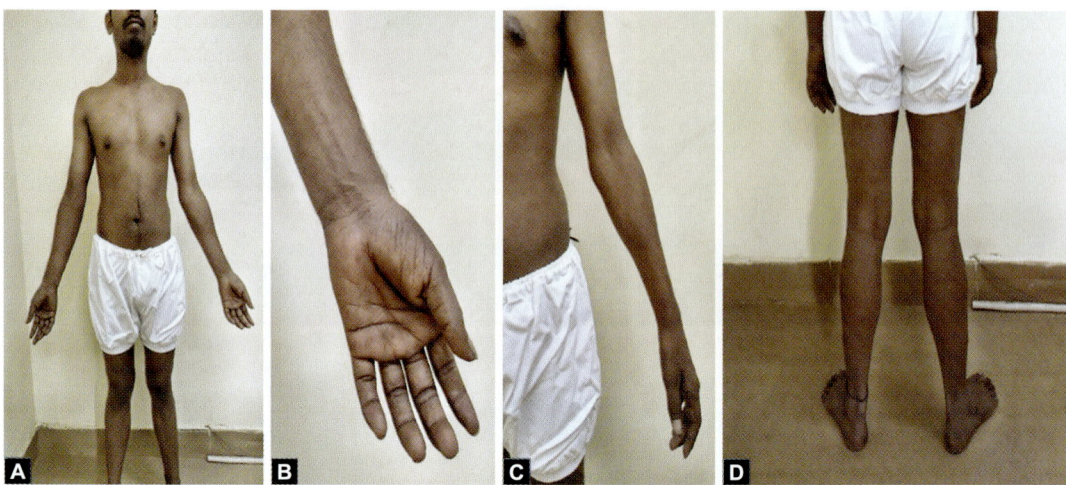

FIGS. 3A TO D: Clinical images of Crural monomelic amyotrophy (MMA). (A to C) Left upper limb progressive distal wasting and weakness with cold paresis; and (D) Left lower limb wasting.

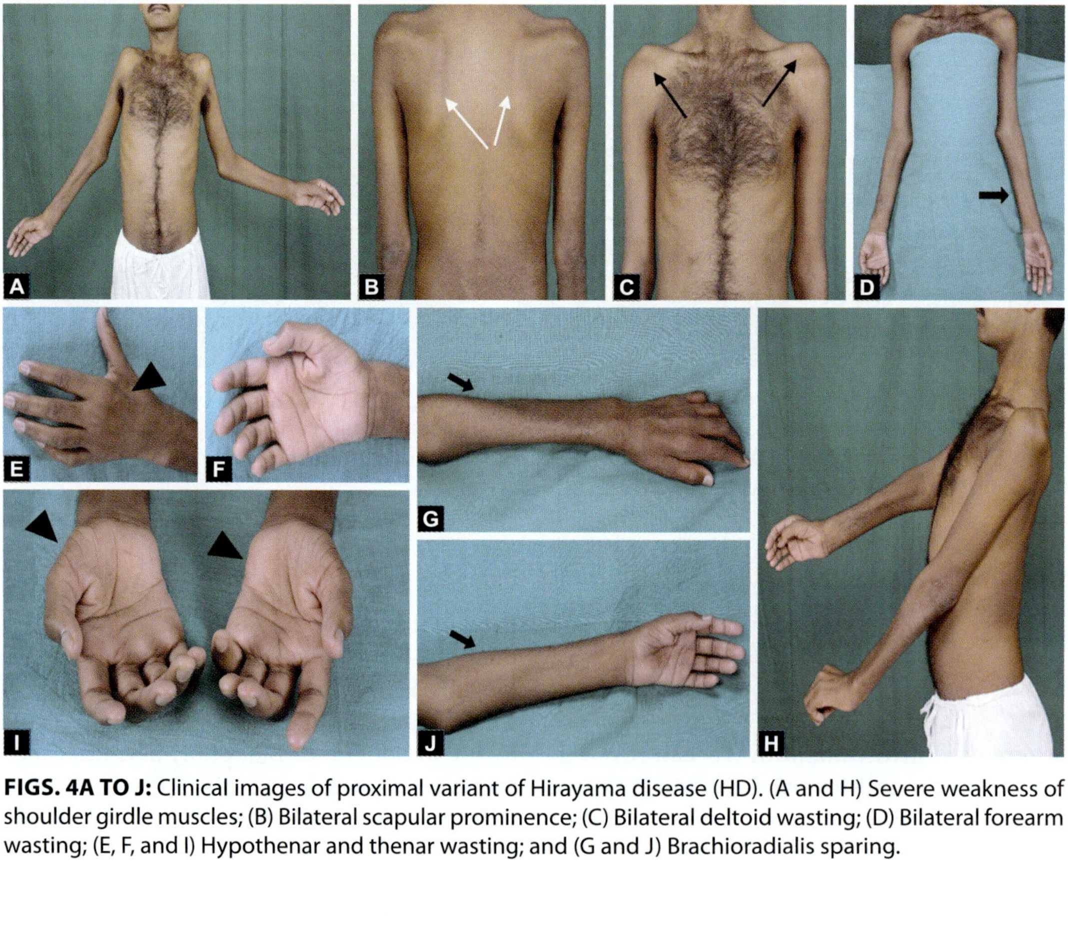

FIGS. 4A TO J: Clinical images of proximal variant of Hirayama disease (HD). (A and H) Severe weakness of shoulder girdle muscles; (B) Bilateral scapular prominence; (C) Bilateral deltoid wasting; (D) Bilateral forearm wasting; (E, F, and I) Hypothenar and thenar wasting; and (G and J) Brachioradialis sparing.

■ DIAGNOSIS

Diagnosis of HD relies on classical and nonclassical manifestations and characteristic observations on spine MRI.

Imaging Features

Imaging studies play an important role in diagnosis of HD. MRI cervical spine plays a pivotal role in diagnosis of HD. The optimal MRI requirements include 1.5T to 3.0T scanner with sequence protocol of sagittal and axial T1-weighted and T2-weighted (T2W) fast/turbo spin echo and T1-weighted fat saturation before and after gadolinium contrast administration and a slice thickness of ideally 3–4 mm.[17] The MRI should be acquired in both neutral and neck flexed position of angle 35–40° preferably in prone position (unpublished data/personal experience).[18] The main findings in MRI can be broadly classified into those obtained in neutral and flexed positions, though flexed neck findings are more sensitive and specific to HD **(Figs. 5 and 6)**.

Neutral position findings include:
- Loss of normal cervical lordosis. In case of proximal variants of HD, the degree of kyphosis is more, especially at C3–C4 and C4–C5 levels while the lower part of cervical spine has retained lordosis resulting in "reverse S" appearance.[19]
- Cord atrophy mostly at C5–C7 levels. Reports of focal cord atrophy resulting in "sand watch" appearance in sagittal view.[20]

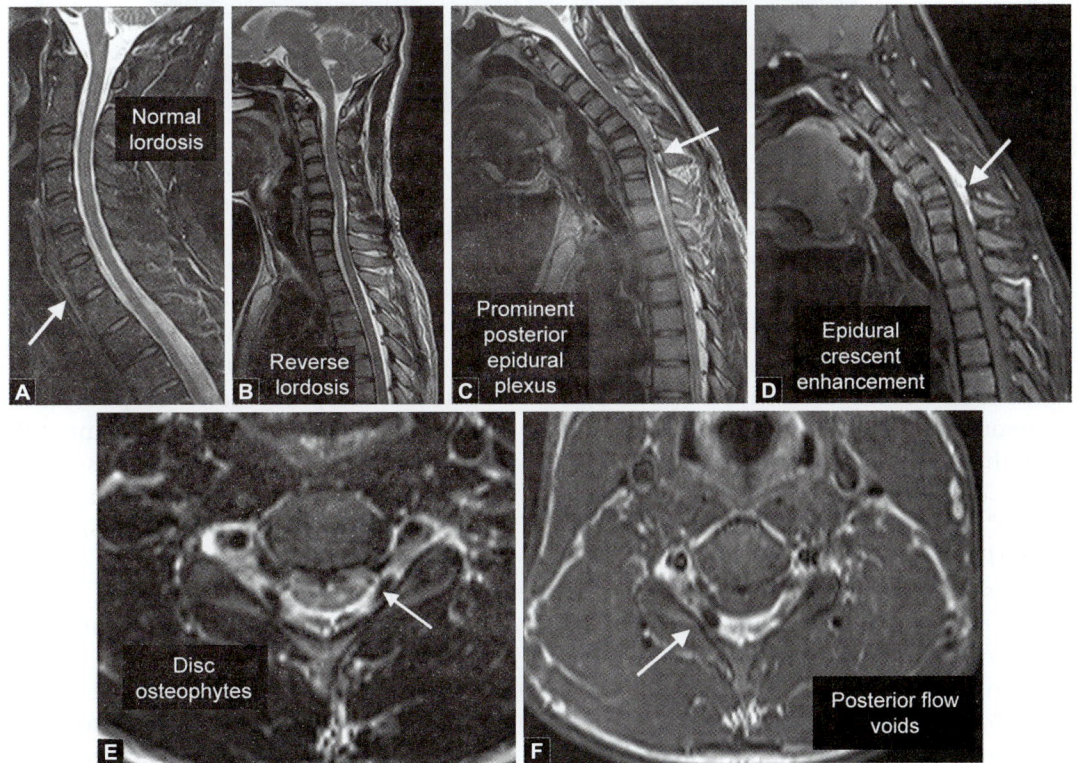

FIGS. 5A TO F: Salient MRI features of Hirayama disease (HD).

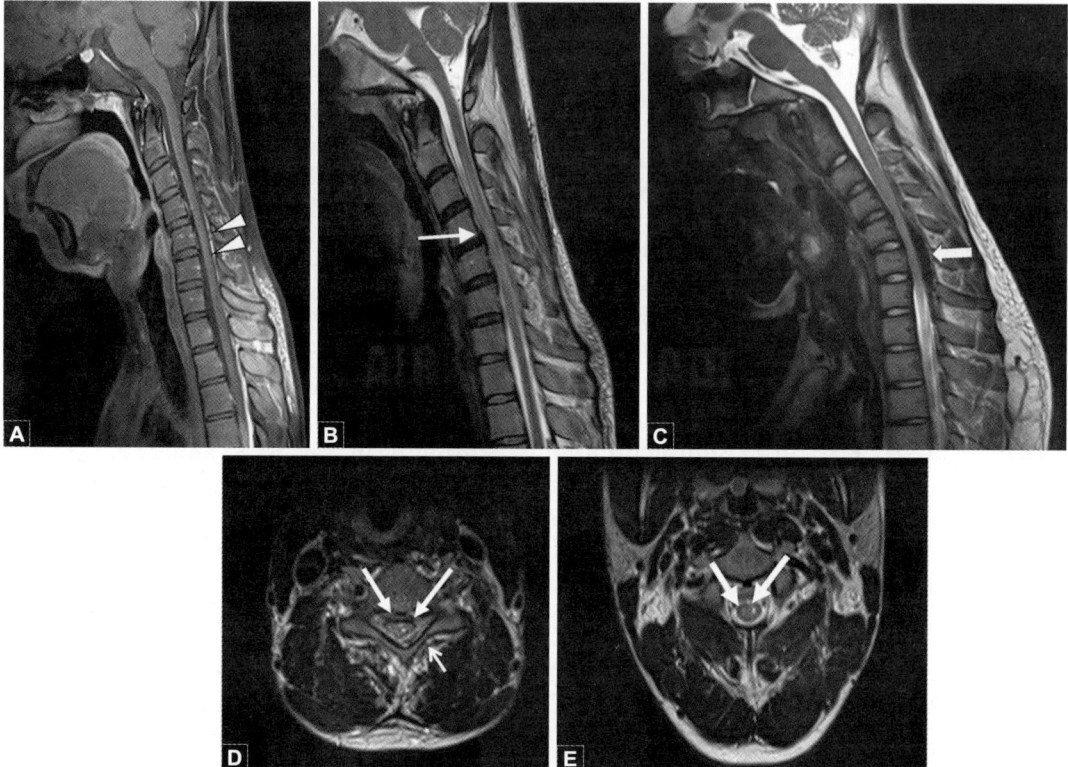

FIGS. 6A TO E: MRI features of Hirayama disease (HD). (A) Postcontrast fat saturation T1-weighted (T1W) in flexion showing epidural soft tissue enhancing (white arrow heads); (B) T2W in flexion showing altered signal intensity (white arrow); (C) T2-weighted (T2W) in flexion showing hypointense epidural tissue with flow voids pushing the cord forward (white arrow); and (D and E) T2W images at the level of C2 and C6 asymmetric gliosis of anterior horn cells.

- Asymmetrical cord flattening in axial images. Cord flattening and atrophy denotes severe cord involvement and poor recovery following surgery.[3,21,22]
- T2 hyperintensity of anterior horns giving the characteristic "snake eye" or "owl's eye" appearance, seen in around 17–77% in HD **(Fig. 7)**.[17,23,24]
- Loss of attachment of posterior dura to the underlying lamina, considered to the most important sign in neutral position with sensitivity and specificity of 93% and 98%, respectively.[25] Loss of attachment is more extensive in proximal group with progression of disease reflecting more severe disease phenotype.[26]

Flexed cervical MRI reveals pathognomonic imaging features as following:
- Anterior displacement of posterior dural sac, the degree of displacement is 6–9 mm as compared to 1–4 mm seen in normal subjects. MRI based spinal ratio between maximum forward displacement of posterior dura and spinal canal diameter is increased in flexed position resulting in significant cord flattening.[27]
- Widening of posterior laminodural space.
- Prominent epidural flow voids seen as T2W hypointense linear structures due to engorgement of posterior epidural venous plexus.

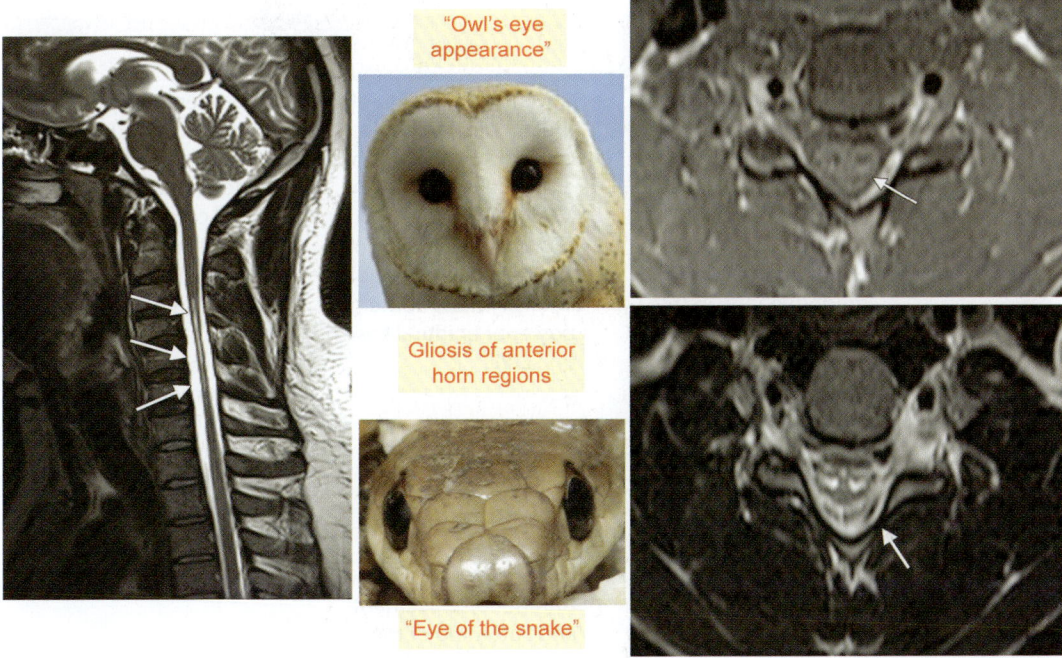

FIG. 7: MRI spine—"snake's eye/owl's eye" appearance.

- Postcontrast enhancement of posterior epidural plexus seen as "crescent-shaped" structure.[14] The enhancement typically disappears on return to neutral position.

The combination of MRI findings on neutral and flexion position has high sensitivity and specificity of 71% and 100%, respectively.[24]

The major shortcoming of conventional dynamic MRI is lack of correlation between degree of cord compression and symptoms and can be partially overcome by diffusion tensor imaging (DTI). The major findings include reduced functional anisotropy and increased apparent diffusion coefficient (ADC) in flexion imaging.[28] These are useful in early stages of HD and to localize level of maximal cord involvement which can guide surgical decisions.

Electrophysiological Features

The major utility of electrodiagnostic studies is to rule out mimics of HD. The electroneuromyography findings reflect segmental neurogenic dysfunction of AHCs of lower cervical cord without sensory involvement.

Evoked potentials can also have changes in HD with sensory evoked potentials (SEPs) being normal or show changes in N9–N13 and N13–N20 interpeak latencies. Motor evoked potentials (MEPs) show changes during neck flexion such as reduced amplitude, longer central motor conduction time, and prolonged latency.[29]

Diagnostic Criteria

Previous criteria relied solely on the clinical features for diagnosis of HD which resulted in misdiagnosis. Hence, updated criteria known as Huashan diagnostic criteria incorporating

TABLE 1: Huashan diagnostic criteria.

Elements for diagnosis	Clinical manifestations	Imaging manifestations	Electrophysiological features
Elements for definite diagnosis	1. Occult onset during puberty, more common in males 2. Localized muscular atrophy and weakness of the upper extremities, predominantly in the ulnar forearms and the intrinsic muscles of the hands unilaterally or mainly on one side 3. Absence of cranial nerve involvement and muscular atrophy in other parts of the body such as the lower limbs	1. Atrophy or thinning of the middle and lower cervical spinal cord on either neutral or flexion MRI 2. LOA or the presence of a crescent-shaped high-intensity mass at the posterior epidural space on T2WI	1. Neurogenic lesions located in anterior horns and/or roots of the middle and lower cervical spinal cord 2. Normal or only mild abnormal conduction velocity in peripheral nerves of the upper limbs 3. Absence of obvious involvement of the cranial nerves and thoracic, lumbar or sacral spinal cord as the third point under electrophysiological features
Other elements	4. Cold paralysis and tremors in fingers when they are stretched 5. Active deep tendon reflex and/or positive pathological signs in parts of patients 6. Mild sensory deficits in the upper limbs in a small number of patients	3. Anterior displacement and flattening of the lower cervical spinal cord and narrowing or absence of the anterior spinal space on neck flexion MRI 4. High-intensity signs located in the anterior horn areas on T2WI in parts of patients	
Definite HD*	Meeting criterion 1, 2, and 3	Meeting criterion 1 and 2	Meeting criterion 1, 2, and 3
Probable HD**	Meeting criterion 2 and 3		Meeting criterion 3

*Definite HD means meeting criterion above, with or without other elements.
**Probable HD means meeting criterion above and lack of 1–5 other elements for definite diagnosis, with or without other elements.
(HD: Hirayama disease; T2WI: T2-weighted imaging; LOA: loss of attachment)

clinical features such as duration of disease, subtle pyramidal and sensory signs, neck flexion MRI, and electrophysiology to increase the sensitivity of diagnosis has been described in **Table 1**.[7]

■ DIFFERENTIAL DIAGNOSIS

The major mimics of HD are conditions which result in muscular atrophy of distal UL muscles and can be classified as follows:

- *Cord lesion*: Cervical spondylotic myelopathy/amyotrophy (CSA), syringomyelia, intramedullary neoplasm, and ossification of posterior longitudinal ligament of cervical spine.
- *Motor neuron disorders*: Early-onset ALS, distal SMA, and flail arm variant of ALS.
- *Neuropathies*: Nerve compression syndromes (carpal tunnel syndrome and thoracic outlet syndrome) and hereditary neuropathies.

None of the mimics will have the classical MRI findings.

MANAGEMENT

Even though HD is traditionally defined as a self-limiting AHC disease, early detection and treatment are crucial since the condition assumes a stationary phase after significant irreversible motor deficits have occurred. For HD, there are no clear-cut accepted treatment recommendations.

Conservative Management

The cervical collar is the most often used initial treatment because it restricts neck flexion and the ensuing progression. Nevertheless, there are a number of drawbacks to using a collar, including low compliance as it has to be worn constantly for at least 3–4.[30] This could be difficult in tropical countries with warm weather. Moreover, cervical collar has predominantly subjective improvement.

Surgical Management

Various surgical procedures are based on the proposed theories in the pathogenesis of HD. Surgical intervention has become the treatment of choice and possible standard of care in recent times.

The major indications for surgery[31] are:
- Progressive course of illness
- Affliction of homologous limb/lower limb(s)
- Noncompliance to cervical collar therapy
- Compressive cord changes in MRI
- Presence of pyramidal signs

The surgical approaches can be classified into anterior and posterior which can further be subclassified into various procedures such as laminectomy, duraplasty, corpectomy, discectomy, decompression, and fusion.[7,32,33]

The various anterior approaches include:
- Anterior cervical corpectomy and discectomy with plate followed by iliac bone graft placement.
- Anterior cervical plating only—consists of fixation of adjacent vertebral segments at the level of spinal cord compression and plating without decompression to restrict movement. There are merits such as ability to remove the plate after stabilization of progression and immobilization of lower cervical spine in lordosis. However, spinal fusion will be required for patients with kyphotic spine alignment or herniated cervical disc with cord compression.
- Anterior cervical discectomy and fusion (ACDF) with or without plating. ACDF with plating has become the most preferred procedure.

The choice of surgical technique is often debated, and it has not been established as to which method is better than the other. Previous pooled analysis has shown a clinical improvement rate of 80% ($n = 489$) with anterior approaches and 81% ($n = 29$) with posterior approaches. Anterior techniques such as ACDF and corpectomy are preferred when there is compression in the ventral aspect of thecal sac. Other merits of anterior approach as compared to posterior include prevention of excessive flexion by post discectomy/corpectomy fixation, less pooled blood loss, and significantly less operative time.[34] There were two kinds of ACDF procedures performed: Single level or two-level ACDF. Single level ACDF is preferred as two-level procedures used longer constructs because of the long level compression seen in T2W sagittal images obtained during flexion **(Figs. 8 and 9)**. However, doing a long construct for a more focal disorder is not ideal. The fulcrum of movement of subaxial cervical spine can be checked on flexion

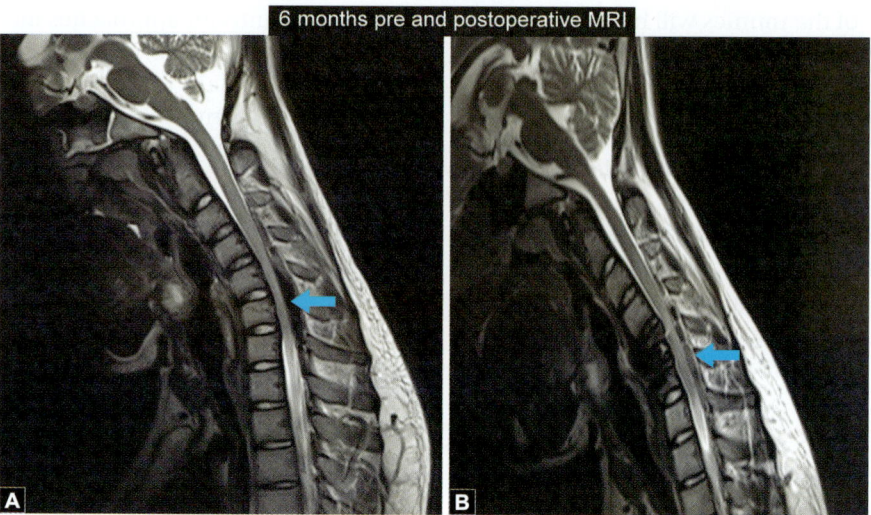

FIGS. 8A AND B: Pre- and postoperative MRI images showing significant reduction in posterior epidural tissue and cord compression.

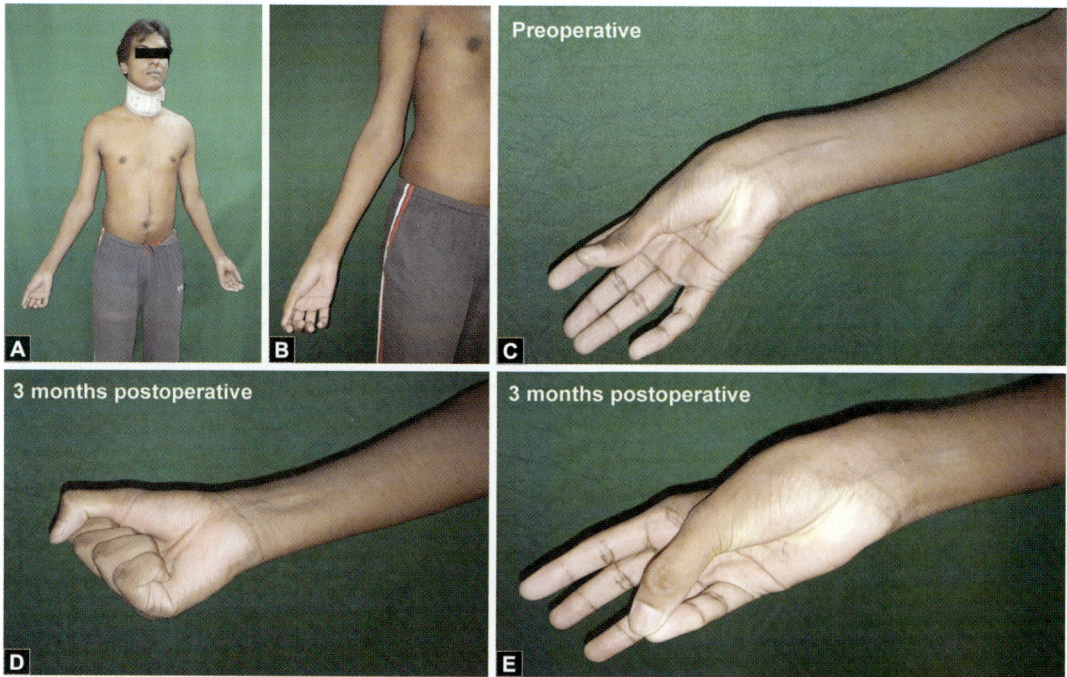

FIGS. 9A TO E: Clinical images showing postoperative motor improvement of distal upper limbs following anterior cervical discectomy and fusion (ACDF).

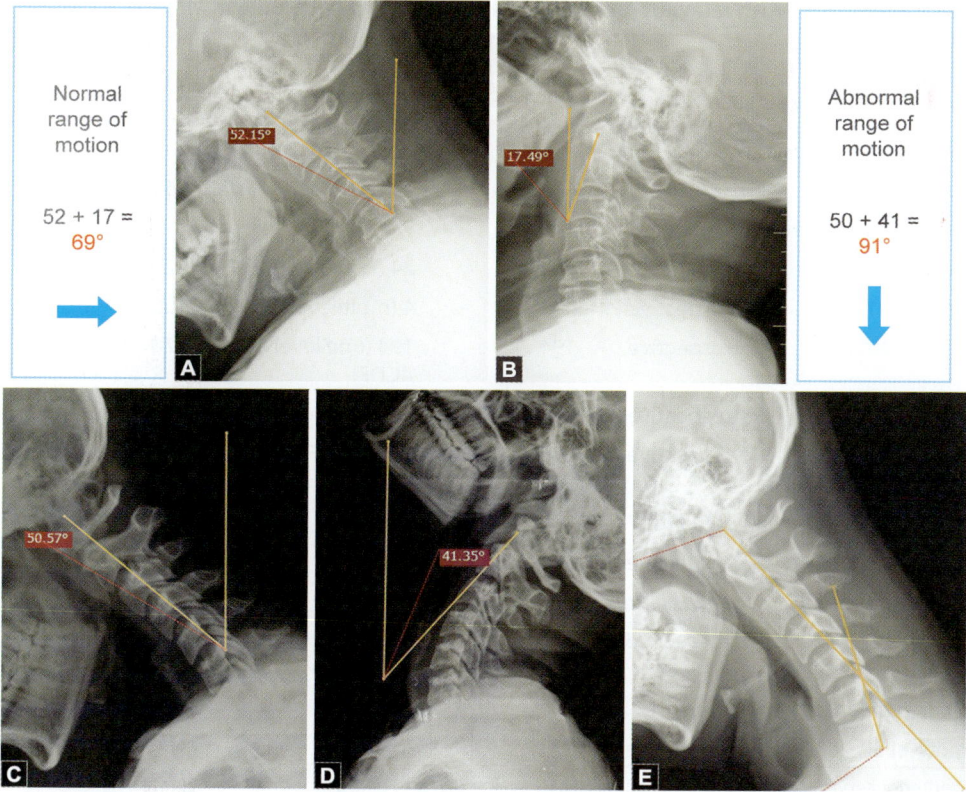

FIGS. 10A TO E: X-ray of cervical spine in flexion showing normal and abnormal range of neck flexion. Level of surgery determined by using the intersection level of two lines drawn along posterior aspect of C2 vertebrae and along posterior aspect of C7 vertebrae.

X-rays of the cervical spine **(Figs. 10A to E)**. This level also corresponds to the maximum level of compression seen on T2W sagittal images acquired during maximum flexion. Thus, single level surgery at this level is considered to minimize the compression in flexion for HD patients.[9] The only advantage with posterior approach is fixation of cervical spine without direct decompression. However, there are several demerits such as risk of excessive bleeding, cerebrospinal fluid (CSF) leakage with risk of meningitis and long operative time.

Comparisons of surgical outcomes of various studies are shown in **Table 2**.

Thus, overall anterior approach is favored over the posterior procedures. The major factors influencing outcome in HD patients include age at onset, duration of symptoms, pathological reflexes, and preoperative motor assessment scores.[9,35]

■ PROGNOSIS

Most of the HD patients are given benign prognosis with arrest of disease after progressing for 3–5 years. The major morbidity lies in the motor disability of the ULs. The immobilization with cervical collar is shown to be effective in 57.2% of cases.[15] Whereas with surgical invention in properly selected, it was seen to be effective in 46.3–87.6% patients, differing with anterior and posterior techniques.[34] Depending on the stage of intervention, some patients may have residual deficits such as amyotrophy and

TABLE 2: Comparison with relevant previous studies on surgical outcome in MMA/HD.

Study	Type of study	Total number of patients	Number of patient underwent surgery	Clinical outcome (% of operated patients with improvement)
Anterior corpectomy and cervical plating				
Lu et al., 2013[37]	Prospective	48	24	66.7
ACDF with anterior cervical plating				
Lu et al., 2013[37]	Prospective	48	24 (two level ACDF)	62.7
Guo et al., 2014[38]	Retrospective	4	4 (multilevel ACDF)	100
Song et al., 2017[35]	Retrospective	194	194 (one level ACDF)	87.6
Zou et al., 2019[22]	Retrospective	40	40 (two level ACDF)	60.4
Vengalil S et al., 2024[9]	Retrospective	136	136 (ACDF at single two and multilevel)	84%
Posterior laminectomy with duraplasty				
Lin et al., 2010[39]	Retrospective	6	1	0
Posterior laminectomy and venous plexus coagulation				
Brandicourt et al., 2018[32]	Retrospective	3	3	100
Posterior laminoplasty and duraplasty				
Fujimoto et al., 2002[34]	Retrospective	23	3	100

(ACDF: anterior cervical discectomy and fusion; HD: Hirayama disease; MMA: monomelic amyotrophy)

cold paresis. Rarely, some patients may have progression following a period of stability[36] and if it continues surgical intervention can be considered.[9]

CONCLUSION

Hirayama disease/monomelic amyotrophy is a flexion induced cervical compressive myelopathy resulting in progressive weakness and atrophy predominantly of distal ULs. Contrast-enhanced dynamic flexion cervical MRI is the main imaging modality for prompt and confirmatory diagnosis of this condition. Treatment of HD aims at preventing neck flexion. Surgical decompression should be considered as the first line and mainstay of management rather than considering conservative treatment with use of cervical collarowing to irreversible deficits as the disease progresses. Surgical outcomes as projected in various studies have shown promising benefit and also reversal of symptoms and signs and objective improvement in the motor disability.

REFERENCES

1. Polavarapu K, Preethish-Kumar V, Nashi S, Vengalil S, Prasad C, Bhattacharya K, et al. Intrafamilial phenotypic variations in familial cases of cervical flexion induced myelopathy/Hirayama disease. Amyotroph Lateral Scler Frontotemporal Degener. 2018;19:38-49.

2. Preethish-Kumar V, Polavarapu K, Singh RJ, Vengalil S, Prasad C, Verma A, et al. Proximal and proximo-distal bimelic amyotrophy: Evidence of cervical flexion induced myelopathy. Amyotroph Lateral Scler Frontotemporal Degener. 2016;17(7-8):499-507.

3. Vitale V, Caranci F, Pisciotta C, Manganelli F, Briganti F, Santoro L, et al. Hirayama's disease: an Italian single center experience and review of the literature. Quant Imaging Med Surg. 2016;6(4):364-73.
4. Ghosh PS, Moodley M, Friedman NR, Rothner AD, Ghosh D. Hirayama disease in children from North America. J Child Neurol. 2011;26(12):1542-7.
5. Kusel K, Warne R, Lakshmanan R, Mason M, Bynevelt M, Shah S. Hirayama disease: the importance of flexion imaging. BJR Case Rep. 2021;8(1):20210105.
6. Tashiro K, Kikuchi S, Itoyama Y, Tokumaru Y, Sobue G, Mukai E, et al. Nationwide survey of juvenile muscular atrophy of distal upper extremity (Hirayama disease) in Japan. Amyotroph Lateral Scler. 2006;7(1):38-45.
7. Wang H, Tian Y, Wu J, Luo S, Zheng C, Sun C, et al. Update on the Pathogenesis, Clinical Diagnosis, and Treatment of Hirayama Disease. Front Neurol. 2022;12:811943.
8. Nalini A, Gourie-Devi M, Thennarasu K, Ramalingaiah AH. Monomelic amyotrophy: clinical profile and natural history of 279 cases seen over 35 years (1976-2010). Amyotroph Lateral Scler Frontotemporal Degener. 2014;15(5-6):457-65.
9. Vengalil S, Pruthi N, Bhat D, Uppar AM, Polavarapu K, Preethish-Kumar V, et al. Monomelic Amyotrophy/Hirayama Disease: Surgical Outcome in a Large Cohort of Indian Patients. World Neurosurg. 2024;183:e88-97.
10. Lim YM, Koh I, Park YM, Kim JJ, Kim DS, Kim HJ, et al. Exome sequencing identifies KIAA1377 and C5orf42 as susceptibility genes for monomelic amyotrophy. Neuromuscul Disord. 2012;22(5):394-400.
11. Foster E, Tsang BK, Kam A, Stark RJ. Mechanisms of upper limb amyotrophy in spinal disorders. J Clinical Neurosci. 2014;21:1209-14.
12. Sawai S, Misawa S, Kanai K, Isose S, Shibuya K, Noto Y, et al. Altered axonal excitability properties in juvenile muscular atrophy of distal upper extremity (Hirayama disease). Clin Neurophysiol. 2011;122(1):205-9.
13. Preethish-Kumar V, Nalini A, Singh RJ, Saini J, Prasad C, Polavarapu K, et al. Distal bimelic amyotrophy (DBMA): Phenotypically distinct but identical on cervical spine MR imaging with brachial monomelic amyotrophy/Hirayama disease. Amyotroph Lateral Scler Frontotemporal Degener. 2015;16(5-6):338-44.
14. Hassan KM, Sahni H, Jha A. Clinical and radiological profile of Hirayama disease: A flexion myelopathy due to tight cervical dural canal amenable to collar therapy. Ann Indian Acad Neurol. 2012;15(2):106-12.
15. Sonwalkar HA, Shah RS, Khan FK, Gupta AK, Bodhey NK, Vottath S, et al. Imaging features in Hirayama disease. Neurol India. 2008;56(1):22-6.
16. Baba Y, Nakajima M, Utsunomiya H, Tsuboi Y, Fujiki F, Kusuhara T, et al. Magnetic resonance imaging of thoracic epidural venous dilation in Hirayama disease. Neurology. 2004;62:1426-8.
17. Khadilkar S, Patel B, Bhutada A, Chaudhari C. Do longer necks predispose to Hirayama disease? A comparison with mimics and controls. J Neurol Sci. 2015;359(1-2):213-6.
18. Hou C, Han H, Yang X, Xu X, Gao H, Fan D, et al. How does the neck flexion affect the cervical MRI features of Hirayama disease? Neurol Sci. 2012;33(5):1101-5.
19. Wang H, Tian Y, Wu J, Sun C, Nie C, Zheng C, et al. The radiological and electrophysiological characteristics of Hirayama disease with proximal involvement: A retrospective study. Front Neurol. 2022;13:969484.
20. Bede P, Walsh R, Fagan AJ, Hardiman O. "Sandwatch" spinal cord: a case of inferior cervical spinal cord atrophy. J Neurol. 2014;261(1):235-7.
21. Liao MF, Chang HS, Chang KH, Ro LS, Chu CC, Kuo HC, et al. Correlations of clinical, neuroimaging, and electrophysiological features in Hirayama disease. Medicine (Baltimore). 2016;95(28):e4210.
22. Zou F, Yang S, Lu F, Ma X, Xia X, Jiang J. Factors Affecting the Surgical Outcomes of Hirayama Disease: A Retrospective Analysis of Preoperative Magnetic Resonance Imaging Features of the Cervical Spine. World Neurosurg. 2019;122: e296-301.
23. Boruah DK, Prakash A, Gogoi BB, Yadav RR, Dhingani DD, Sarma B. The Importance of Flexion MRI in Hirayama Disease with Special Reference to Laminodural Space Measurements. AJNR Am J Neuroradiol. 2018;39(5):974-980.
24. Lehman VT, Luetmer PH, Sorenson EJ, Carter RE, Gupta V, Fletcher GP, et al. Cervical spine MR imaging findings of patients with Hirayama disease in North America: a multisite study. AJNR Am J Neuroradiol. 2013;34(2):451-6.
25. Chen CJ, Hsu HL, Tseng YC, Lyu RK, Chen CM, Huang YC, et al. Hirayama flexion myelopathy: neutral-position MR imaging findings—importance of loss of attachment. Radiology. 2004;231(1):39-44.
26. Shao M, Yin J, Lu F, Zheng C, Wang H, Jiang J. The Quantitative Assessment of Imaging Features

27. Lai V, Wong YC, Poon WL, Yuen MK, Fu YP, Wong OW. Forward shifting of posterior dural sac during flexion cervical magnetic resonance imaging in Hirayama disease: an initial study on normal subjects compared to patients with Hirayama disease. Eur J Radiol. 2011;80(3):724-8.
28. Singh NA, Viswanathan VK, Shetty AP, Kanna RM, Rajasekaran S. Diffusion Tensor Imaging Characteristics in Hirayama Disease: Case Report and Review of the Literature. World Neurosurg. 2020;140:180-7.
29. Abraham A, Gotkine M, Drory VE, Blumen SC. Effect of neck flexion on somatosensory and motor evoked potentials in Hirayama disease. J Neurol Sci. 2013;334(1-2):102-5.
30. Fu Y, Qin W, Sun Q, Fan D. Investigation of the compliance of cervical collar therapy in 73 patients with Hirayama disease. Natl Med J China. 2016;96:3485-8.
31. Lyu F, Zheng C, Wang H, Nie C, Ma X, Xia X, et al. Establishment of a clinician-led guideline on the diagnosis and treatment of Hirayama disease using a modified Delphi technique. Clin Neurophysiol. 2020;131:1311-9.
32. Brandicourt P, Sol JC, Aldéa S, Bonneville F, Cintas P, Brauge D. Cervical laminectomy and micro resection of the posterior venous plexus in Hirayama disease. Neurochirurgie. 2018;64(4):303-9.
33. Zhang H, Wang S, Li Z, Shen R, Lin R, Wu W, et al. Anterior Cervical Surgery for the Treatment of Hirayama Disease. World Neurosurg. 2019;127:e910-8.
34. Bohara S, Garg K, Mishra S, Tandon V, Chandra PS, Kale SS. Impact of various cervical surgical interventions in patients with Hirayama's disease—a narrative review and meta-analysis. Neurosurg Rev. 2021;44(6):3229-47.
35. Song J, Wang HL, Zheng CJ, Jiang JY. Risk factors for surgical results of Hirayama disease: a retrospective analysis of a large cohort. World Neurosurg. 2017;105:69-77.
36. Moglia C, Calvo A, Cammarosano S, Ilardi A, Canosa A, Gallo S, et al. Monomelic amyotrophy is not always benign: a case report. Amyotroph Lateral Scler. 2011;12(4):307-8.
37. Lu F, Wang H, Jiang J, Chen W, Ma X, Ma X, et al. Efficacy of anterior cervical decompression and fusion procedures for monomelic amyotrophy treatment: a prospective randomized controlled trial: clinical article. J Neurosurg Spine. 2013;19:412-9.
38. Guo X, Lu M, Xie N, Guo Q, Ni B. Multilevel anterior cervical discectomy and fusion with plate fixation for juvenile unilateral muscular atrophy of the distal upper extremity accompanied by cervical kyphosis. J Spinal Dis Techn. 2014;27:E241-6.
39. Lin MS, Kung WM, Chiu WT, Lyu RK, Chen CJ, Chen TY. Hirayama disease. J Neurosurg Spine. 2010;12(6):629-34.

Recent Classification and Emerging Therapies in Charcot–Marie–Tooth Disease

Ritu Shree, Manoj Kumar Goyal

ABSTRACT

Charcot–Marie–Tooth (CMT) disease is the most common hereditary neuropathy worldwide. Traditionally, CMT was classified on the basis of electrophysiological findings and can be divided into demyelinating and axonal subtypes with intermediate form described later. Recently, there has been attempt to classify them such that their name should include all the three important features of the disease—(1) phenotype, (2) mode of inheritance, and (3) gene responsible. The new classification is particularly helpful for research trials and epidemiological studies. Even after decades of in vitro and in vivo studies, we lack specific therapy for CMT. This is mainly because CMT is a heterogeneous disease with wide phenotypic and genetic variation. Gene therapy has emerged as one of the most promising tools for treating genetic disorders. Existing data of successful therapies for other genetic diseases such as spinal muscular atrophy and adrenoleukodystrophy has suddenly boosted the use of gene therapy in ongoing preclinical trials in CMT. Viral vector-mediated gene therapy using adeno-associated virus (AAV) is regarded as the best choice delivery of gene therapy. The following chapter discusses the recent classification along with recent advances in the treatment of CMT.

Keywords: CMT, Classification, Newer therapies, Management.

■ INTRODUCTION

Ever since the initial descriptions in 1886 by Charcot and Marie[1] and further by Tooth[2] in his thesis, our knowledge about Charcot-Marie-Tooth (CMT) disease has distinctly evolved. What was initially described as "peroneal muscular atrophy" with similarly affected family members[1,3] is now known to be the most frequent form of hereditary neuropathy all over the world.[4] CMT is an inherited disorder affecting peripheral nerves which is genetically heterogenous with phenotypic variations such as other neurogenetic diseases. The disease is characterized by weakness and wasting of distal lower limbs followed by upper limbs with foot deformities **(Figs. 1A and B)**.[5] Numerous implicated genes have now been discovered with many new reported every year in the world literature.[6]

Due to this growing list of responsible genes and their numerous mutations, the current knowledge of understanding the

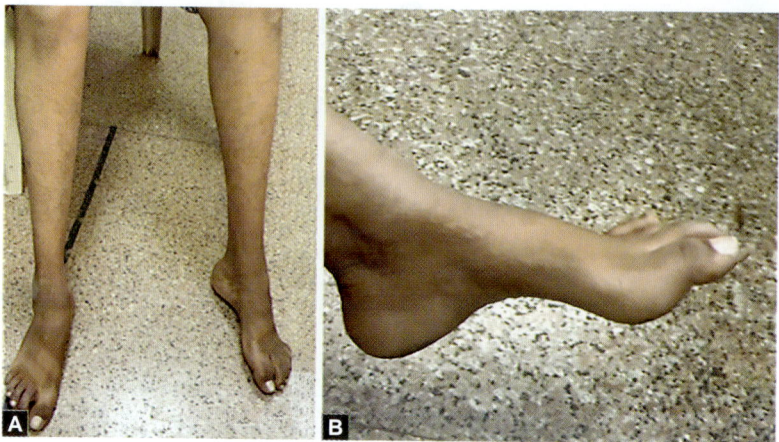

FIGS. 1A AND B: (A) The wasting of bilateral legs giving the appearance of "Champagne Bottle" characteristically seen in Charcot–Marie–Tooth (CMT) disease. (B) The presence of pes cavus and hammer toes.

specific presentations of each subtype is limited and thus classifying it is much more difficult than before.

CLASSIFICATION OF CHARCOT– MARIE–TOOTH—HISTORICAL PERSPECTIVE

The initial attempt to classify CMT can be seen in seminal work by Dyck and Lambert[3] in their paper *"Lower Motor and Primary Sensory Neuron Diseases with Peroneal Muscular Atrophy"* where they made three groups on the basis of natural course of disease, electrophysiological findings, biopsy characteristics, and inheritance pattern. The first group hypertrophic neuropathy of CMT type (dominant inheritance) was characterized by demyelinating neuropathy with low motor conduction velocities (MCVs) (<38 m/s in median nerves) with autosomal dominant (AD) inheritance. The second group was hypertrophic neuropathy of CMT type with either sporadic, dominant with poor expressivity or recessive inheritance. The third type was hypertrophic neuropathy of Dejerine–Sottas type which was infantile onset with delayed motor development milestones and had very low conduction velocities in the range of 3–5 m/s in ulnar nerves.[3] Subsequently, axonal forms were recognized and therefore, CMT were classified based on MCVs of median nerves into demyelinating and axonal groups called as hereditary motor and sensory neuropathy (HMSN type I)/hypertrophic form of CMT and HMSN type II/neuronal form of CMT, respectively.[7] An intermediate group was further defined with MCV between 25 and 45 m/s.[8] HMSN III group included patients who belonged to infantile onset Dejerine–Sottas syndrome (DSS). The further list went on to include other subtypes **(Table 1)**.[9]

The terminology was changed from HMSN to CMT over the years and therefore terms were changed to CMT1, CMT2, etc. CMT1 is among the most common CMT diseases and has demyelinating pattern with AD inheritance along with CMT4 which is autosomal recessive (AR). CMT2 has primarily axonal pattern with AD and AR patterns.[10] "CMT plus" was also proposed for associated signs other than peripheral nervous system (CMT5 and CMT6) and is still used by many

TABLE 1: Old classification with terminology HMSN.

Subtypes	Clinical characteristics
HMSN I	Hypertrophic neuropathy with dominant inheritance
HMSN II	Neuronal form of peroneal muscular atrophy
HMSN III	Hypertrophic neuropathy of infancy/DSS
HMSN IV	Refsum disease
HMSN V	Neuropathy with spastic paraplegia
HMSN VI	Neuropathy with optic atrophy
HMSN VII	Neuropathy with retinitis pigmentosa

(HMSN: hereditary motor sensory neuropathy; DSS: Dejerine–Sottas syndrome)

clinicians. CMTX represented X-linked (XL) inherited CMT and its further subtypes were labeled as CMTX1 to CMTX6.[11]

The classification has been challenged repeatedly as our knowledge improved with the discovery of genes responsible for the specific subtypes. It is specifically criticized in research and is considered not appropriate for use. It lacks a particular schematic pattern part from differentiation of demyelinating and axonal forms. The basis of classification has been electrophysiological findings in conduction studies only. The inheritance pattern was not included at that time and AD and AR can be seen in many CMT subtype. There is also lack of uniformity. CMTX subtypes are not given alphabets such as CMT1A and CMT2A, but they are numbered from CMTX1 to CMTX6.[11] Traditional classification was made on the basis of limited knowledge of the disease at that time, but currently due to expanding phenotypes and numerous genotypes, the alphabets for CMT has reached 'Z' in CMT2Z.[12] The single gene can have different phenotypes, e.g., PMP22 duplication leads to CMT1A but PMP22 deletion leads to hereditary neuropathy with liability to pressure palsies (HNPP).[6] The name of the disease or its position in the classification does not clarifies whether it is the gain or loss of function. MPZ mutation can cause AD CMT1B which is demyelinating form, also AD CMT2I/J which is an axonal form and sometimes as DSS which has infantile onset with severe disease phenotype. The classification has no clarifications on the numerical sequence of the disease. HMSN I and II are CMT1 and CMT2, respectively but there is no CMT3 corresponding to HMSN III. CMT4 does not correspond to HMSN IV. HMSN IV is Refsum disease as per classification which is a neurometabolic disorder with cerebellar ataxia (CA), anosmia, hearing loss as other symptoms[13] while CMT4 presents with severe hypomyelinating neuropathy.[14] We know that single gene can cause different phenotypes, e.g., GDAP1 mutation can cause CMT2K, CMT4A, CMT2H, CMT2K, and CMTRIA.[10] There is no clear classification of distal hereditary motor neuropathy (dHMN) and hereditary sensory and autonomic neuropathy (HSAN).

To update the knowledge about the disease and genetic data, a new and simplified classification system was proposed by Mathis et al. in 2015.[4] The classification system used a simplified three step module—(1) mode of inheritance (AD, AR, XL, and mitochondrial) followed by (2) generic term of disease (CMT) and electrophysiological category. "De" and "Ax" for demyelinating and axonal forms, respectively. For intermediate forms, "In" is to be used. "1" in CMT1 has been replaced by "De" and "2" in CMT2 is replaced by "Ax". (3) The third and the most important step is the name of the gene affected. As per this classification, CMT2H becomes "AR-CMTAx-GDAP1" and CMRIA becomes AR-CMTIn-GDAP1.

Authors did an international internet survey in 2016 including >300 CMT experts worldwide via a questionnaire.[15] They proposed their classification system for all inherited neuropathies. Based on the results of this questionnaire, the classification was modified as given in three steps:

- *Step 1—phenotype*: The clinical presentation will be mentioned first as CMT or dHMN or HSAN or spastic paraplegia (SPG) or CA.
- *Step 2—mode of transmission*: Inheritance will be mentioned as AD, AR, XL, and sporadic (Spo-) and mitochondrial inheritance (Mit).
- *Step 3—gene*: This is the most important step because this indicated the gene responsible for the disease, e.g., "PMP22" or "MPZ". If the gene is not yet known or not yet discovered, the status has to be shown as "unknown".

The classification system is also used in the same way for other neuropathies. The authors have mentioned many advantages of this new classification. The main strength is defining the kind of genetic mutation with the name of the gene. However, many neurologists and CMT experts still use the old alphabetical classification of CMT and the term CMT1A is still used in all the research and publications worldwide.

EMERGING THERAPIES IN CHARCOT–MARIE–TOOTH

Genetic disorders have never been an era for research as it is currently because of revolutionary technologies which provide quick diagnosis thus emerging treatment trials. It is said that the next decade will be dominated by the treatment with the gene therapy. Currently, there is no definite disease modifying pharmacological or genetic treatment available for CMT, however, numerous studies done in mice and primates have paved the way and promise to bring therapies sooner.[16-21] We are going to discuss the major undergoing areas of research and future aspects which can be used to develop therapies in patients with CMT. Before getting the knowledge of the areas of research, it is important to know why it is so complex to develop curative/preventive therapies in CMT. The major challenges faced are due to:

- Genetic and phenotypic heterogeneity of the disease is the major issue. Numerous genes have been discovered with their several mutations with vast phenotype. Single therapy developed for one type of genetic mutation will target that specific subtype only and not others.
- The number of patients belonging to a specific mutation is few.
- Another problem is to monitor response of the therapy which is challenging because of slowly progressing natural course. There is high need to develop an ideal biomarker for measuring the efficacy of management strategies.
- Translation of therapy from mice to primates into human trials is the too complex and is the most puzzling step.

The basis for developing treatment strategies in CMT is the knowledge toward the involved genes, mutations, and their basic pathophysiology. The neuropathies which are primarily demyelinating have their corresponding mutation in the genes which are highly expressed in myelin forming Schwann cells. Axonal types of CMT will have mutated genes which are involved in the functioning of the axon/neuron. However, it has been found that a specific gene can cause demyelinating as well as axonal type of disease because of different kinds of mutation leading to distinct phenotypes and different inheritance pattern.[15] As a result of all these obstacles, developing treatment for genetic disorders has always been problematic. If we intend to gain useful results, we need to understand the exact molecular basis and the cellular changes of each specific mutation.

There has to be an understanding of the exact pathophysiological process which is still advancing. Additionally, it is believed that axonal neuropathies affect only the distal most part of the sensory and motor nerves and demyelinating neuropathies affect the whole neuron from roots to distal part owing to the fact that the myelin is affected. Mode of treatment would differ accordingly from intravenous to intrathecal to intramuscular. The number of doses would vary as per the type of delivery of route. The route of administration would influence the number of dosing required, the immunogenetic property of the vector and the host, toxicity, and expected adverse effects.

Gene Therapy (Table 2)

Gene therapy is the usage of viral vectors or nonviral methods to edit, silence, repair, or replace genetic material in order to modify the disease phenotype.[17] Developing gene therapies differs as per the type of genetic mutation. Gene replacement is the modality of choice in diseases with loss of function mutation. In contrast, disorders with gain of toxic function, oversurplous gene, dominant inheritance, gene silencing, or gene editing would be beneficial.

- *Viral vector-based therapy*: Viral vectors are used to deliver the genetic material inside the cells. Viruses which are used

TABLE 2: Overview of gene therapy for various Charcot–Marie–Tooth (CMT) disease.

Subtype	Target gene	Mode of delivery of gene therapy	Stage of research
CMT1A	PMP22	AAV9	In vivo
		LV	In vivo
		ASO	In vivo
		CRISPR/Cas9	In vivo
		siRNA	In vivo
		miRNA	In vivo
		Squalene NP	In vivo
	NT-3	AAV1	Phase I trial
CMT1X	GJB1	AAV9	In vivo
		LV	In vivo
	MPZ	AAV9	In vivo
		LV	In vivo
	NT-3	AAV1	In vivo
CMT1B	MANF	LV	In vivo
CMT2A	SARM1	AAV8	In vivo
CMT2D	GARS	AAV9	In vivo
	NT-3	AAV1	In vivo
CMT2E	NEFL	CRISPR/Cas9	In vivo
CMT2S	IGHMBP2	AAV9	Phase I trial
CMT4C	SH3TC2	LV	In vivo
CMT4J	FIG4 and CBA	AAV9	In vivo

must be able to pass blood–brain barrier as well as blood-nerve barrier and should be less immunogenic. The technique is mainly used in diseases with loss of function mutation. Viral vector-based gene therapy has revolutionized the medical field after successful treatment in children with spinal muscular atrophy (SMA) with the use of *SMN* gene through adeno-associated virus 9 (AAV9) in 2018.[22] The engineered virus used is devoid of its own genetic material and is a protein-based carrier which can penetrate the plasma membranes of the host cells and deliver the specific DNA into the nucleus.[23] Lentiviruses were the first to be successfully used as a vector for stem cell gene therapy in patients with adrenoleukodystrophy (ALD).[24] Injecting hematopoietic stem cells with lentiviral vector carrying ABCD1 DNA in these patients has shown cessation of further central demyelination.[25] The biggest therapeutic challenge is the presence of preexisting immunity with induction of natural antibodies against the viral antigens which can led to failure of therapeutic response or adverse effects.[23] The mode of delivery is another challenge which needs to be explored. The viral vectors have been used intravenous, directly to the central nervous system (CNS) by intrathecal route, intramuscular, or into the specific targets (cardiac and pulmonary).[23]

Gene replacement therapy has been tried in CMT only in animal studies currently. CMT1A is the most common CMT and is a prototype of Schwann cell disease. Neurotrophin-3 (NT-3) expressed by Schwann cells and is required for their survival and differentiation. Preclinical study of intramuscular gene therapy of AAV. NT-3 in Trembler^J mice suggests sustained NT-3 levels through muscle secretion.[26] However, efficacy of any trial on the basis of studies done in mice cannot be predicted. CMT1X which is an XL disorder with GJB1 mutation encoding connexin32 (Cx32) resulting in myelin gaps in Schwann cells. Intrathecal delivery of viral derived CX32 in Cx32 knockout mouse models has shown functional and electrophysiological recovery.[27] Same group also examined the effect of delayed effectiveness of intrathecal gene therapy after the neuropathy has started. It was checked on GJB1-null mouse model.[28] The mice showed increased conduction velocities in sciatic nerves with increased plasma NEFL levels.[28]

- *Antisense oligonucleotide (ASO)*: ASO has clearly changed the management of SMA in infants and children and has been shown effective in various randomized clinical trials.[29,30] CMT1A results from excess of PMP22 expression.[9] The more the number of copies of PMP22, the more severe is the neuropathy.[31] Sometimes, missense mutation can also result in CMT1A.[9] Thus, gene silencing with use of ASO could be the modality of choice in treating the patients with CMT1A. Zhao et al., evaluated effect of engineered ASO in mouse with severe demyelinating neuropathy (C22 mouse) and another CMT1A rat model with mild neuropathy (3 murine PMP22 copies). They demonstrated that ASO treatment improved grip strength, CMAP amplitudes in both mice and rats.[32] They also demonstrated that there was decreased expression of PMP22 Schwann cells in skin biopsies of foot pads of rats who were treated with ASO.[32] It was noted that gene therapy with ASO does not prevent secondary axonal degeneration, thus to be used before starting of neuropathy. There were concerns about thrombocytopenia with ASO therapy in SMA, but long-term safety trials including large number of patients from Europe have now cleared the doubts about safety of use at least in patients with SMA.[33] Route of administration is still controversial and need to be explored in CMT. Because Schwann cell proliferation became better after intrathecal route of administration in studies by Kagiava et al.,[27] intrathecal route should be preferred over intramuscular or intravenous is debatable.

- *CRISPR/Cas9*: CRISPR/Cas9 technology works by editing a specific sequence of gene called gene editing. This method was used by Lee et al., in C22 mice to downregulate PMP22 expression by deleting the TATA box of the gene. It resulted in reduced expression of *PMP22* gene followed by reduced concentration of PMP22 mRNA in the Schwann cells. *CRISPR/Cas9* gene editing looks promising in mice models with CMT1A which has excess copies of *PMP22* genes.[19]
- *RNA interference (RNAi)*: RNAi is the normal physiological mechanism by which cells control gene expression. It involves silencing gene complex with the help of small interfering RNA (siRNA), short hairpin RNA (shRNA), and microRNA (miRNA). Posttranscriptional gene silencing has been proven beneficial in the first ever RNA-based therapy in hereditary transthyretin mediated amyloidosis.[34] RNAi has been used in animal studies to reverse CMT1A phenotype. Because CMT1A is a disease with excess of gene copies, siRNA theoretically must be the best method used to develop therapy for CMT1A patients. In vivo targeting mutation in *PMP22* gene in Trembler[J] mice by intraperitoneal injection of allele specific siRNA resulted in significant increase in motor function and muscle mass.[20] Serfecz et al., demonstrated that transfection of seed sequence of miR-29a binding site of *PMP22* gene in CMT1A mouse models leads to almost 50% decrease in PMP22 mRNA levels which is equal to 20% decrease in PMP22 protein levels.[35] Boutary et al. further used siRNA and conjugated them with squalene nanoparticles to make them stable and intravenously gave them to mutated mice models of CMT1A. It resulted in a decrease in PMP22 levels and improved motor function. The effect lasted only 3 weeks and recurrent doses were needed. They concluded that the PMP22 levels are dose sensitive and thus decrease when specific dose of siRNA is used.[36] These studies show emerging role of RNAi in the management of genetic disorders specially when there is gain of function mutation.
- *VM202 (Engensis)*: VM202 is plasmid DNA that encodes two isoforms of hepatocyte growth factor and is used as nonviral vector-based gene therapy which stimulates regeneration and Schwann cell repair.[37] The safety and tolerability of VM202 were tested in genetically proven patients with CMT1A (NCT05361031, results not yet reported). The drug has been evaluated in diabetic neuropathy as a nonviral gene therapy in phase 3 study.[38]

Drug Therapy

Numerous drug compounds have been explored in the treatment of CMT but none of them so far have succeeded in providing effective results. **Table 3** provides detailed outline of the drugs compounds used and currently being evaluated. Authors will discuss few of the important ones in this subsection. Majority of them were tried for CMT1A subtype.

Amongst all of the pharmacological compounds, ascorbic acid has been used on a very large scale in many trials. It reduces PMP22 expression via inhibition of cAMP (cyclic adenosine monophosphate) pathway. Mouse model study suggested its therapeutic

TABLE 3: Potential targets and pharmacological compounds in treatment of CMT.

Final target mechanism	Compound	Mechanism of action	Subtype	Data to support potential application in humans
To decrease PMP22 expression	Ascorbic acid	cAMP mediated reduction in PMP22 expression	CMT1A	No efficacy seen in phase II and III trials
	PXT3003	*Baclofen*: GABA receptor agonist *Naltrexone*: Increases baclofen activity *D-sorbitol*: Stabilizes misfolded protein	CMT1A	Phase II trial followed by phase III RCT (PLEO-CMT): High-dose demonstrates significant change in ONLS
	Progesterone antagonist	Epigenetic regulation of gene expression	CMT1A	Preclinical trials No human studies
To improve clearance of PMP22 aggregates	Rapamycin	mTORC1 inhibitor leading to PMP22 aggregates clearance	CMT1A	Preclinical trials
	NVP-AUY922	HSP90 inhibitor	CMT1A	Preclinical trials
To improve Schwann cell differentiation	P2X7 inhibitor	Decreased calcium influx and reduced demyelination	CMT1A	Preclinical studies
	Neuregulin (NRG-1)	Myelin thickness preservation	CMT1A, CMT1B, CMT4B1, CMT4H, HNPP	Preclinical studies
	Lipid supplementation	Improved myelin biosynthesis	CMT1A	Preclinical studies
To reduce protein misfolding	Curcumin	SERCA inhibitor: Reduces UPR marker expression	CMT1A, CMT1E, CMT1B	Preclinical studies
	IFB-088/Sephin1/ Icerguestat	UPR modulator	CMT1B, CMT1A	Phase I trials completed, also trials in ALS and MS
Improve axonal transport	HDAC6 deacetylase inhibitors	Axonal, mitochondrial and microtubular transport	CMT2F, CMT1A, CMT2A, CMT2D	Preclinical studies
Prevent axonal degeneration	SARM1 inactivation	Prevents NAD+ depletion	All CMT	Preclinical studies
Restoring MFN2	MiM111	Improves mitochondrial trafficking	CMT2A	Preclinical studies
To reduce sorbitol accumulation	Aldolase reductase inhibitors	Reduces production of sorbitol from glucose in *SORD* gene deficiency	CMT-SORD-Ax	Phase II-III trials ongoing

(cAMP: cyclic adenosine monophosphate; CMT: Charcot–Marie–Tooth disease; GABA: gamma-aminobutyric acid; HDAC6: histone deacetylase 6; HNPP: hereditary neuropathy with pressure palsies; HSP90: heat shock protein 90; MFN2: mitofusin 2; NAD: nicotinamide adenine dinucleotide; ONLS: overall neuropathy limitation score; RCT: randomized controlled trial; SARM1: sterile a and TIR motif containing 1; SORD: sorbitol dehydrogenase; UPR: unfolded protein response) use in CMT1A;[39] however, double blind randomized trial (RT) (CMT-TRAUK and CMT-TRIAAL) in CMT1A patients found no significant effectiveness after 2 years of therapy as compared to placebo.[40]

PXT3003 drug is a form of polytherapy with combination of three drugs—baclofen, naltrexone hydrochloride, and D-sorbitol. Baclofen is a gamma-aminobutyric acid (GABA) agonist; naltrexone potentiates the effect of baclofen and D-sorbitol stabilizes misfolded protein. PXT3003 has been found to improve myelination both in vitro and in vivo testing in rodent models.[41] The compound was explored in double-blind placebo-controlled RT in CMT1A in 1:1:1 ratio of high dose versus low dose PXT3003 versus placebo. It was concluded that the compound is safe and well tolerated with improvement in the primary endpoint—Overall Neuropathy Limitation Score (ONLS) as compared to placebo.[42] The change in ONLS score was highest in the high-dose group (mean effect: −0.37 points, $p = 0.008$). It is important to note here that high-dose formulations were found to have crystallization inside the bottle because of which 62 patients have to be discontinued from the study. There was no difference between low-dose drug versus placebo.[42]

Other drug compounds have also been evaluated but in preclinical studies in CMT1A animal models, but did not yield promising results. Progesterone antagonists were used with the hypothesis that steroid hormones regulate the epigenetic induced expression of genes. Onapristone was used in CMT1A rat models and has been noted to cause significant motor improvement but safety concern did not allow for trials in patients.[21] Ulipristal is another progesterone antagonist used in phase III trial, but suspended in between.[17] Rapamycin and heat shock protein inhibitors were found to increase the clearance of PMP22 aggregates and improve Schwann cell function in preclinical studies, but the role is not clear.[21] P2X7 inhibitors (A438079) work by inhibition of calcium influx into the Schwann cells which is found to be in excess in CMT1A rats due to overexpression of PMP22. Affected rats treated with 3 mg/kg of A438079 showed improvement in motor power as compared to placebo.[43] ACE-083 is another compound which was studied in patients with CMT1 and CMTX, but the trial have been terminated as secondary endpoints were not achieved.[44]

Recently promising results have been expected from sorbitol dehydrogenase (SORD) inhibitors.[45] SORD mutations have been found in axonal form of CMT2 and dHMN.[18] SORD encodes the enzyme responsible for conversion of glucose to fructose. If enzyme is deficient, then there is accumulation of sorbitol leading on to neuropathy.[18] Aldolase reductase inhibitors inhibits the enzyme aldolase reductase which is involved in conversion of glucose to sorbitol, thus decreasing the neurotoxicity. Already human trials are underway in this field (NCT05397665).[45] Many other compounds are being explored, most of them were proven effective in animal models but the research could not be translated to human subjects.

■ CONCLUSION

The next decade is expected to take off the "no effective treatment" label from the inherited disorders. We have come so far in research and the target is not distant. The advantage of collective knowledge of causative genes and their mutation has changed the understanding of the pathological mechanisms of every subtype of CMT. Despite the challenges ahead, development of adequate therapies with biomarkers will be available sooner.

REFERENCES

1. Charcot JM, Marie P. Sur une forme particuliere d'atrophie musculaire progressive souvent familial debutant par les pieds et les jambes et atteignant plus tard les mains. Rev Med (Paris). 1886;6:97-138.
2. Tooth HH. The Peroneal Type of Progressive Muscular Atrophy, thesis. London: H K Lewis & Co, Ltd.; 1886.
3. Dyck PJ, Lambert EH. Lower motor and primary sensory neuron diseases with peroneal muscular atrophy. II. Neurologic, genetic, and electrophysiologic findings in various neuronal degenerations. Arch Neurol. 1968;18(6):619-25.
4. Mathis S, Goizet C, Tazir M, Magdelaine C, Lia AS, Magy L, et al. Charcot-Marie-Tooth diseases: an update and some new proposals for the classification. J Med Genet. 2015;52(10):681-90.
5. Vallat JM, Goizet C, Magy L, Mathis S. Too many numbers and complexity: time to update the classifications of neurogenetic disorders? J Med Genet. 2016;53(10):647-50.
6. Ferese R, Campopiano R, Scala S, D'Alessio C, Storto M, Buttari F, et al. Cohort Analysis of 67 Charcot-Marie-Tooth Italian Patients: Identification of New Mutations and Broadening of Phenotype Expression Produced by Rare Variants. Frontiers in Genetics. 2021;12:682050.
7. Bouche P, Gherardi R, Cathala HP, Lhermitte F, Castaigne P. Peroneal muscular atrophy: Part 1. Clinical and electrophysiological study. J Neurol Sci. 1983;61(3):389-99.
8. Bradley WG, Madrid R, Davis CJ. The peroneal muscular atrophy syndrome. Clinical genetic, electrophysiological and nerve biopsy studies. Part 3. Clinical, electrophysiological and pathological correlations. J Neurol Sci. 1977;32(1):123-36.
9. Shy ME LJ, Chance PF, Klein CJ, Dyck PJ. Hereditary Motor and Sensory Neuropathies: An Overview of Clinical, Genetic, Electrophysiologic, and Pathologic Features. In Peripheral Neuropathy. Expert Consult Basic Elsevier. 2005;2:1623-58.
10. Braathen GJ. Genetic epidemiology of Charcot–Marie–Tooth disease. Acta neurologica Scandinavica. 2012;126(s193):iv-22.
11. Wang Y, Yin F. A review of X-linked Charcot-Marie-Tooth disease. J Child Neurol. 2016;31(6):761-72.
12. Sancho P, Bartesaghi L, Miossec O, García-García F, Ramírez-Jiménez L, Siddell A, et al. Characterization of molecular mechanisms underlying the axonal Charcot-Marie-Tooth neuropathy caused by MORC2 mutations. Hum Mole Genet. 2019;28(10):1629-44.
13. Wills AJ, Manning NJ, Reilly MM. Refsum's disease. QJM. 2001;94(8):403-6.
14. Othmane KB, Hentatl F, Lennon F, Hamida CB, Blel S, Roses AD, et al. Linkage of a locus (CMT4A) for autosomal recessive Charcot-Marie-Tooth disease to chromosome 8q. Hum Mole Genet. 1993;2(10):1625-8.
15. Magy L, Mathis S, Le Masson G, Goizet C, Tazir M, Vallat JM. Updating the classification of inherited neuropathies: Results of an international survey. Neurology. 2018;90(10):e870-e6.
16. Bai Y, Treins C, Volpi VG, Scapin C, Ferri C, Mastrangelo R, et al. Treatment with IFB-088 Improves Neuropathy in CMT1A and CMT1B Mice. Mol Neurobiol. 2022;59(7):4159-78.
17. Pisciotta C, Pareyson D. Gene therapy and other novel treatment approaches for Charcot-Marie-Tooth disease. Neuromusc Dis. 2023;33(8):627-35.
18. Liu X, He J, Yilihamu M, Duan X, Fan D. Clinical and genetic features of biallelic mutations in SORD in a series of chinese patients with Charcot-Marie-Tooth and distal hereditary motor neuropathy. Front Neurol. 2021;12:733926.
19. Lee JS, Lee JY, Song DW, Bae HS, Doo HM, Yu HS, et al. Targeted PMP22 TATA-box editing by CRISPR/Cas9 reduces demyelinating neuropathy of Charcot-Marie-Tooth disease type 1A in mice. Nucleic Acids Res. 2020;48(1):130-40.
20. Lee JS, Chang EH, Koo OJ, Jwa DH, Mo WM, Kwak G, et al. Pmp22 mutant allele-specific siRNA alleviates demyelinating neuropathic phenotype in vivo. Neurobiol Dis. 2017;100:99-107.
21. Bolino A, D'Antonio M. Recent advances in the treatment of Charcot-Marie-Tooth neuropathies. J Peripher Nerv Syst. 2023;28(2):134-49.
22. Mendell JR, Al-Zaidy S, Shell R, Arnold WD, Rodino-Klapac LR, Prior TW, et al. Single-Dose Gene-Replacement Therapy for Spinal Muscular Atrophy. N Engl J Med. 2017;377(18):1713-22.
23. Naso MF, Tomkowicz B, Perry WL, 3rd, Strohl WR. Adeno-associated virus (AAV) as a vector for gene therapy. BioDrugs. 2017;31(4):317-34.
24. Cartier N, Hacein-Bey-Abina S, Bartholomae CC, Veres G, Schmidt M, Kutschera I, et al. Hematopoietic stem cell gene therapy with a lentiviral vector in X-linked adrenoleukodystrophy. Science (New York, NY). 2009;326(5954):818-23.
25. Eichler F, Duncan C, Musolino PL, Orchard PJ, Oliveira SD, Thrasher AJ, et al. Hematopoietic stem-

cell gene therapy for cerebral adrenoleukodystrophy. N Engl J Med. 2017;377(17):1630-8.
26. Sahenk Z, Galloway G, Clark KR, Malik V, Rodino-Klapac LR, Kaspar BK, et al. AAV1.NT-3 gene therapy for Charcot-Marie-Tooth neuropathy. Mol Ther. 2014;22(3):511-21.
27. Kagiava A, Karaiskos C, Richter J, Tryfonos C, Lapathitis G, Sargiannidou I, et al. Intrathecal gene therapy in mouse models expressing CMT1X mutations. Human molecular genetics. 2018;27(8):1460-73.
28. Kagiava A, Richter J, Tryfonos C, Karaiskos C, Heslegrave AJ, Sargiannidou I, et al. Gene replacement therapy after neuropathy onset provides therapeutic benefit in a model of CMT1X. Hum Mole Genet. 2019;28(21):3528-42.
29. Finkel RS, Mercuri E, Darras BT, Connolly AM, Kuntz NL, Kirschner J, et al. Nusinersen versus Sham Control in Infantile-Onset Spinal Muscular Atrophy. N Engl J Med. 2017;377(18):1723-32.
30. Mercuri E, Darras BT, Chiriboga CA, Day JW, Campbell C, Connolly AM, et al. Nusinersen versus Sham Control in Later-Onset Spinal Muscular Atrophy. N Engl J Med. 2018;378(7):625-35.
31. Pareyson D, Testa D, Morbin M, Erbetta A, Ciano C, Lauria G, et al. Does CMT1A homozygosity cause more severe disease with root hypertrophy and higher CSF proteins? Neurology. 2003;60(10):1721-2.
32. Zhao HT, Damle S, Ikeda-Lee K, Kuntz S, Li J, Mohan A, et al. PMP22 antisense oligonucleotides reverse Charcot-Marie-Tooth disease type 1A features in rodent models. J Clin Invest. 2018;128(1):359-68.
33. Günther R, Wurster CD, Brakemeier S, Osmanovic A, Schreiber-Katz O, Petri S, et al. Long-term efficacy and safety of nusinersen in adults with 5q spinal muscular atrophy: a prospective European multinational observational study. Lancet Reg Health Eur. 2024;39:100862.
34. Adams D, Gonzalez-Duarte A, O'Riordan WD, Yang CC, Ueda M, Kristen AV, et al. Patisiran, an RNAi therapeutic, for hereditary transthyretin amyloidosis. N Engl J Med. 2018;379(1):11-21.
35. Serfecz J, Bazick H, Al Salihi MO, Turner P, Fields C, Cruz P, et al. Downregulation of the human peripheral myelin protein 22 gene by miR-29a in cellular models of Charcot–Marie–Tooth disease. Gene Therapy. 2019;26(12):455-64.
36. Boutary S, Caillaud M, El Madani M, Vallat JM, Loisel-Duwattez J, Rouyer A, et al. Squalenoyl siRNA PMP22 nanoparticles are effective in treating mouse models of Charcot-Marie-Tooth disease type 1 A. Commun Biol. 2021;4(1):317.

37. Ko KR, Lee J, Lee D, Nho B, Kim S. Hepatocyte growth factor (HGF) promotes peripheral nerve regeneration by activating repair Schwann cells. Sci Rep. 2018;8(1):8316.
38. Perin E, Loveland L, Caporusso J, Dove C, Motley T, Sigal F, et al. Gene therapy for diabetic foot ulcers: Interim analysis of a randomised, placebo-controlled phase 3 study of VM202 (ENGENSIS), a plasmid DNA expressing two isoforms of human hepatocyte growth factor. Int Wound J. 2023;20(9):3531-9.
39. Passage E, Norreel JC, Noack-Fraissignes P, Sanguedolce V, Pizant J, Thirion X, et al. Ascorbic acid treatment corrects the phenotype of a mouse model of Charcot-Marie-Tooth disease. Nat Med. 2004;10(4):396-401.
40. Pareyson D, Reilly MM, Schenone A, Fabrizi GM, Cavallaro T, Santoro L, et al. Ascorbic acid in Charcot-Marie-Tooth disease type 1A (CMT-TRIAAL and CMT-TRAUK): a double-blind randomised trial. Lancet Neurol. 2011;10(4):320-8.
41. Chumakov I, Milet A, Cholet N, Primas G, Boucard A, Pereira Y, et al. Polytherapy with a combination of three repurposed drugs (PXT3003) down-regulates Pmp22 over-expression and improves myelination, axonal and functional parameters in models of CMT1A neuropathy. Orphanet J Rare Dis. 2014;9(1):201.
42. Attarian S, Young P, Brannagan TH, Adams D, Van Damme P, Thomas FP, et al. A double-blind, placebo-controlled, randomized trial of PXT3003 for the treatment of Charcot-Marie-Tooth type 1A. Orphanet J Rare Dis. 2021;16(1):433.
43. Sociali G, Visigalli D, Prukop T, Cervellini I, Mannino E, Venturi C, et al. Tolerability and efficacy study of P2X7 inhibition in experimental Charcot-Marie-Tooth type 1A (CMT1A) neuropathy. Neurobiol Dis. 2016;95:145-57.
44. NIH. (2022). An Open-Label Extension Study to Evaluate the Long-Term Effects of ACE-083 in Patients With Facioscapulohumeral Muscular Dystrophy (FSHD) Previously Enrolled in Study A083-02 and in Patients With Charcot-Marie Tooth (CMT) Disease Types 1 and X Previously Enrolled in Study A083-03. [online] Available from https://clinicaltrials.gov/study/NCT03943290 [Last accessed August, 2024].
45. NIH. (2023). A RandomIzed, Double-Blind, Placebo-CoNtrolled, Two-Part Study to Evaluate the Pharmacodynamic EffIcacy and Clinical Benefit of AT 007 in Patients With SoRbitol Dehydrogenase (SORD) DEficiency. [online] Available from: https://clinicaltrials.gov/study/NCT05397665 [Last accessed August, 2024].

Genetics of Amyotrophic Lateral Sclerosis and Implications for Therapy

Saranya B Gomathy, Seena Vengalil, Atchayaram Nalini

ABSTRACT

Amyotrophic lateral sclerosis (ALS) is a rare disease which presents with degeneration of motor neurons leading to muscle wasting, bulbar involvement, and death within 3–5 years due to respiratory involvement. About 10% of ALS is familial. Recent advances in gene sequencing technologies have led to substantial progress in identifying the genetic basis of ALS. This, in turn, has led to the development of various genetic treatments. In this chapter, we outline the major and minor genes of ALS, indications for genetic testing, and the current molecular therapeutic approaches.

Keywords: *C9orf72, FUS, SOD1*, Gene therapy, Antisense oligonucleotides.

■ INTRODUCTION

Amyotrophic lateral sclerosis (ALS) is a rare disease which presents with degeneration of motor neurons with onset in late middle age, manifesting with progressive muscle wasting, associated with weakness, and respiratory involvement affecting survival.[1] Currently available treatments are symptomatic and supportive. The only Food and Drug Administration (FDA) approved treatment options are riluzole and edaravone, and they subserve very less benefits. Around 10% cases are associated with genetic factors, referred to as familial ALS (fALS).[2] These genetic discoveries have paved way to a better understanding of pathomechanisms of ALS and have the potential to aid in developing gene therapies. This chapter reviews the genetic landscape of ALS and throws light on the pathomechanisms, apart from the various genetic treatment aspects.

■ GENETICS OF AMYOTROPHIC LATERAL SCLEROSIS

Clinical and translational research studies in ALS have suggested a variety of causes for ALS, with important but varied genetic components. fALS accounts for 10%, most of which are inherited in an autosomal dominant fashion. ALS cases occurring in individuals without a family history constitute 90–95%, and are considered to have sporadic ALS (sALS). Genome wide association studies and next-generation sequencing techniques have advanced our knowledge of the genetic causes of ALS. Mutations in *C9ORF72, TARDBP, SOD1,* and *FUS* contribute to 70% fALS cases.

MAJOR AMYOTROPHIC LATERAL SCLEROSIS GENES

Superoxide Dismutase 1

Superoxide dismutase 1 (SOD1) (Cu/Zn-*SOD*) was the first gene identified in 1993 with over 200 mutations, which are associated with different age of onset and survival.[3] Most cases present with a lower motor neuron (LMN) involvement of lower limbs (LLs). G37R and L38V mutations have been associated with an earlier age of onset, whereas A4V mutation was found to be associated with limb onset, and aggressive progression with reduced survival.[4,5] The D90A variant is the most common worldwide, associated with bulbar, upper, and/or LL onset with rapid progression.[6]

A toxic gain of function mechanism is implicated in *SOD1* ALS pathogenesis. Mechanisms include excitotoxicity, oxidative stress, mitochondrial defect, and prion-like transfer. Protein aggregation leading to cellular toxicity is implicated in causing degeneration.[7,8]

TAR DNA-binding Protein *(TDP43)*

Microscopic examination of spinal cord showed cytoplasmic ubiquitinated neuronal inclusion bodies in patients with ALS. The main component of the inclusion was identified in 2006 as TAR DNA-binding protein (*TARDBP*).[9] Accumulation of this protein is encountered in 97% cases. *TDP43* is a nuclear protein that binds to DNA or RNA and shuttles to and fro between the nucleus and cytoplasm. It has a role in messenger ribonucleic acid (mRNA) presplicing, mRNA stability and transport, and protein synthesis. *TDP43* pathology is also seen in 50% frontotemporal dementia (FTD) cases. Both loss and gain of function mutations have been found to cause degeneration.[10] A prion-like spreading mechanism may also be operating in *TDP43* ALS.

TARDBP mutation is more associated with limb-onset phenotype and can be encountered in a wide age group. The p.G376D mutation progresses rapidly with death within 1.5 years of onset.[11] The p.G298S mutation is also short-lived, while the p.A315T mutation has a smoldering course of around 10 years.[12,13]

Fused in Sarcoma

Identified in 2009, fused in sarcoma *(FUS)* is an RNA-binding protein and patients almost always present early in their life (<35 years).[14] *FUS* gene encodes a FET protein responsible for nucleocytoplasmic transport. It is also involved in gene transcription, pre-mRNA splicing, translation, DNA repair, and cellular defense against stresses. More than 50 missense mutations in this gene have been identified. Loss of function mutations cause pathologic cytoplasmic redistribution of *FUS* making it unable to perform its nuclear functions.[15] Gain of function mechanisms have also been postulated; a transgenic mouse model with wild-FUS was shown to develop aggressive neurodegeneration as evidenced by accumulation of *FUS* in cytoplasm.

Chromosome 9 Open Reading Frame 72

Chromosome 9 open reading frame 72 *(C9orf72)* is the most common genetic cause in Europeans and this hexanucleotide expansion (GGGGCC) in the noncoding region was identified in 2011.[16] A large number of repeats are seen in ALS patients, seen in 34% fALS and 5% sALS in Europeans. The exact function of *C9orf72* is still not known and is pointed toward endosomal trafficking regulation, immune function, and autophagy. The principal pathogenic mechanisms include loss of function of *C9orf72* protein, toxic gain of function of GGGGCC repeats, and dipeptide repeat proteins produced by non-ATG translation.[17,18] Bulbar onset is frequently observed in C9orf72 ALS. Other phenotypes such as FTD, sensory neuropathy, and parkinsonism have also been associated.[19-21] Shamim et al., described 3.2% GGGGCC expansion-positive ALS patients from India from a total of 593 cases. Two lineages of GGGGCC-associated haplotypes were found in Indian patients. This study established the Indian prevalence of C9orf72 ALS.[22]

■ GENES WITH MINOR ROLES IN AMYOTROPHIC LATERAL SCLEROSIS

Next-generation sequencing has paved way for the discovery of rare mutational ALS variants. These genes influence RNA processing, proteostasis, and cytoskeletal dynamics. **Table 1** details the genes associated with ALS and their postulated mechanisms and functions. Novel *ALS* genes such as *TBK1, NEK1, CCNF,* and *C21orf2* have been identified late which have paved way to new research avenues.

■ PROPOSED PATHOPHYSIOLOGIC MECHANISMS IN AMYOTROPHIC LATERAL SCLEROSIS

Despite decades of extensive research, the pathophysiology of ALS is elusive, especially in sALS. Multiple factors are implicated leading to the initiation and progression of ALS. The pathogenetic mechanisms are summarized in **Figure 1**. These include RNA metabolism defects, impaired proteostasis, defects in nucleocytoplasmic transport, excitotoxicity, mitochondrial defects, DNA repair defects, oxidative stress, inflammation, autophagy, cell-to-cell transmission (prion-like), and vesicular transport defects.[23]

The mostly implicated genes, *C9orf72, TARDBP,* and *FUS* cause aberrant RNA metabolism; *C9orf72, TARDBP,* and *SOD1* lead to abnormal protein accumulation.[24,25] *SOD1* mutation also can cause mitochondrial defects and oxidative stress.[26] *C9orf72* repeats can lead to mutated protein and haploinsufficiency from the wild-type allele; also, the RNA transcripts accumulate into toxic foci, sequestering the RNA-binding proteins and affecting RNA metabolism. This generates proteotoxic dipeptide repeats.[27] Mislocalized *TDP43* affects RNA splicing and reduce microtubule stability.[10] The pathomechanisms of other *ALS* genes are given in **Table 1**.

■ GENETIC ASPECTS OF JUVENILE AMYOTROPHIC LATERAL SCLEROSIS

Almost 40% cases of juvenile amyotrophic lateral sclerosis (JALS) have a genetic basis, and the most common gene involved is FUS. The pathogenetic mechanisms are similar to adult onset ALS; however, JALS has overlap with many neurodegenerative disorders such as hereditary spastic paraplegia, Charcot–Marie–Tooth disease, and autosomal recessive cerebellar ataxia. FTD is usually not an accompaniment. The most common genes implicated include *FUS, ALS2, SETX,* and *SPG11*; genes with minor involvement are *SIGMAR1, SOD1, SPTLC1, ERLIN1, GNE, TARDBP,* etc. Rapidly progressive disease course is usually encountered in patients with *FUS* or *SOD1* variants with an LMN phenotype. Slowly progressive disease course is seen in predominant upper motor neuron (UMN) forms of disease mediated by *ERLIN1, TARDBP,* and *SPG11* variants. Ataxia is seen in *SETX-*and *SYNE1-*related ALS. Autonomic instability and sensory neuropathy are seen in association with *VRK1-*related JALS and *SPG11*.[28]

TABLE 1: Minor genes in ALS and their possible functions and other disease associations.

Genes	Function	Inheritance	Pathophysiology	Overlap with other diseases
ANXA11 (annexin A11)	Calcium-dependent protein that binds to phospholipid with a role in vesicle transport	AD	Annexin inclusions; impaired binding to calcyclin	FTD, IBM, white matter changes in brain
C21orf2	DNA repair	Not known	Cytoskeletal distortion	–
CCNF (cyclin F)	Cell cycle regulation, part of E3-ubiquitin ligase	AD	Defective proteostasis	FTD
DNAJC7 (DNAJ heat shock protein C7)	Heat shock protein	Not known	–	None
GLT8D1 (glycosyltransferase 8 domain containing 1)	Not known	AD	Not established; localized to the Golgi apparatus	None
KIF5A (kinesin family member 5A)	Kinesin tubule protein	AD	Cytoskeletal defects, impaired axonal transport	CMT2, HSP
HFE (hereditary hemochromatosis)	Iron homeostasis	Not known	–	Alzheimer's disease, Parkinson's disease
NEK1 (NIMA-related kinase 1)	Cell cycle regulation, DNA repair	Not known	DNA damage accumulation	Short rib, thoracic dysplasia
TBK1 (TANK binding kinase 1)	Serine-threonine kinase; innate immunity, cell cycle regulation	AD	Autophagy, inflammation	FTD
TIA1	RNA-binding protein	AD	Aberrant RNA metabolism	–
ALS2 (amyotrophic lateral sclerosis 2)	Guanine-nucleotide exchange factor	AR	Defects in vesicular trafficking	Juvenile PLS, infantile HSP
ATXN2 (ataxin 2)	RNA-binding protein	AD	Defects in ribostasis	–
CHCHD10 (coiled-coil-helix-coiled-coil-helix domain containing 10)	Mitochondrial protein	AD	Energy metabolism defects	FTD; ataxia; isolated mitochondrial myopathy, SMA
CHMP2B (charged multivesicular body protein 2B)	ESCRT-III complex component	AD	Proteostasis and vesicular trafficking defects	FTD

Continued

Continued

Genes	Function	Inheritance	Pathophysiology	Overlap with other diseases
DCTN1 (dynactin 1)	Dynactin microtubule protein	AD	Defects in axon transport	Distal hereditary motor neuropathy VIIB, Perry syndrome
HNRNPA1 (heterogeneous nuclear ribonucleoprotein A1)	RNA-binding protein	AD	Ribostasis defects	Inclusion body myopathy; Paget's disease, FTD
MATR3 (matrin 3)	RNA-binding protein	AD	Ribostasis defects	FTD; distal myopathy with vocal cord and pharyngeal myopathy
NEFH (neurofilament heavy polypeptide)	Neurofilament protein	AD	Defects in axon transport	Axonal CMT 2C
SPG11 (spatacsin)	Transmembrane protein	AR	DNA damage	HSP; CMT2X
SQSTM1 (sequestosome 1)	Ubiquitin-binding protein regulating NF-κB	AD	Autophagy, inflammation	FTD, distal myopathy, dystonia, Paget's disease
TUBA4A (tubulin alpha 4A chain)	Microtubule protein	AD	Cytoskeletal defects	FTD
VAPB (VAMP-associated protein B)	Plasma and intracellular vesicle binding protein	AD	Defects in proteostasis	Finkel type SMA
VCP (valosin-containing protein)	ATPase that regulates protein degradation	AD	Proteostasis defects and inflammation	FTD, CMT 2Y, IBM with early Paget's disease
OPTN (optineurin)	Golgi maintenance, membrane trafficking, autophagy	AD, AR	Autophagy, inflammation	FTD; primary open angle glaucoma
ERLIN1 (endoplasmic reticulum lipid raft-associated protein 1)	Protein complex degrading inositol 1,4,5-triphosphate intracellular receptor ion channels	AR	Calcium release disruption from endoplasmic reticulum; synaptic dysfunction	HSP, Huntington's disease

(AD: autosomal dominant; ALS: amyotrophic lateral sclerosis; AR: autosomal recessive; ATP: adenosine triphosphate; CMT: Charcot–Marie–Tooth disease; DNA: deoxyribonucleic acid; ESCRT: endosomal sorting complexes required for transport; FTD: frontotemporal dementia; HSP: hereditary spastic paraplegia; IBM: inclusion body myopathy; PLS: primary lateral sclerosis; RNA: ribonucleic acid; SMA: spinal muscular atrophy)

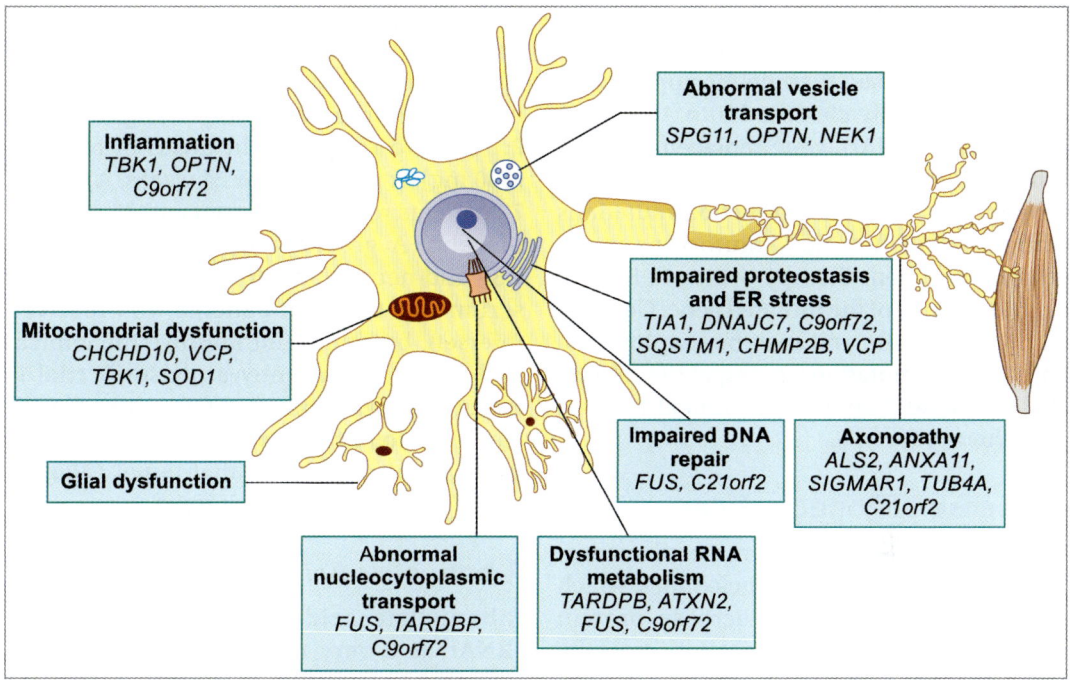

FIG. 1: Amyotrophic lateral sclerosis (ALS) pathogenesis.

Genetic testing is routinely advised in JALS, in both sporadic and familial cases. Negative gene testing does not rule out JALS. Very limited data is available on disease modifying treatments in JALS-antisense oligonucleotides (ASOs) are in the pipeline for *SOD1, FUS, and ATXN2* gene variants.

■ INDICATIONS FOR GENETIC TESTING IN AMYOTROPHIC LATERAL SCLEROSIS

Despite the advances in the genetic discovery, and an extensive array of testing options, genetic testing to all ALS patients is not considered the standard of care and most who actually need access to testing are not offered the same. Evidence-based consensus for genetic testing in ALS and counseling was put forth by Roggenbuck and colleagues. A total of 35 statements were made. Guidelines recommend that all ALS patients should be offered genetic testing with a panel of genes that comprises at a minimum *C9orf72, SOD1, FUS, TARDBP*, any gene to which FDA approves targeted treatment, and genes strongly associated with ALS by ClinGen. The guidelines also recommend provision of genetic counseling and education to all ALS cases, and that it should precede the testing. A three generation-spanning family tree should be noted; pedigree should confirm ALS and associated motor neuron disorders, FTD, other dementias, movement disorders, and psychiatric disease.[29]

Gene-based Therapeutic Strategies

Till date there is no cure for ALS. The FDA approved treatment is riluzole, which inhibits presynaptic glutamate release by blocking sodium channels and thereby reduce excitotoxicity. There is only a modest beneficial effect with Riluzole.[30] The multitude of risk genes for ALS with gain-of-function and loss-of-function mutations calls for gene-based therapeutic approaches. These are broadly classified into ASO, RNA interference (RNAi), gene replacement, and genome editing. ASO or RNA interference can be employed for gain-of-function mutations while loss-of-function mutations need gene replacement therapy, which delivers a functional copy of the mutated gene. Genome editing is specific and may be employed in both types of mutations, to target the mutant allele.[31] **Table 2** shows the clinical trials of gene therapy for ALS.

Antisense Oligonucleotides

These are single-stranded molecules comprising about 20 modified nucleotides, which attach to the mRNA to decrease protein expression. These molecules cannot cross the blood–brain barrier and need to be delivered intrathecally. In ALS patients, ASOs can be employed to target *C9orf72, TARDBP, SOD1,* or *FUS* RNA.[32]

Tofersen, an ASO targeting *SOD1* was found safe and lower *SOD1* levels in cerebrospinal fluid (CSF) in a phase 1/2 trial in high dose group, but was unable to attain primary outcome in a phase III randomized trial. In this trial, ALS patients with *SOD1* mutation were randomly assigned in a 2:1 ratio to receive eight doses of tofersen (100 mg) or placebo over 24 weeks. A total of 72 patients received tofersen and 36 received placebo. A greater reduction of *SOD1* in CSF and neurofilament light (NFL) chain in serum was found in patients who received tofersen, but it did not improve the clinical end points.[33] Currently a phase III trial is recruiting asymptomatic *SOD1* carriers with elevated blood NFL levels.[34] Multiple phase I trials are also going on that target *C9orf72, and ATXN2 and FUS* (Jacifusen).

Ribonucleic Acid Interference

Ribonucleic acid-mediated interference (RNAi) is a very rapid technique of gene silencing. The small interfering RNAs (siRNAs) are double-stranded duplexes having around 20 nucleotide base pairs. The siRNA strand complementary to the target gene binds to the endoribonuclease and target mRNA, forming a silencing complex. The complex further breaks the target mRNA and lead to

TABLE 2: Gene therapy trials in ALS.

Modality	Target	Name of the trial	Drug	Phase	Delivery route
Antisense oligonucleotides					
	SOD1	VALOR[33]	Tofersen	III	Intrathecal
	Asymptomatic *SOD1*	ATLAS[34]	Tofersen	III	Intrathecal
	C9orf72	245AS101	IONIS-C9	I	Intrathecal
	C9orf72	FOCUS-C9	WVE-004	I/II	Intrathecal
	C9orf72	TBD	ASO5-2	NA	Intrathecal
	ATXN-2	275AS101	ION541	I/II	Intrathecal
	FUS	ION363-CS1	Jacifusen	III	Intrathecal
	Stathmin-2	TBD	QRL-201	I	Intrathecal
Delivery mediated by AAV					
	SOD1	TBD	APB-102	I	Intrathecal

(AAV: adeno-associated virus; ALS: amyotrophic lateral sclerosis)

silencing of the gene.[35] The RNAi technique is the FDA approved for hereditary transthyretin amyloidosis, but is being tested currently in ALS trials. A few animal studies led to a trial in two humans with fALS employing a single *AAV-miR-SOD1* infusion intrathecally; one developed meningoradiculitis and second did not have any adverse effects. Even though reduced *SOD1* levels were seen on first patient's autopsy, there was no decrease in the levels of *SOD1* in CSF in both at two weeks. Second patient had a fairly stable ALS Functional Rating Scale (ALSFRS) score at 1 year.[36]

Gene Replacement Therapy

This technique uses viral vectors to deliver functional copy of a gene in patients having loss of function mutations. These can be administered intravenously and have the ability to cross the blood–brain barrier. Lentivirus and adeno-associated viruses (AAVs) are usually employed. Onasemnogene abeparvovec, an AAV9-mediated gene replacement treatment for spinal muscular atrophy (SMA) received FDA approval and is currently being used in the treatment of children below 2 years of age with SMA.[37] The most common mutations causing ALS (*C9orf72, FUS, SOD1, and TARDBP*) ensue due to gain-of-function mutation, and hence cannot be targeted by this technique.

Genome Editing

This technique employs the RNA-guided CRISPR-Cas9 (clustered regularly interspaced short palindromic repeats and CRISPR-associated protein) technology which acts by targeting the gene by simple base pairing. This technique can do targeted changes compared to the rest of the techniques, and modulate transcription and edit RNA. This technology is being tested in experimental *C9orf72* models. A 2017 animal study employed the CRISPR targeting *SOD1* gene employing modified AAV9. The viral vector delivered *Staphylococcus aureus*-derived Cas9 and a single-guide RNA (sgRNA) against the *SOD1* gene and it was administered into the facial vein to neonatal mice. Reduced motor neuron death and increased survival of mice was noted.[38]

■ INDIAN REPORTS ON AMYOTROPHIC LATERAL SCLEROSIS GENES

NIMHANS Experience (Unpublished Data)

Whole exome sequencing of 700 ALS patients showed genetic mutations in 113. The mean age at presentation was 51.9 years + 11.2 years (19–72) years, male:female ratio was 71:42. The most common genetic variants identified were in *SETX* and *SOD1* (12) followed by *DCTN1, FUS, NEFH,* and *OPTN*.

Faheem Arshad et al. (2022)

Reported a patient having FTD-ALS syndrome due to a new loss of function mutation (c.1810G>T) in the *TBK1* gene. Brain MRI revealed asymmetric frontotemporal atrophy and hypometabolism. Segregation analysis of the genetic variant demonstrated its presence in multiple asymptomatic members in the family.[39]

■ CONCLUSION

A lot of advances have been made toward a better understanding of *ALS* genes and disease mechanisms, and this has led to the clinical application of molecularly driven treatments. Ongoing genetic testing will identify new *ALS* genes. Given the varied and innumerable genetic variants and the molecular pathways, there is likely a large amount of heterogeneity between patients. Using patient-derived models from large cohorts with ALS may help in more accurately developing beneficial treatments. As gene delivery methods improve, there is immense hope that better treatments for ALS will gradually emerge.

■ CASE VIGNETTES

A case of flail leg syndrome with positive family history

A 54-year-old man presented with insidious onset weakness of left LL for 8 months associated with thinning of left leg and a high-stepping gait. There was a significant positive history of similar complaints in three family members, with age of onset in the sixth decade. On examination, power of left ankle dorsiflexor was 3/5 while plantar flexor was 4/5. Bilateral upper limb reflexes and bilateral knee jerks were brisk, with absent bilateral ankle reflexes. Fasciculations were seen over the left vastus medialis, bilateral deltoids, and biceps brachii. Nerve conduction study showed nonrecordable left tibial and left peroneal motor amplitudes, along with normal sensory conduction parameters. Electromyography (EMG) revealed active denervation and chronic reinnervation in cervical and lumbosacral segments. Whole-exome sequencing (WES) revealed a heterozygous missense pathogenic mutation in the *SOD1* gene (c.10A.G; p.Lys4Glu), in chromosome 21. Riluzole and edaravone were introduced. We counseled the patient for tofersen, but it could not be administered because of financial constraints.

Patient with gynecomastia and progressive bulbar weakness

A 51-year-old male, with history of hypertension, presented with progressive bulbar palsy and bifacial weakness since 5 years without any limb weakness or sensory disturbances in limbs with no family history of similar illness. On examination, he had gynecomastia; a clinical possibility of bulbar-onset motor neuron disease (MND) versus Kennedy syndrome was considered. WES revealed *OPTN* mutation (c.1465A>G) in the exon 13 **(Figs. 2A and B)**.

Fatigable ptosis mimicking myasthenia

A 25-year-old man presented with progressive proximodistal weakness and atrophy of left LL for 12 months, proximal weakness of right LL followed by right upper limb (RUL) for 2 months, generalized fasciculations for 5 months. On examination, he had bilateral asymmetrical fatigable ptosis, proximal LL weakness with fatigability, with ptosis in multiple family members. Serum creatine phosphokinase (CPK) was 600 IU/L and repetitive nerve stimulation test showed a decremental pattern. WES showed pathogenic *FUS* mutation (c.1561C>T) **(Figs. 3A to D)**.

Patient with Proximal weakness, sensory abnormalities, with family history of dementia and parkinsonism

A 68-year-old woman presented with pain and proximal weakness of LLs for 12 years and upper limbs for 8 years. She also had itchy blackish discoloration around eyes and limbs for 12 years **(Fig. 4)**. Her sister and mother had similar skin discoloration around the eyes. Her father, two elder brothers, and an

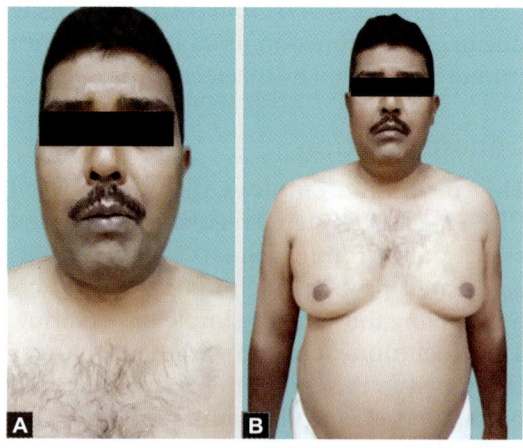

FIGS. 2A AND B: Patient with progressive bulbar weakness and gynecomastia.

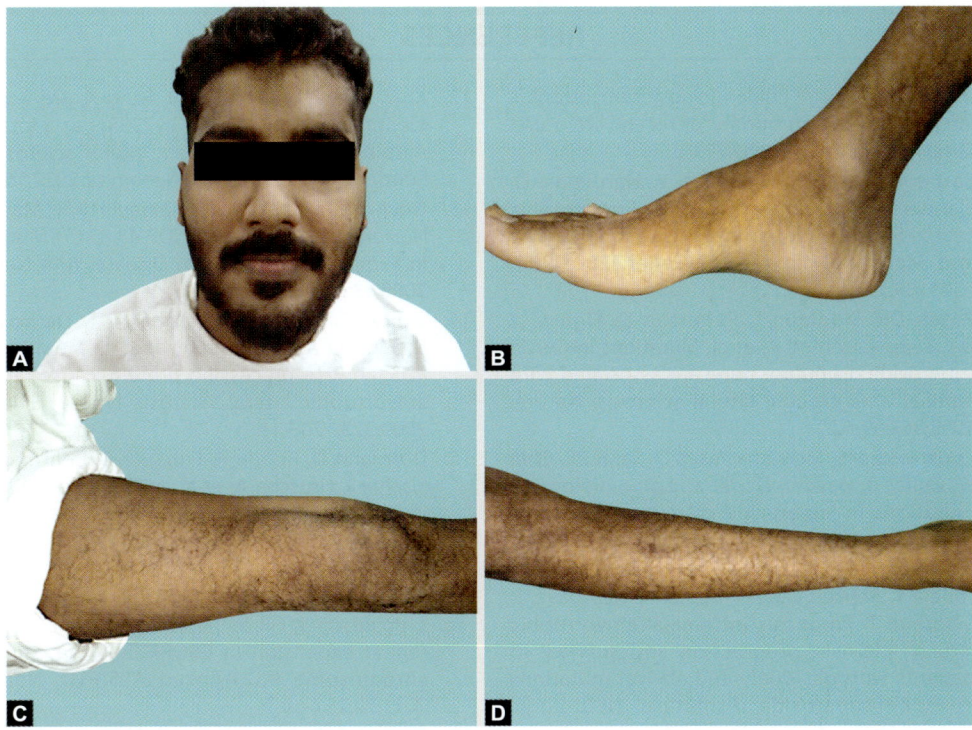

FIGS. 3A TO D: Patient presenting with fatigable ptosis and distal lower limb weakness.

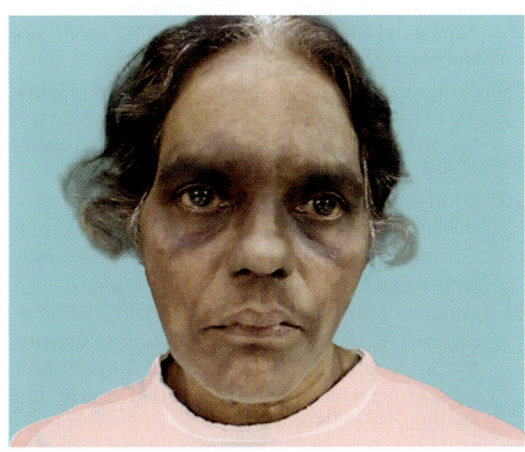

FIG. 4: Patient with blackish discoloration around eyelids.

elder sister had features of parkinsonism with cognitive dysfunction. She scored 93/100 on Addenbrooke's Cognitive Examination III (ACE-III). Eye movements showed mildly restricted upward and downward gaze with broken pursuits. There was mild rigidity in left and right LLs, bradykinesia in LLs, bilateral postural tremors, and small muscle atrophy of hands, forearm, and leg muscles. There was impaired pinprick sensation up to mid legs and impaired vibration at the malleoli. The tendon reflexes in upper limbs were brisk; the knee jerks were sluggish and ankle jerks were absent, and she had a spastic gait. WES revealed a likely pathogenic mutation in the *VCP* gene (c.290G>A) in exon 3.

REFERENCES

1. Longinetti E, Fang F. Epidemiology of amyotrophic lateral sclerosis: an update of recent literature. Curr Opin Neurol. 2019;32:771-6.
2. Barberio J, Lally C, Kupelian V, Hardiman O, Flanders WD. Estimated Familial Amyotrophic Lateral Sclerosis Proportion: A Literature Review and Meta-analysis. Neurol Genet. 2023;9(6):e200109.
3. Rosen DR, Siddique T, Patterson D, Figlewicz DA, Sapp P, Hentati A, et al. Mutations in Cu/Zn superoxide dismutase gene are associated with familial amyotrophic lateral sclerosis. Nature. 1993;362:59-62.
4. Cudkowicz ME, McKenna-Yasek D, Sapp PE, Chin W, Geller B, Hayden DL, et al. Epidemiology of mutations in superoxide dismutase in amyotrophic lateral sclerosis. Ann Neurol. 1997;41:210-21.
5. Juneja T, Pericak-Vance MA, Laing NG, Dave S, Siddique T. Prognosis in familial amyotrophic lateral sclerosis: progression and survival in patients with glu100gly and ala4val mutations in Cu,Zn superoxide dismutase. Neurology. 1997;48:55-7.
6. Robberecht W, Aguirre T, Van den Bosch L, Tilkin P, Cassiman JJ, Matthijs G. D90A heterozygosity in the SOD1 gene is associated with familial and apparently sporadic amyotrophic lateral sclerosis. Neurology. 1996;47:1336-9.
7. Kaur SJ, McKeown SR, Rashid S. Mutant SOD1 mediated pathogenesis of Amyotrophic Lateral Sclerosis. Gene. 2016;577:109-18.
8. Berdyński M, Miszta P, Safranow K, Andersen PM, Morita M, Filipek S, et al. SOD1 mutations associated with amyotrophic lateral sclerosis analysis of variant severity. Sci Rep. 2022;12:103.
9. Chen-Plotkin AS, Lee VMY, Trojanowski JQ. TAR DNA-binding protein 43 in neurodegenerative disease. Nat Rev Neurol. 2010;6:211-20.
10. Prasad A, Bharathi V, Sivalingam V, Girdhar A, Patel BK. Molecular Mechanisms of TDP-43 Misfolding and Pathology in Amyotrophic Lateral Sclerosis. Front Mol Neurosci. 2019;12:25.
11. Mitsuzawa S, Akiyama T, Nishiyama A, Suzuki N, Kato M, Warita H, et al. TARDBP p.G376D mutation, found in rapid progressive familial ALS, induces mislocalization of TDP-43. eNeurologicalSci. 2018;11:20-2.
12. Xu F, Huang S, Li XY, Lin J, Feng X, Xie S, et al. Identification of TARDBP Gly298Ser as a founder mutation for amyotrophic lateral sclerosis in Southern China. BMC Med Genomics. 2022;15:173.
13. Gitcho MA, Baloh RH, Chakraverty S, Mayo K, Norton JB, Levitch D, et al. TDP-43 A315T Mutation in Familial Motor Neuron Disease. Ann Neurol. 2008;63:535-8.
14. Vance C, Rogelj B, Hortobágyi T, De Vos KJ, Nishimura AL, Sreedharan J, et al. Mutations in FUS, an RNA processing protein, cause familial amyotrophic lateral sclerosis type 6. Science. 2009;323:1208-11.
15. Dormann D, Rodde R, Edbauer D, Bentmann E, Fischer I, Hruscha A, et al. ALS-associated fused in sarcoma (FUS) mutations disrupt Transportin-mediated nuclear import. EMBO J. 2010;29:2841-57.
16. Renton AE, Majounie E, Waite A, Simón-Sánchez J, Rollinson S, Gibbs JR, et al. A hexanucleotide repeat expansion in C9ORF72 is the cause of chromosome 9p21-linked ALS-FTD. Neuron. 2011;72:257-68.
17. Braems E, Swinnen B, Bosch LVD. C9orf72 loss-of-function: a trivial, stand-alone or additive mechanism in C9 ALS/FTD? Acta Neuropathol (Berl). 2020;140:625-43.
18. Freibaum BD, Taylor JP. The Role of Dipeptide Repeats in C9ORF72-Related ALS-FTD. Front Mol Neurosci. 2017;10:35.
19. Cooper-Knock J, Kirby J, Highley R, Shaw PJ. The Spectrum of C9orf72-mediated Neurodegeneration and Amyotrophic Lateral Sclerosis. Neurotherapeutics. 2015;12:326-39.
20. Bourinaris T, Houlden H. C9orf72 and its Relevance in Parkinsonism and Movement Disorders: A Comprehensive Review of the Literature. Mov Disord Clin Pract. 2018;5:575-85.
21. Pegat A, Bouhour F, Mouzat K, Vial C, Pegat B, Leblanc P, et al. Electrophysiological Characterization of C9ORF72-Associated Amyotrophic Lateral Sclerosis: A Retrospective Study. Eur Neurol. 2019;82:106-12.
22. Shamim U, Ambawat S, Singh J, Thomas A, Pradeep-Chandra-Reddy C, Suroliya V, et al. C9orf72 hexanucleotide repeat expansion in Indian patients with ALS: a common founder and its geographical predilection. Neurobiol Aging. 2020;88:156.e1-156.e9.

23. Mejzini R, Flynn LL, Pitout IL, Fletcher S, Wilton SD, Akkari PA. ALS Genetics, Mechanisms, and Therapeutics: Where Are We Now? Front Neurosci. 2019;13:1310.
24. Donnelly CJ, Grima JC, Sattler R. Aberrant RNA homeostasis in amyotrophic lateral sclerosis: potential for new therapeutic targets? Neurodegener Dis Manag. 2014;4:417-37.
25. Zhou W, Xu R. Current insights in the molecular genetic pathogenesis of amyotrophic lateral sclerosis. Front Neurosci. 2023;17:1189470.
26. Vehviläinen P, Koistinaho J, Gundars G. Mechanisms of mutant SOD1 induced mitochondrial toxicity in amyotrophic lateral sclerosis. Front Cell Neurosci. 2014;8:126.
27. Mackenzie I, Arzberger T, Kremmer E, Troost D, Lorenzl S, Mori K, et al. Dipeptide repeat protein pathology in C9ORF72 mutation cases: Clinicopathological correlations. Acta Neuropathol (Berl). 2013;126:859-79.
28. Souza PVS de, Serrano P de L, Farias IB, Machado RIL, Badia B de ML, Oliveira HB de, et al. Clinical and Genetic Aspects of Juvenile Amyotrophic Lateral Sclerosis: A Promising Era Emerges. Genes. 2024;15:311.
29. Roggenbuck J, Eubank BHF, Wright J, Harms MB, Kolb SJ, ALS Genetic Testing and Counseling Guidelines Expert Panel. Evidence-based consensus guidelines for ALS genetic testing and counseling. Ann Clin Transl Neurol. 2023;10:2074-91.
30. Saitoh Y, Takahashi Y. Riluzole for the treatment of amyotrophic lateral sclerosis. Neurodegener Dis Manag. 2020;10:343-55.
31. Goutman SA, Hardiman O, Al-Chalabi A, Chió A, Savelieff MG, Kiernan MC, et al. Emerging insights into the complex genetics and pathophysiology of amyotrophic lateral sclerosis. Lancet Neurol. 2022;21:465-79.
32. Boros BD, Schoch KM, Kreple CJ, Miller TM. Antisense Oligonucleotides for the Study and Treatment of ALS. Neurotherapeutics. 2022;19:1145-58.
33. Miller TM, Cudkowicz ME, Genge A, Shaw PJ, Sobue G, Bucelli RC, et al. Trial of Antisense Oligonucleotide Tofersen for SOD1 ALS. N Engl J Med. 2022;387:1099-110.
34. Benatar M, Wuu J, Andersen PM, Bucelli RC, Andrews JA, Otto M, et al. Design of a Randomized, Placebo-Controlled, Phase 3 Trial of Tofersen Initiated in Clinically Presymptomatic SOD1 Variant Carriers: the ATLAS Study. Neurotherapeutics. 2022;19:1248-58.
35. Agrawal N, Dasaradhi PVN, Mohmmed A, Malhotra P, Bhatnagar RK, Mukherjee SK. RNA Interference: Biology, Mechanism, and Applications. Microbiol Mol Biol Rev. 2003;67:657-85.
36. Mueller C, Berry JD, McKenna-Yasek DM, Gernoux G, Owegi MA, Pothier LM, et al. SOD1 Suppression with Adeno-Associated Virus and MicroRNA in Familial ALS. N Engl J Med. 2020;383:151-8.
37. Naveed A, Calderon H. Onasemnogene Abeparvovec (AVXS-101) for the Treatment of Spinal Muscular Atrophy. J Pediatr Pharmacol Ther. 2021;26:437-44.
38. Gaj T, Ojala DS, Ekman FK, Byrne LC, Limsirichai P, Schaffer DV. In vivo genome editing improves motor function and extends survival in a mouse model of ALS. Sci Adv. 2017;3:eaar3952.
39. Arshad F, Vengalil S, Nalini A, Polavarapu K, Shamim U, Jabeen S, et al. Novel TBK1 variant associated with Frontotemporal Dementia overlap syndrome. Acta Neurol Scand. 2022;145:399-406.

Index

Page numbers followed by *f* refer to figure, *fc* refer to flowchart, and *t* refer to table.

A

Abatacept 48
ABC008 49*t*
Abdominal muscle weakness 54*f*
Abduction sign 53*f*
Abscesses 145
Acetazolamide 29
Acetyl coenzyme A 21
Acetylcholine receptor deficiency 27
Acetylcholinesterase 22
 inhibitor 23, 28, 29
Acid maltase deficiency 41
Acute inflammatory
 demyelinating
 polyneuropathy 120
Acylcarnitine profile 100
 mimics 98
Acyl-coenzyme A 98
Adductors 149
Adenine-thymine 3
Adeno-associated virus 172, 184, 185
Adenosine triphosphate 182
Adrenal sufficiency 104
Adrenocorticotropic hormone 48
Adrenoleukodystrophy 167, 172
Aerobic exercise 81
Alanine aminotransferase 40
Albuterol 28
Aldolase 40
Alemtuzumab 49
Alpers–Huttenlocher syndrome 109
Alpha-dystroglycan, restored glycosylation of 61
Alternate conventional agents 12
Amino acids 108
Amyotrophic lateral sclerosis 64, 68, 76, 146, 153, 180, 182-184
 genes 185
 genetics of 178
 pathogenesis 183*f*
Anakinra 48

Anecdotal evidence 15
Anechoic regions 145
Angiotensin-converting enzyme
 inhibitors 6
Ankle contracture 53*f*
Anosmia 169
Anterior cervical
 corpectomy and discectomy 161
 discectomy and fusion 161, 162*f*, 164
Anterior horn cells 2, 95, 152, 158*f*
Antibody-mediated neurological
 diseases, treatment-refractory 120
Anti-CNTN1 antibodies 116
Antigen presenting cell 16
Antimyelin-associated
 glycoprotein 144
Antisense oligonucleotide 2, 6, 172, 184
Antisynthetase syndrome 33, 34, 36, 38, 41, 43, 48
Apabetalone 84
Apparent diffusion coefficient 159
Apremilast 48
Arimoclomol 49
Arm muscles, normal appearance
 of 138*f*
Arthritis 37, 140
Arthrogryposis 22
Aseptic meningitis 127
Aspartate aminotransferase 40
Asymmetric cord atrophy 154*f*
Asymmetrical cord flattening 158
Ataxia 106, 107
ATXN2 gene 183
Autoantibody, inhibition of 126
Autoimmune
 nodoparanodopathies 115
 nodopathy, therapeutic
 advances in 117*t*

Autophagy 180
Autosomal dominant 76, 182
 disorders 65
 inheritance 23
Autosomal recessive 76, 182
 cerebellar ataxia 180
 disease 73
 disorders 65
Axial weakness 40
Axonal neuropathy 106
Azathioprine 12, 46, 116, 130

B

Baricitinib 48
Basal ganglia 107
B-cell
 activating factor 48
 depleting therapies 120
 depletion strategies 115
Becker's muscular dystrophy 6, 53, 66
Belimumab 48
Beta-2 adrenergic receptor
 agonists 83
Beta-2 laminin 23
Biallelic variants 99
Bicep
 bulge sign 54*f*
 normal 137*f*
Bifacial weakness, severe 97*f*
Bifid median nerve at wrist,
 ultrasound axial image of 140*f*
Bilevel positive airway pressure 25*f*
Bimagrumab 49
Biological agents, novel 16*f*
Biotinidase deficiency 108
Blackish discoloration around
 eyelids 187*f*
Blocking sodium channels 183
Blood-nerve barrier 172
Boltshauser syndrome 98

Brachial monomelic amyotrophy, typical 154f
Brachialis muscle 137f
Brachioradialis, sparing of 154f
Brain
  involvement 1
  parenchyma 97f
Brainstem 107
  auditory evoked response 95
BRD4 inhibitor 83
Bromodomain inhibitors 84
Brown–Vialetto–Van–Laere
  disease 95t
  syndrome 93
Bruton kinase inhibitors 120
Bulbar symptoms 10, 25f

C

C2 vertebrae 163f
C20orf54 gene 93
C7 vertebrae, posterior aspect of 163f
C9orf72
  function of 179
  protein, function of 179
Calcinosis cutis 38
Calf
  atrophy 54f
  hypertrophy 25f, 53, 53f
Calpain 73
Calpainopathy 53f, 54f, 61
Carbon dioxide 147
Carcinoma metastasis 143
Cardiac arrhythmias 105
Cardiac care, advances in 6
Cardiac toxicity 59
Care and ethical concerns, advances in standards of 7
Carpal tunnel syndrome 139, 139f, 160
Cas9-nickase 88
CD20+ B cells 13
Cell-to-cell transmission 180
Cellular toxicity 179
Central nervous system 119, 172
  defects 22
Cerebellar ataxia 30, 169
Cerebellar nuclei with gliosis 95
Cerebellum 107
Cerebrospinal fluid 163
Cervical
  collarowing, use of 164
  lordosis, loss of 154f
  spinal cord, expansion of 97f
  spine
    lower part of 157
    X-ray of 163f
Champagne bottle 168f
  appearance of 168f
Charcot–Marie–Tooth disease 68, 107, 167, 168f, 170, 171t, 174, 182
  classification of 168
  subtype of 175
  treatment of 174t
Childhood myocerebrohepatopathy spectrum 109
Childhood-onset biotin responsive peripheral motor neuropathy 76
Chills 126
Chimeric antigen receptor T cell 15, 16
Chimeric autoantibody receptor T cell therapies 15
Choline 21
  acetyltransferase, mutations of 21
Chromatin modifier genes 81
Chromosomal microarray techniques 70
Chromosome 80, 179
Chronic inflammatory demyelinating polyneuropathy 114, 119
  first-line therapies for 125
  therapy 133
  treatment 125
polyradiculoneuropathy 124, 125, 127, 128, 130, 131
  therapy 132fc
  treatment of 130
Chronic progressive external ophthalmoplegia 104
  plus 105
  syndromes 104
Coenzyme Q10 deficiency 106
Cold paresis 156f
Combined annotation dependent depletion 73
Common inherited myopathies 66t
Common neurogenic disorders 67t
Comparative genomic hybridization 77
Comparative genomic hybridization arrays 68

Complement inhibitors 14
Compound muscle action potentials 23
Congenital myasthenic syndrome 11, 20, 24, 27, 29, 30t, 64, 67, 74, 75
  diagnosis of 26
  genetic defects causing 21f
  types of 25f
Congenital myopathies 147
Connective tissue disease, mixed 36
Connexin32 172
Consanguineous marriages 55
Conservative management 161
Contactin-associated protein-1 119
Contraction stress test 119
Conventional gene therapy 7
CoQ10 deficiency 106
Cord
  compression 162f
  lesion 160
Corpectomy 161
Corticosteroids 10, 124, 128
COVID-19 34
COXIII mutations 104
Creatine 108
  kinase 24, 39, 71, 108
CREB-binding protein 84
CRISPR/Cas9 gene 173
Crural monomelic amyotrophy 154, 156f
Cryptogenic neuropathies 146
Cyclic adenosine monophosphate 174
Cyclophosphamide 12, 17, 17t, 47, 116
Cyclosporine 12, 17, 130
  A 47
  effectiveness of 12
Cytochrome C oxidase 41, 45, 109
Cytoplasmic bodies 45
Cytotoxic T-lymphocyte associated protein 48

D

D4Z4 macrosatellite 80
Daratumumab 120
Dejerine–Sottas syndrome 169
Delivery of route, type of 171
Deltoid muscle 149
Deltoid wasting, bilateral 156f
Dementia 106
  family history of 186

Index

Dendritic cells 41
Deoxyribonucleic acid 58, 64, 182
Depressed nasal bridge 97f
Dermatomyositis 34, 37, 41, 43, 44f, 48, 147f
　adult 36
　mild-to-moderate 46
Diabetes 105
　mellitus 106
Diabetic neuropathies 146
Diamond sign 53f
Diarrhea 14
Digitorum brevis muscles 60
Discectomy 161
Disease, in vitro models of 96
Disease-modifying
　therapeutics 2
　therapies 1
　treatment 80
Distal acquired demyelinating sensorimotor neuropathy 130, 131
Distal bimelic amyotrophy 154, 155f
Distal forearm 142f
Distal hereditary motor neuropathy 169
Distal lower limb weakness 187f
Distal muscular dystrophy 52
Distal upper
　extremity 152
　limbs 153, 162f
Diverse genes 149
Dosing weight, concept of 125
Drug therapy 173
Dry itchy skin 37
Duchenne and Becker muscular dystrophy 68
Duchenne muscular dystrophy 1, 5, 6, 66, 147
　analysis of 69f
　gene 6
　therapy 7, 8
　mutation 6
Dural sac theory 153
Dural structural abnormality 153
Duraplasty 161
DUX4
　expression 82
　gene 80
　messenger 81
　polyadenylation 88
　protein inhibition 84
　related transcription 82
　transcripts 88

Dynamic cord compression, pathogenesis of 153
Dysferlin 73
Dysferlinopathy 53f, 54f, 59, 61, 148f
Dysphagia 37, 105
Dystrophin 73
　gene 5
Dystrophinopathy 1, 66, 71

E

Eculizumab 14, 17, 48
Efgartigimod 17
Electromyography 40
Electrophysiological category 169
Emerging therapies 167
Endocrine abnormalities 30
Endomysial inflammation 45f
Endosomal sorting complexes required for transport 182
Enlarged brachial plexus trunks 144f
Enlarged median nerve 139f, 146f
Entrapment neuropathy 139
Enzyme histochemistry 41
Ephedrine 28
Epicondyle, medial 145f
Epidermolysis bullosa 30
Epidural soft tissue enhancing 158f
Epilepsy 30, 106
Episodic apnea 21, 30
ERLIN1 variant 180
Erythematous
　rash 37
　scaly papules 37
Escobar syndrome 30
Etanercept 48
Eteplirsen 6
Etiopathogenesis 153
Excitotoxicity 179
Exercise intolerance 105
Exertional myalgia 60
Exocrine pancreatic insufficiency 106
Exome sequencing 27
Extensor digitorum brevis hypertrophy 53f
Eyelid crutches 110

F

Facioscapulohumeral dystrophy 66, 72, 77, 80, 147

Facioscapulohumeral muscular dystrophy 54, 80, 81, 81f, 82, 105
　pathogenesis of 80
　therapeutics 83t, 86t, 88t
Familial amyloid polyneuropathy 68
Fascicular enlargement 144f
Fasciculations 97f
Fatigable ptosis 187f
Fatigable ptosis mimicking myasthenia 186
Fatty infiltration
　degree of 139
　severe 148f
Fazio–Londe syndrome 93
Fc receptor 13
　inhibitors 13
Fetal akinesia deformation sequence 23
Fever 126
Fibro-osseous canals 145
First-line therapies 125
FKRP gene 61
Flail leg syndrome 186
Fluid-attenuated inversion recovery 95
Fluorine 18-fluorodeoxyglucose 41
Fluoxetine 28
Focal peripheral neuropathies 139
Folic acid 81
Follistatin gene therapy 49
Foot drop, bilateral 97f
Foot muscles, severe wasting of 97f
Forearm
　oblique atrophy of 154f
　wasting, bilateral 156f
Forehead and facial hyperpigmentation 37f
Fragments, ladder of 74f
Frontotemporal dementia 179, 182
FTD-ALS syndrome 185
Functional rating scale 185

G

Gain-of-function mutation 184, 185
Gamma-aminobutyric acid 174, 175
Ganglion cysts 140

Ganglioside antibodies 115, 120
Gastrointestinal dysmotility 105
Gastrointestinal symptoms 106
Gene
  editing 87, 88*t*
  replacement 184
    therapy 185
  therapy 52, 58, 61, 171, 171*t*, 184*t*
    developing 178
    principles of 58
Gene-based therapeutic strategies 183
Gene-editing strategies 88
Genetic 99
  analysis 101
  basic concepts in 64
  basis 180
  counseling, provision of 183
  disorders 170
  heterogeneity 65, 170
  mutation's severity 53
  spectrum and management 20
  techniques 58*fc*
  test 64, 68, 77*fc*, 109, 183
    strategies 71
  variant
    classification of 72
    segregation analysis of 185
Genome editing 185
Genotype-phenotype correlation 99
Gingival telangiectasias 37
Glass cut injury 142*f*
Glaucoma 106
Gliomedin 114
Glutamine-fructose-6-phosphate transaminase 1 24
Glutathione 108
Glycosylation 2 homolog 24
Glycosylation defects 24
GNT0006, immunogenicity of 61
Golodirsen 7
Gomori trichrome, modified 44, 45*f*
Gottron's papules 37, 37*f*
Granular basophilic material 44
Ground glass appearance 147, 148*f*
Growth hormone insufficiency 104
Guanine-cytosine 3
Guillain–Barré syndrome 114, 144

GYM329 82
Gynecomastia 186, 186*f*

H

Hammer toes 168*f*
Hamstrings 149
Hand contractures 37*f*
Hansen's disease 145*f*
Headache 14, 126
Hearing
  impaired 105
  impairment 100
  history of 96
  loss 96
Heart 104
Heat shock protein 90 174
Heliotrope rash 37*f*
Hematoma 140
Hematopoietic stem cell transplantation 14, 16
Hepatic dysfunction 104
Hereditary diseases 58
Hereditary motor
  neuropathy 76
  sensory neuropathy 169
Hereditary neuropathy 68
  with pressure palsies 174
Hereditary spastic paraplegia 182
Heterogeneous disease 167
Heterozygous 73
Hip splaying 53*f*
Hirayama disease 152, 156*f*-158*f*, 160, 164
  diagnosis of 157
  treatment of 164
  variants of 153
Histone deacetylase 2, 174
Holster sign 37
Homozygous alleles 74
Honeycomb 137
Huashan diagnostic criteria 159, 160*t*
Human cells 85
Human gene mutation database 73
Human leukocyte antigen 37
Hyperthyroidism 11
Hypertrophic neuropathy 168
Hypointense epidural tissue 158*f*
Hypokalemic periodic paralysis 65
Hypomyelinating neuropathy, severe 169
Hypophonia 95

I

Idiopathic inflammatory myopathy 33, 35*t*, 36, 42*t*
  classification of 34
  cutaneous manifestations of 37*f*
  immunotherapy for 46*t*
  subtypes of 37
  treatment of 45
Illness, course of 98
Immune
  checkpoint inhibitor 34, 40
  function 179
Immune-mediated
  demyelinating polyneuropathy, chronic 144, 144*f*
  necrotizing myopathy 34, 36, 38, 41, 43, 46
  neuropathy 144
Immunoglobulin 13
  G 11, 126
  M 130, 144
Immunohistochemistry 41
Immunopathology behind refractory myasthenia gravis 11
Immunoprecipitation technique 36
Immunosuppressive agents, development of 10
Immunotherapy 45, 129
Impaired cognition 106
Inclusion body
  myopathy 182
  myositis 43, 45*f*, 148
Inflammation 180
Inflammatory arthritis 36
Inflammatory cells 41, 44
Inflammatory myopathy 147
Inflammatory neuropathy cause and treatment 116, 127
Inflammatory Rasch-built overall disability scale 127
Infliximab 48
Infraspinatus muscle 149
Inherited myopathy 64, 66
Inherited neuromuscular disorders 71
Inherited neuropathy 75, 76*fc*, 143
Interleukin 48
Interosseous nerve, enlarged posterior 141*f*
Interstitial edema 44*f*

Index

Interstitial lung disease 36, 48
Intervening connective tissue 137
Intraneural ganglion 141, 142
Intravenous 49
   methylprednisolone 46
Intravenous immunoglobulin 12,
   47, 98, 114, 119, 124-126, 129*f*,
   130-132
   after 128*f*
   therapy
     adverse effects of 126
     drawbacks of 126
     usage, real-life 125
Intronic splicing silencer N1 3

J

Janus kinase 48
Joint 34
Juvenile
   amyotrophic lateral sclerosis
     180
   asymmetric segmental spinal
     muscular atrophy 152
   dermatomyositis 36
   muscular atrophy 152
   nonprogressive monomelic
     amyotrophy 152

K

Kearns–Sayre syndromes 104
Kennedy disease 73
KIAA1377 153
Kidneys 104
Killer cell 45
Killer cell lectin-like receptor G
   45, 49
Knee jerks, bilateral 186

L

Lactate 108
   dehydrogenase 40
Lactic acidosis 104, 105
Lambert–Eaton like myasthenic
   syndrome 22
Laminectomy 161
Leber's hereditary optic
   neuropathy 107
Left lower limb wasting 156*f*
Left upper limb 156*f*
Left upper trunk and roots 145*f*
Leigh syndrome 107
Lenabasum 48

Lentivirus 185
Leprosy 145
Leyden classified muscular
   dystrophies 52
Limb
   fatigue 25*f*
   weakness of 124
Limb-girdle
   dystrophy 52
     treatment of 58
   muscle dystrophy, gene
     therapy for 58, 59
   muscular dystrophy 52, 53*f*,
     54, 54*f*, 55, 56*f*, 58-61, 66,
     71, 149
     classification of 61
     treatment of 58*fc*
   myasthenia 23, 75
   syndrome 30
   weakness 34, 40
Lipid droplets 109
Lithium 49
Liver 104
Local muscle function 60
Loss-of-function mutations 65,
   184
Lower cervical
   and thoracic cord, atrophy
     of 97*f*
   spine 161
Lower cranial nerve nuclei 95
Lower limb 95, 152, 179
   asymmetrical bilateral 155
   muscles 149
Lower motor neuron 179
   diseases 168
Lumbar lordosis 54*f*
Lung 34
Lymphocytes 44, 45
Lymphomatosis 146

M

Machine learning 148
Madras motor neuron disease
   95, 95*t*
Major amyotrophic lateral
   sclerosis genes 179
Major histocompatibility complex
   43
Malondialdehyde 108
MAPK inhibitors 83
Maternally inherited leigh
   syndrome 107
McArdle disease 67

Mechanic's foot 37*f*
Median nerve at wrist, normal
   appearance of 137*f*, 143*f*
Membrane attack complex 16,
   41, 43
Memory B cells 11
Mental subnormality 25*f*, 30
Messenger ribonucleic acid 58
Metabolic myopathies 67, 77
Metabolic stress, period of 107
Methionine 81
Methotrexate 12, 17, 46, 130
   use of 12
Might influence DUX4 levels 84
Migraine 106
Mitochondria, abnormal 108
Mitochondrial abnormality 39
Mitochondrial cocktail 110
Mitochondrial cytopathy 75
Mitochondrial defect 179
Mitochondrial disorders 103, 108
   diagnosis of 108
Mitochondrial DNA 103
Mitochondrial
   encephalomyopathy 105
Mitochondrial homeostasis 103
Mitochondrial myopathies
   103-105, 111
   biomarkers of 108
Mitochondrial
   neurogastrointestinal
   encephalomyopathy 75, 106
Mitochondrial peripheral
   neuropathies 107
Mitofusin 2 174
Monomelic amyotrophy 152,
   164
Morton's neuromas 142
Motor chronic inflammatory
   demyelinating
   polyneuropathy variant 129
Motor evoked potentials 159
Motor neuron
   disease 136, 186
   disorders 160
Motor neuropathy 131
MT-TK gene 106
Mucopolysaccharidosis 146*f*
Multifocal acquired
   demyelinating sensory 131
Multifocal motor neuropathy
   114, 131, 144
Multiple acyl-CoA dehydrogenase
   deficiency 67
Multiple mutations 103

Multiplex ligation-dependent probe amplification 68, 76, 77
Multisystem and cancer complications, management of 45
Muscle
 atrophy 154
 biopsy 41, 44f, 45f, 108
 bulk 139
 cells, parts of 52
 diseases 74
 echogenicity 139, 147
 enzymes 40
 fascicles 137
 fibers 147
  deficient 109
 imaging 40, 139
 pseudohypertrophy of 54
 specific antibodies 33, 35t
 ultrasound 147
 weakness 103
Muscular dystrophies 41, 64, 108
Mutations, types of 184
Myasthenia gravis 10, 16, 104
 treatment 12
  strategies for 11
Mycophenolate 116, 130
 mofetil 12, 47
Myelin-associated glycoprotein antibodies 130
Myelin-dependent organization 114
Myeloma 15
Myocarditis 37, 40
Myoclonic epilepsy 106
 myopathy sensory ataxia 109
Myoclonus 106
Myofibrillar myopathy 58, 149
Myopathy 103, 106, 136, 147
 distal 67, 75
 subacute sever 38
Myositis 34, 35
 associated antibodies 35, 36t
 specific antibodies 35
Myostatin inhibitors 82
Myotonic dystrophy 66, 74f, 149
Myxovirus resistance protein A 43

N

N-acetylglucosamine phosphotransferase 1 24
Naltrexone potentiates 175
Nasopharyngitis 14

Nathalie syndrome 98
Neck
 flexion, range of 163f
 weakness 37
Needle electromyogram 71
Neisseria meningitidis 14
Nerve
 and muscle imaging 139
 biopsy 95
 conduction velocity 132
 imaging 139
 inherently 137
 root theory 153
 sheath tumors, malignant peripheral 142
 tumors 142
Neural lipomatosis 142
Neuralgic amyotrophy 146
Neurofascin neuropathies 116
Neurofascin-155 113, 119
Neurofascin-186 113
Neurofibroma 142, 143, 143f
Neurogenetic diseases 167
Neurological examination 95
Neurolymphomatosis 143
Neuroma 140, 142, 142f
 traumatic 142
Neurometabolic disorder 136, 169
Neuromuscular disorders
 genetic diagnosis of 74
 genetic testing in 64
Neuromuscular imaging, basic principles of 136
Neuromuscular junction 66
Neuropathology 95
Neuropathy 66, 136, 160
 limitation score 174
 severe demyelinating 172
 traumatic 141
Newer therapies 120
Next-generation sequencing 27, 70, 109, 180
Nicotinamide adenine dinucleotide 174
Nodal antigen 114f
Node of Ranvier 113
Nodoparanodopathy 113
 therapeutic advances in 113
 therapy of 115
Non-necrotic fibers 44
Nonsense mutations 77
Normal cervical lordosis, loss of 157
Novel disease-related genes 73
Nucleocytoplasmic transport 179, 180

Nusinersen 4
Nystagmus 96

O

Ochlear implantation 100
Ocrelizumab 120
Oculopharyngeal distal myopathy 67, 73
Oculopharyngeal muscular dystrophy 67, 73
Ofatumumab 120
Old classification 169t
Oligonucleotide therapeutics 85
Oligotherapeutic drugs 86t
Onapristone 175
Onasemnogene, drawback of 5
Ophthalmoplegia 104, 106
 external 24
Optic atrophy 106, 107
Optic disk hyperemia 107
Oral prednisolone 46
Oral pulse dexamethasone 46
Overlap myositis 48
Overlap syndrome 39
Owl's eye appearance 158, 159f
Oxandrolone 49
Oxidative phosphorylation 103
Oxidative stress 179, 180

P

P2X7 inhibitors 175
P300 histone acetyltransferase inhibitors 82
P38 inhibitors 82
Paranodal antigen 114f
Paraproteinemia 144
Parkinsonism, family history of 186
Patchy hyperechogenicity 147f
Perifascicular atrophy 44f
Periorbital bluish–purplish rash 37
Peripheral nerve 139
 injuries 141
Peripheral nervous system 168
Perivascular epimysial inflammation 44f
Peroneal muscular atrophy 168
Peroneal neuropathy 141
Pes cavus 168f
Phenotype
 severe 104
 variety of 60
Phenotypic heterogeneity 109, 170

Phosphorodiamidate morpholino oligomer 6
Pierson syndrome 30
Pigmentary retinopathy 106
Plasma
   cells 11
   exchange 12, 13, 115, 124, 130, 132
   gelsolin 108
Plectin 24
Pluripotent stem cells 94
PMP22
   copies 172
   gene 173
Poikiloderma 38
POLG1 mutations 109
Polymerase chain reaction 68
Polymyositis 34, 40, 48
Polyneuropathy 143
Pompe disease 67, 77, 147
Positive plasma cells 115
Posterior epidural
   plexus 159
   tissue 162f
   venous plexus 158
Potassium channel blocker 27
Potentially treatable disorders 93
Prednisolone 131
   oral daily 129
Predominantly sensory 130
Preeclampsia 119
Preferential adductor weakness 53f
Presynaptic congenital myasthenic syndrome 21
Primary sensory neuron diseases 168
Prion-like transfer 179
Progesterone antagonist 175
Progressive bulbar weakness 186, 186f
Progressive multifocal leukoencephalopathy 14
Prolyl-endopeptidase 21
   like-CMS gene 22
   like-gene mutations 22
Protein expression, advances in 2
Protrudent abdomen 54f
Proximal bimelic amyotrophy 155
Pseudo refractoriness 11
Pseudotumors 142
Ptosis 25f, 106, 110
   mild 25f
Pulsed oral dexamethasone 129
Pure sensory 131
Pyramidal dysfunction 106
Pyridostigmine 28
Pyruvate 108
   carboxylase deficiency 108

Q

Quinidine 29

R

RAAV9 mediated 61
Radial neuropathy 141
Ragged blue fibers 109
Ragged red fibers 106
Randomized controlled trial 48, 119, 174
Rapamycin, mammalian target of 49
Ravulizumab 14, 17
Raynaud's phenomenon 37
Rectus femoris, sparing of 40
Refractory cases, management of 133
Refractory idiopathic inflammatory myopathies 48t
Refractory myasthenia 10
   gravis 12
   treatment of 13
Renal dysfunction 104
Renal failure 127
Repeat expansion disorders 73
Repetitive nerve stimulation 22, 26f
Reproductive health 16
Respiratory distress 25f
Respiratory failure 22, 40
Respiratory tract infection 14
Reverse transcription-polymerase chain reaction, triplet-primed 74f
Rheumatoid arthritis 36
Riboflavin 100
   transporter deficiencies 76
Riboflavinopathies 93
Ribonucleic acid 58, 64, 77, 182
   interference 173, 184
   mediated interference 184
Risdiplam 4
Rituximab 13, 17, 47, 115, 119, 130
Rozanolixizumab 17
Ruxolitinib 48

S

Salbutamol 28
Sand watch appearance 157
Sarcoglycan 73
   complex 59, 60
Sarcoglycanopathy 53f, 59, 61
Sarcolemma 41, 44, 59
Sarcoma 179
   fused in 179
   mutation, fused in 186
Scapular prominence, bilateral 156f
Scapular winging 54, 54f
Scapulothoracic arthrodesis 82
Scar tissue 140
Schwann cells 173
Schwannoma 140-143
Sciatic nerve, normal appearance of 138f
Sclerosis, primary lateral 182
Segmental cytochrome C oxidase deficiency 109
Seizures 25f, 106, 107
Sensorineural deafness 107
Sensorineural hearing loss 106, 110
Sensory
   abnormalities 186
   ataxic neuropathy, dysarthria, and ophthalmoplegia, syndrome of 107
   evoked potentials 159
Serum
   creatine phosphokinase 186
   immunoglobulin G 125, 128f
   neurofilament light chain 119
Severe autoimmune disorders 12
Shawl sign 37, 37f
Short hairpin ribonucleic acid 173
Shoulder girdle muscles, severe weakness of 156f
Sifalimumab 48
Simple sequence length polymorphisms 81
Single nucleotide
   substitutions 65
   variants 70
Single-fiber electromyography 26
Single-nucleotide polymorphism 70
Sirolimus 49
Sjögren's syndrome 39
Skeletal muscle 103
   ability 5

Skin
- rash, severe 38
- vasculopathy with weakness 38

SLC52A2
- alleles 99
- gene 93, 99

SLC52A3 gene 93, 94*f*, 100
Slow channel syndrome 75
Small molecule drugs 82, 83*t*
Small muscles of hands, severe wasting of 97*f*
SMN gene 172
SMN1 gene 4
SMN2 gene 3, 4, 4*f*c
- mature 4

Snake eye appearance 158, 159*f*
Sodium channel 24
Sorbitol dehydrogenase 174
- inhibitors 175

SPG11 variant 180
Spinal bulbar muscular atrophy 68
- Kennedy disease 68

Spinal cord, microscopic examination of 179
Spinal muscular atrophy 1, 2, 4, 67, 68, 152, 182, 185
- classification of 3*t*
- types of 2

Spinraza, mechanism of action of 3
Sporadic disorders 65
Sporadic inclusion body myositis 34, 36, 39, 44, 49*t*
SRP-9003, efficacy of 60
Steroid 115, 129, 129*f*
- sparing agent 12, 130
- use of 130

Stroke-like episodes 105, 107
Subcutaneous 38
- immunoglobulin 13, 124, 127
- therapy 128*f*

Subscapularis muscle 149
Succinate dehydrogenase 45
Supraspinatus muscle 149
Sural nerve 146
Survival motor neuron 4*f*c
- gene 2

Synaptotagmin 22
Syndrome of arthrogryposis multiplex congenita 23
Systemic autoimmune diseases 35

Systemic lupus erythematosus 36, 39
Systemic sclerosis 39

T

T1-gadolinium sequences 138
T2 short tau inversion recovery 40
T2-weighted imaging 160
Tacrolimus 12, 13, 17, 47
TAR DNA-binding protein 179
- mutation 179

TARDBP variant 180
Targeted gene panels 70
Tarsal tunnel syndrome 141
TBK1 gene 185
T-cells 41
Textural analysis 148
Thalami 107
Therapeutic drug monitoring 17
Third-generation sequencing 72
Thoracic outlet syndrome 160
Thromboembolism 127
Thrombotic thrombocytopenic purpura 5
Thymectomy 15
Thymic lesion 15
Tibial nerve, posterior 144*f*, 145*f*
T-lymphocyte-associate protein 4 40
Tocilizumab 48
Tofacitinib 48
Tongue atrophy 25*f*, 97*f*
- severe 97*f*

Toxic gain of function 179
Tracheostomy 8
Transcriptome sequencing 72
Transfer ribonucleic acid 38
Transmembrane protein 99
Treatabolome, developing 27
True remission, less chance of 126
Truncal muscle 54*f*
Tumors 140
- benign 142
- malignant 142
- necrosis factor 48

U

Ulnar nerve
- at elbow, discrete enlargement of 140*f*
- enlarged 145*f*
- right 142*f*

Ulnar neuropathy 140
Ultrasonography 136
Uncertain significance, variants of 72
Unfolded protein response 174
Upper limb 127
- muscles 149
- reflexes 186
- right 186

Upper motor neuron 155, 180

V

Vasculitic ulcers 37, 37*f*
Vasculitis neuropathies 146
Venous engorgement, abnormal 153
Vesicle-associated membrane protein 1 22
Vesicular acetylcholine transporter 21
Viltolarsen 7
Viral vector-based therapy 171
Viral vector-mediated gene therapy 58
Viruses 171
Vision 100
Visual evoked potentials 95
Visual impairment 100
Vocal cord paralysis 30
V-sign 37

W

Weakness 186
- severe 129

Whole exome sequencing 76, 77, 185
Whole genome sequencing 72
Whorls bodies 45
Wolff–Parkinson–White syndrome 105
Wrist 139*f*

X

X-linked spinobulbar muscular atrophy 98

Z

Zanubrutinib 120
Zilucoplan 14, 17
Zolgensma 5